ASCP QUICK COMPENDIUM

COMPANION

FOR

CLINICAL PATHOLOGY

Dedication

I would like to dedicate this book to my wife, Kate, and daughter, Audrey, both of whom were very patient with my constant writing and typing for the last few months. Also, thanks to my mom for her encouragement and to my dad because I know that he would have liked this.

GL

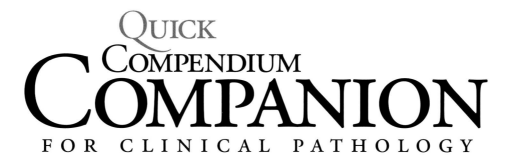

QUICK COMPENDIUM COMPANION
FOR CLINICAL PATHOLOGY

George Leonard, MD, PhD
MAJ, MC, USA

Medical Director of Transfusion Services
Surgical Pathologist, Department of Pathology and Area Laboratory Services
Walter Reed Army Medical Center
Washington, DC

Daniel D Mais, MD

Medical Director of Hematopathology
Surgical Pathologist, Department of Pathology
St. Joseph's Mercy Hospital and Warde Medical Laboratory
Ann Arbor, MI

American Society for
Clinical Pathology
Press
Chicago

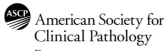 American Society for
Clinical Pathology
Press

Publishing Team

Tae Moon (design)

Joshua Weikersheimer (publishing direction)

Table of

Contents

Making Things Memorable

Pathology residency training is notoriously sparse with the teaching of clinical pathology. Many times it is relegated to self-directed instruction. In addition the clinical pathology board exam is a formidable foe. Subjects as diverse as hematopathology, clinical chemistry, immunology, microbiology, and transfusion medicine are lumped together in what many consider the single most difficult exam of their lives. For these reasons and many others the Quick Compendium of Clinical Pathology owes its success. A lean epitome of a protean collection of information is much appreciated by residents as they try to prepare for the board exam. And the need for a text such as the Quick Compendium will only grow as all newly-minted pathologists and many practicing pathologists will be required to pass the Maintenance of Certification exam every 10 years.

However, with a subject so vast and a book so small the value of each word skyrockets. Space is a premium and text is worth gold. For this reason it becomes important that the reader absorb each word. There is no filler material to skip over. How does one remember it all?

We all have our different styles of learning. For me the three most helpful techniques are flashcards, mnemonics, and question writing/answering. I will discuss in turn each of these techniques and explain how to get them to work for you. In addition I hope to offer examples of each of these on the website for your download and review.

Flashcards

For the purposes of discussion a flashcard is defined as a two-sided card with information on one side of the card that the learner is trying to associate with information on the other side of the card. For years these have been used to learn simple associative facts. Building foreign language vocabulary is one popular example. The use of spaced repetition of flash cards was popularized by an Austrian educator named Sebastian Leitner. His text "How to Learn to Learn" (I love that title) first described the use of interval repetition as a means of increasing the efficiency of learning. His technique involves the use of categories or boxes into which one sorts "cards" of information. Each box is defined by the degree to which the student self-rates their knowledge of the information on the card. If the student knows the information on the card well the card is placed in a higher box, if the student does not know the information it is placed in a lower box. An

algorithm then presents the well-known cards at a longer spaced interval than the less well-known cards. Several popular foreign language courses use this technology to great effect. Flashcards are an extraordinarily effective means of learning, but there are limitations and rules to be followed:

1. **The cards must be made properly.** They must be simple and not overloaded with information. For example on one side of the card one could write - "Preferred growth medium for Bordetella" and on the other side "Regan-Lowe medium" (I do realize there are other suitable media, but it's just an example). An example of a poorly written card would be to have "Bordetella" on one side and a slew of facts, such as media, gram stain, species, diseases, antibiotic sensitivities, etc. on the other. Cards must be simple to be effective.

2. **Certain types of information are not "flashable".** There is information that does not lend itself to flashcards. For this reason it is important to be selective in the construction of flashcards. I would find it difficult to learn syndromic associations with flash cards. It would be too difficult to keep these cards simple, thus violating our first rule.

3. **One must honestly grade their performance.** You aren't doing anyone any favors by upgrading or downgrading your ability to remember a card. For spaced repetition to work there must be an accurate accounting of whether you know the information or not.

If one follows these rules flashcards are an efficient means to learn vast amounts of information. At least in the short-term. For longer term memorization a technique involving deep association is necessary. Which brings me to the next technique, mnemonics.

Mnemonics

Named after Mnemosyne, the Greek mother of the Muses and the personification of memory, mnemonics involve the association of a fact or concept with which one is already familiar with another to be learned. This is the key of using mnemonics - one must associate the unknown quantity with a known one. The Roman orator, Cicero, described the method of loci as a means to remember long speeches. With this technique one imagines walking around a familiar location, such as one's home. At each part of the home one associates a portion of the speech. For example the front door is visualized as the opening of the speech. This is followed by the front hallway, perhaps the hall closet, the kitchen, the living room, the dining room, etc. There are numerous mnemonic techniques and the discussion of each is beyond the scope of this text. The publication of this book will be supported by an online adjunct where I will be able to discuss mnemonics in more depth. One technique, however, does deserve a brief introduction because I will use it throughout the text.

You can learn the technique, but it takes practice to make it work well. The technique has many names: phonetic numbers, sound numbers, the major system, and number words, among others. The basic premise is simple - we can remember words better than numbers. Additionally, there are 10 basic consonantal sounds in the english language, which helps with the assignation of one number to one sound for numbers 0 through 9. Arbitrarily, I use the most popular mapping scheme as demonstrated below:

Number	Sound
0	S or Z
1	T or D
2	N
3	M
4	R
5	L
6	SH, TH, CH
7	K
8	F or V
9	P or B

Since the technique is based on the sounds rather than actual letters there is leeway to create words. Once you create a word (or words) from the number (or numbers) it is a simple task to use another mnemonic technique to memorize the words. A simple associative technique is useful to link two sets of numbers together. For example, I imagine a tot in a tire of a bicycle weighed down with a heavy chain on the mantle of a fireplace. To translate - tot = 11, tire =14; bicycle = the cyclin D1 gene, the heavy chain is the immunoglobulin heavy chain gene, mantle = mantle cell lymphoma. This is how I remember that the t(11;14) translocation of cyclin D1 and Ig

heavy chain is associated with mantle cell lymphoma. I have subsequently further expanded the image by placing a fishing pole hanging from the mantle to remind me that the FISH assay is the preferred molecular technique for diagnosis.

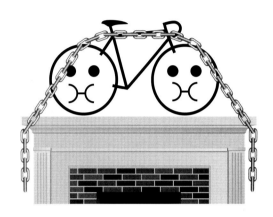

Question Writing/Answering

While I was in graduate school a friend noticed my tendency to sleep in lecture. He taught me the trick of actively listening to the lecture and formulating two questions to ask the speaker. That trick is applicable to reading with the added benefit of increasing retention of the material. When I read I write questions to review later. Repetition is an effective means of reinforcing memories. Repetition is an effective means of reinforcing memories. Try this: read the material, come up with a question, write down the question, type up the question and answer, then later review. This cycle of repetition wears a rut in your mind and aids in "knee-jerk" responses (similar to flash cards). I have found a variety of technologies to use when typing up the questions - making an electronic presentation or a web page helps. From time to time I will post more information on the online forum for this book on newer technologies and potential applications.

Suggestions for reading this book

When reading this book I encourage you to choose a single answer for each question. The action of making a decision will reinforce the information whether you are correct or not. Narrow down choices then choose a single best answer (if applicable). If you get it correct you are reinforcing it in your mind. If you do not get it correct you are indexing it for further study. There are a lot of questions in this book. That is by design. It can be picked up at random and reviewed or you can go over the book from cover to cover. Do not get discouraged if you are getting questions wrong - this isn't a real test! Hopefully, it will point out areas for further study and you can come back later and try again. A review technique that I recommend is the one put forth by Supermemo creator, Piotr Wozniak on his website (http://www.supermemo.com/articles/paper.htm). Starting with the preformed questions in this book, utilize the algorithmic approach to maximize retention.

Summary

I hope the information presented in this introduction will help you to best utilize the resources presented both in the text and online. In addition I hope that you use these techniques to create your own unique means of studying for the boards or the maintenance exam. The more you practice and the more personal your study routines are the more success you will enjoy!

A special thanks to Joshua Weikersheimer, PhD for pushing when he knew he could, to Dan Mais, MD for encouraging me, to Bart Wacek, JD for making sure all the legal ducks were in a row, and Patrick Voorhees, MD for partial proofreading.

Please contact me with any questions or suggestions at QCCP2Companion@gmail.com - George

Chapter 1

Clinical Chemistry

1. Which statement best describes Michaelis-Menten enzyme kinetics?
    A. Substrate concentration is inversely related to reaction rate at concentrations below saturation.
    B. Rate of enzyme activity varies linearly with substrate concentration when enzyme is fully saturated.
    C. Saturation of enzyme by substrate leads to logarithmic increases in reaction rate.
    D. Rate of enzyme activity varies logarithmically with substrate concentration when enzyme is fully saturated.
    E. Rate of enzyme activity is independent of substrate concentration when enzyme is fully saturated.

2. What differential property of NADH allows it to be measured in a coupled enzyme assay?
    A. NADH does not precipitate from the reaction; NAD does.
    B. NADH differentially precipitates out of the reaction; NAD does not.
    C. NADH does not absorb light at 340nm, while NAD does.
    D. NADH absorbs light at 340nm, while NAD does not.
    E. none of the above.

3. The production of N-nitrophenyl and phosphate from p-nitrophenyl phosphate can be catalyzed by two different enzymes at two different pHs. Match the enzyme and pH.
    A. alkaline phosphatase, pH 10; acid phosphatase, pH 5.
    B. alkaline phosphatase, pH 5; acid phosphatase, pH 10.
    C. nitrophenyl phosphatase, pH 5; nitrophenyl kinase, pH 10.
    D. nitrophenyl phosphatase, pH 10; nitrophenyl kinase, pH 5.
    E. None of the above.

4. While enzyme concentration and enzyme activity are commonly used interchangeably, what's the most common discordance between them?
    A. immunoassay measurement of enzyme concentration is always equal to enzyme activity
    B. immunoassay measurement of enzyme concentration is never equal to enzyme activity
    C. enzyme activity is usually measured in a different manner and therefore cannot be coordinated
    D. immunoassay underestimates activity
    E. activity underestimates immunoassay

5. What is the BEST definition of a macroenzyme and what is the effect?
    A. an enzyme multimer; creating a new active site
    B. a zymogenic form of an enzyme; inhibiting enzyme activity
    C. an enzyme bound to an antibody; inhibiting enzyme and preventing it from being cleared
    D. an enzyme larger than 300kDa; can only function in a specific subcellular location
    E. a multistep enzyme; converts reagents to products in a successive, stepwise fashion

6. What is plotted on a Lineweaver-Burke plot?
    A. [enzyme] versus 1/v
    B. 1/[enzyme] versus 1/v
    C. Vmax versus [substrate]
    D. 1/[S] versus 1/v
    E. v versus [enzyme]

1: Clinical Chemistry Questions

7. What is the x-intercept and the y-intercept, respectively, on a Lineweaver-Burk plot?
    A. substrate-max versus Vmax
    B. Km versus 1/Vmax
    C. 1/S versus -1/Km
    D. -1/Km versus 1/Vmax
    E. -1/Km versus Vmax

8. Which of the following types of inhibition can be overcome by increasing substrate concentration?
    A. competitive inhibition
    B. noncompetitive inhibition
    C. uncompetitive inhibition
    D. A & B
    E. B & C

9. How is the International Unit (IU) defined?
    A. amount of enzyme that catalyzes the conversion of 1 mole of substrate per second.
    B. amount of enzyme that catalyzes the conversion of 1 micromole of substrate per minute.
    C. the normalized ratio based on accepted standards.
    D. moles per liter of enzyme.
    E. gram molecular weight of enzyme.

10. Of the two following enzymes, which one is more liver-specific?
    A. AST
    B. ALT

11. What are the effects of heparin and renal failure on AST and ALT, respectively?
    A. higher, higher
    B. lower, lower
    C. lower, higher
    D. higher, lower
    E. no change

12. Which lactate dehydrogenase (LDH) isoenzyme is at the highest concentration in serum and what is the significance of a "flipped LD ratio," respectively?
    A. LD1, chronic alcoholism
    B. LD2, acute MI, hemolysis, or renal infarction
    C. LD3, liver damage
    D. LD4, skeletal damage
    E. LD5, liver congestion

13. Which LD isoenzyme that migrates cathodal to LD5 is indicative of hepatic vascular insufficiency?
    A. LD1
    B. LD3
    C. LD4
    D. LD5
    E. LD6

1: Clinical Chemistry Questions

14. Of the following which is not one of the major sources of acid phosphatase?
    A. placenta
    B. prostate
    C. red blood cells
    D. bone
    E. all of the above are major sources of acid phosphatase

15. Which alkaline phosphatase isoenzyme is most sensitive to inhibition by heat or urea treatment?
    A. bile duct
    B. intestine
    C. placenta
    D. bone
    E. kidney

16. Which of the following cell types produces bone alkaline phosphatase?
    A. osteoclasts
    B. osteoblasts
    C. chondrocytes
    D. macrophages
    E. megakaryocytes

17. Which of the following conditions is associated with mildly increased alkaline phosphatase?
    A. non-fasting Lewis (+) type B or O secretors after a meal
    B. unrecognized pregnancy
    C. congestive heart failure
    D. hepatic metastases
    E. all of the above are associated with mild increases in alkaline phosphatase.

18. Which two tests are the best tests to confirm that an elevated alkaline phosphatase is from the biliary tree (pick 2)?
    A. ALT
    B. GGT
    C. AST
    D. AFP
    E. 5' nucleotidase

19. Elevated serum ammonia (hyperammonemia) is nearly always due to failure of this organ:
    A. liver
    B. kidney
    C. heart
    D. spleen
    E. pancreas

20. What modification converts unconjugated bilirubin to conjugated bilirubin?
    A. sulfonylation
    B. ubiquitination
    C. methylation
    D. glucuronidation
    E. phosphorylation

1: Clinical Chemistry Questions

21. What is the significance of direct and indirect bilirubin (choose the single BEST answer)?
    A. direct can be excreted directly in the urine, while indirect can't
    B. direct is directly measured in a diazo-colorimetric assay, while indirect is calculated
    C. direct can be visualized by spectroscopy, indirect cannot
    D. direct comes straight from the liver, indirect doesn't
    E. direct is equal to 1/2 of the total, while indirect is equal the other half

22. Which of the following is a cause of conjugated hyperbilirubinemia?
    A. cirrhosis
    B. Gilbert syndrome
    C. Crigler-Najjar syndrome
    D. hemolysis
    E. Dubin-Johnson syndrome

23. Which coagulation factor has the shortest *in vitro* half-life and which test is commonly used to measure it?
    A. Factor V, Factor V Leiden
    B. Factor II, PTT
    C. Factor VII, PT
    D. Factor XIII, D-dimer
    E. Protein C, serum albumin

24. What is the leading cause of neonatal jaundice?
    A. physiological jaundice due to hepatic enzymes not being up to capacity
    B. hemolysis secondary to hemoglobinopathies
    C. sepsis due to TORCH infections
    D. metabolic disorders, such as glycogen storage diseases
    E. breast milk jaundice

25. Which of the following is NOT associated with benign physiological jaundice?
    A. jaundice that appears within 24 hours of birth
    B. jaundice that appears 2-3 days after birth
    C. bilirubin rises at a rate of 2 mg/dL/day
    D. bilirubin levels of 10 mg/dL
    E. all of the above are associated with benign physiological jaundice

26. At what bilirubin level should exchange transfusion be first considered over phototherapy?
    A. >10mg/dL before 12 hours of age
    B. 12 mg/dL before 18 hours of age
    C. 14 mg/dL before 24 hours of age
    D. 18 mg/dL before 48 hours of age
    E. 20 mg/dL at any time

27. Which of the following alternatives to measuring serum bilirubin in newborns has been proposed as a screen for hyperbilirubinemia?
    A. transcutaneous bilirubin levels
    B. umbilical vein whole blood bilirubin levels
    C. superior sagittal sinus Doppler
    D. percutaneous liver biopsy
    E. plasmon laser resonance bilirubin diffraction

1: Clinical Chemistry Questions

28. Which of the following causes of acute hepatitis is LEAST likely to lead to a complete recovery?
    A. HAV
    B. HBV
    C. HCV
    D. drugs
    E. all of the above usually experience a complete recovery

29. Which of the following acute hepatitis viruses are sensitively detected by serological testing?
    A. HAV
    B. HBV
    C. HCV
    D. A & B
    C. B & C

30. Which of the following produces the most profound elevations in transaminases?
    A. HAV
    B. HBV
    C. HCV
    D. ischemia
    E. autoimmune

31. How does the AST:ALT ratio help in distinguishing toxic, ischemic, and alcoholic hepatitis from viral hepatitis?
    A. AST:ALT <1, implies viral hepatitis
    B. AST:ALT >1, implies viral hepatitis
    C. AST:ALT <2, implies toxic, ischemic, or alcoholic hepatitis
    D. AST:ALT >2, implies toxic, ischemic, or alcoholic hepatitis
    E. A & D
    F. B & C

32. Which are among the most common causes of jaundice?
    A. HAV
    B. HBV
    C. HCV
    D. alcoholic hepatitis
    E. toxic hepatitis
    F. A & C
    G. A & D

33. What is the single best prognostic test in acute hepatic injury?
    A. viral titers
    B. bilirubin
    C. AST:ALT ratio
    D. protime (PT)
    E. GGT (gamma-glutamyl transpeptidase)

1: Clinical Chemistry Questions

34. What are the two isoenzymes of serum amylase and what is the effect of wheat germ lectin, *Triticum vulgaris*, on each (pick 2)?
    A. salivary, inhibited
    B. salivary, uninhibited
    C. pancreatic, inhibited
    D. pancreatic, uninhibited
    E. biliary, inhibited

35. Persistent elevations of serum amylase after an initial onset of acute pancreatitis are worrisome for which of the following?
    A. serous cystadenoma
    B. metastatic carcinoma
    C. pseudocyst
    D. parotid tumor
    E. chronic pancreatitis

36. What is the most common cause of acute pancreatitis associated with normal serum amylase levels?
    A. hypertriglyceridemia
    B. Trinidad scorpion venom
    C. smoking
    D. alcohol
    E. estrogen

37. What's the best explanation for the elevated serum amylase with low urine amylase seen in macroamylasemia?
    A. increased production in the pancreas of proenzyme forms of amylase
    B. decreased cleavage of pro-amylase to make amylase
    C. antibody bound to amylase, leading to decreased renal clearance
    D. toxic injury to renal glomeruli
    E. pancreatic ductal adenocarcinoma

38. Which of the following is one of the many advantages of lipase over amylase for the diagnosis of acute pancreatitis?
    A. lipase is more pancreas-specific
    B. lipase is less reliant on renal clearance
    C. lipase rises in parallel to amylase, but remains elevated for longer.
    D. all of the above are advantages of lipase
    E. none of the above are advantages of lipase

39. Which of the following is NOT considered one of the Ranson criteria for the assessment of acute pancreatitis at hospital admission?
    A. age
    B. hematocrit
    C. serum glucose
    D. AST
    E. LDH

40. How long does it take to assign a Ranson score to a patient presenting with acute pancreatitis?
    A. one can assign a score based on the initial evaluation at admission
    B. at least 1 hour
    C. at least 24 hours
    D. at least 48 hours
    E. at least one week

1: Clinical Chemistry Questions

41. Which of the following genes has NOT been implicated as a cause of recurrent pancreatitis?
    A. *TSC1*
    B. *PRSS-1*
    C. *PSTI*
    D. *CFTR*
    E. all of the above genes are associated with recurrent pancreatitis

42. Of the following tests, which is the most sensitive and specific test of pancreatic exocrine function?
    A. fecal fat
    B. chymotryspin
    C. elastase-1
    D. D-xylose
    E. trypsinogen

43. Match the cyst fluid associated with each of the following pancreatic cysts:
    1. pseudocyst
    2. serous cystadenoma
    3. mucinous cystadenoma
    4. intraductal papillary mucinous neoplasm
    5. solid-pseudopapillary tumor

    A. low amylase, low CEA, low CA 19-9
    B. high amylase, high CEA, normal to high CA 19-9
    C. low amylase, high CEA, normal to high CA 19-9
    D. low amylase, low CEA, low CA 19-9
    E. high amylase, low CEA, high CA 19-9

44. Which of the creatinine kinase isozymes is most widely distributed?
    A. CK-MM
    B. CK-MB
    C. CK-BB
    D. CK-BM
    E. CK-DB

45. What creatinine kinase isozyme composes nearly 100% of normal serum CK?
    A. CK-BB
    B. CK-MB
    C. CK-MM
    D. CK-BM
    E. CK-DB

46. Which creatinine kinase isozyme migrates slightly slower than MM and whose appearance is associated with disseminated malignancies and poor prognosis?
    A. CK-MB
    B. CK-BB
    C. macro-CK
    D. mitochondrial CK
    E. CK-MB3

1: Clinical Chemistry Questions

47. Which of the following troponins has both a cardiac and skeletal muscle isoform?
    A. TnT
    B. TnI
    C. TnC
    D. A & B
    E. A, B, C

48. Which of the following is the most cardiac-sensitive enzyme isoform with a commercially-available assay?
    A. cTnT
    B. cTnI
    C. cTnC
    D. CK-MB
    E. myoglobin

49. Which of the following descriptions best fits myoglobin?
    A. most sensitive, least specific marker of acute myocardial infarction
    B. most specific, least sensitive
    C. earliest marker of acute myocardial infarction
    D. A & C
    E. B & C

50. Ischemia-modified albumin reflects myocardial ischemia, rising within minutes of ischemic damage and returning to baseline within a few hours. The assay is based on the altered binding of albumin to which of the following elements?
    A. calcium
    B. cobalt
    C. phosphorus
    D. oxygen
    E. iron

51. Which of the following natriuretic peptides provides the most longitudinal information about congestive heart failure?
    A. atrial (A-type) natriuretic peptide (ANP)
    B. brain (B-type) natriuretic peptide (BNP)
    C. pro-BNP
    D. N-terminal pro-BNP
    E. C-type natriuretic peptide

52. All of the following are included in the definition of acute coronary syndrome (ACS), <u>except</u>:
    A. stable angina
    B. unstable angina
    C. congestive heart failure
    D. acute myocardial infarction
    E. sudden cardiac death

53. What is the purpose of serial measurements of elevated troponins in suspected acute myocardial infarction?
    A. increased sensitivity
    B. increase negative predictive value
    C. increased specificity
    D. A & B
    E. A, B, C

1: Clinical Chemistry Questions

54. What is the purpose of measuring CK-MB in the presence of elevated troponin in a patient with a suspected acute myocardial infarction (AMI)?
     A. troponin is less sensitive than CK-MB for AMI
     B. troponin is less specific than CK-MB for AMI
     C. troponin is not helpful in determining the time course of AMI
     D. CK-MB is more stable than troponin and stays elevated longer
     E. CK-MB can provide additional information about congestive heart failure

55. In the quantitation of protein by the Kjedahl technique, what is actually measured?
     A. spectrophotometry
     B. colorimetric assay
     C. refractometry
     D. ammonium nitrogen released by acid digestion

56. What is the usual net charge on proteins and toward which pole do they migrate?
     A. negative, anode
     B. negative, cathode
     C. positive, anode
     D. positive, cathode
     E. no charge, it depends

57. Which represents the fastest migrating band on standard serum protein electrophoresis performed at pH 8.6?
     A. albumin
     B. alpha-1
     C. alpha-2
     D. beta
     E. gamma

58. All of the following techniques are used to characterize a suspected monoclonal band, except:
     A. immunofixation electrophoresis
     B. immunotyping
     C. immunoelectophoresis
     D. immunoprecipitation
     E. all of the above are routinely used

59. Which of the following condition(s) account for the most significant changes in serum albumin levels?
     A. protein-losing enteropathy
     B. nephrotic syndrome
     C. liver disease
     D. A & B
     E. A, B, C

60. All of the following are functions of pre-albumin, except:
     A. binding thyroid hormones, T3 & T4
     B. bind and carry retinol-binding protein:vitamin A complex
     C. amyloid precursor in senile cardiac amyloidosis
     D. maintenance of serum osmotic pressure
     E. all of the above are functions of pre-albumin

1: Clinical Chemistry Questions

61. Transferrin may be elevated with iron deficiency and resemble an M-spike on serum protein electrophoresis. Where does the transferrin band migrate?
    A. pre-albumin
    B. albumin
    C. alpha-1
    D. alpha-2
    E. beta-1

62. This protein is elevated in serum with renal or hepatic disease:
    A. ceruloplasmin
    B. alpha-2-macroglobulin
    C. haptoglobin
    D. transferrin
    E. fibrinogen

63. The asialated form of this protein is also known as tau protein and can be found in cerebrospinal fluid:
    A. pre-albumin
    B. albumin
    C. transferrin
    D. alpha-1-antitrypsin
    E. ceruloplasmin

64. This protein should not normally be found in serum, but when it is, it runs with the beta-globins:
    A. C-reactive protein
    B. fibrinogen
    C. haptoglobin
    D. ceruloplasmin
    E. alpha-2-macroglobulin

65. What is the clinical significance of a twin albumin band?
    A. M-spike
    B. normal variant
    C. acute inflammation
    D. starvation
    E. high cholesterol

66. In non-selective proteinuria, all of the bands on serum protein electrophoresis are decreased, except:
    A. albumin
    B. alpha-1
    C. alpha-2
    D. beta
    E. gamma

67. Beta-gamma bridging is most commonly seen in which of the following situations?
    A. monoclonal gammopathy
    B. cirrhosis
    C. starvation
    D. non-selective proteinuria
    E. selective proteinuria

1: Clinical Chemistry Questions

68. All of the following are potential causes of apparent hypogammaglobulinemia, <u>except</u>:
    A. congenital hypogammaglobulinemia
    B. lymphoma
    C. nephrotic syndrome
    D. myeloma
    E. all of the above are potential causes of hypogammaglobulinemia

69. All of the following are characteristic features of normal CSF protein electrophoresis relative to serum protein electrophoresis, except:
    A. oligoclonal gamma bands
    B. prominent pre-albumin band
    C. dim albumin band
    D. double beta-transferrin band
    E. dim alpha-2 band

70. Which of the following types of proteinuria presents with a strong albumin band on urine protein electrophoresis?
    A. tubular proteinuria
    B. glomerular proteinuria
    C. tubulointerstitial proteinuria
    D. overflow proteinuria
    E. none of the above patterns exhibit a strong albumin band

71. Which of the following types of cryoglobulins is most commonly associated with Waldenstrom macroglobulinemia?
    A. Type I
    B. Type II
    C. Type III
    D. Type IV
    E. Type V

72. What's the most common cause of mixed cryoglobulinemia?
    A. chronic liver disease
    B. lupus
    C. hepatitis C virus
    D. lymphoproliferative disorders
    E. chronic infections

73. What's the most common renal pathology associated with mixed cryoglobulinemia?
    A. membranoproliferative glomerulonephritis, type II
    B. membranoproliferative glomerulonephritis, type I
    C. membranous glomerulonephritis
    D. focal segmental glomerulosclerosis
    E. minimal change disease

74. What is the most common adverse effect of correcting hyponatremia too <u>slowly</u>?
    A. central pontine myelinolysis
    B. cerebral edema
    C. cardiac arrhythmias
    D. anesthesia
    E. reflex hypoglycemia

1: Clinical Chemistry Questions

75. All of the following are potential causes of hypervolemic hyponatremia, <u>except</u>:
    A. cardiac failure
    B. nephrotic syndrome
    C. cirrhosis
    D. renal tubular acidosis, type I
    E. all of the above lead to hypervolemic hyponatremia

76. Which of the following are potential causes of hypokalemia?
    A. GI potassium losses
    B. renal potassium losses
    C. transcellular shifts
    D. all of the above
    E. none of the above

77. Which of the following causes of acidosis is associated with hypokalemia?
    A. renal tubular acidosis, type I
    B. renal tubular acidosis, type II
    C. renal tubular acidosis, type IV
    D. A & B
    E. A, B, C

78. What is the cause of primary hyperparthyroidism?
    A. excess parathyroid hormone
    B. CASr gene mutation
    C. thiazide diuretics
    D. sarcoidosis
    E. hyperthyroidism

79. Which of the following causes of hypercalcemia is least likely to be associated with kidney stone formation?
    A. sarcoidosis
    B. hypervitaminosis D
    C. primary hyperparathyroidism
    D. milk-alkali syndrome
    E. squamous cell carcinoma-associated PTHrP

80. What accounts for the majority of cases of hypercalcemia?
    A. hyperparathyroidism
    B. malignancy
    C. hypervitaminosis D
    D. A & B
    E. A, B, C

81. What is the corrected calcium in a patient with a measured calcium of 10.4 mg/dL and an albumin of 2.0 g/dL?
    A. 8 mg/dL
    B. 10.4 mg/dL
    C. 12.0 mg/dL
    D. 12.8 mg/dL
    E. it cannot be calculated from the information provided.

1: Clinical Chemistry Questions

82. What is the most common cause of secondary hyperparathyroidism?
    A. parathyroid adenoma
    B. parathyroid hyperplasia
    C. parathyroid carcinoma
    D. peripheral resistance to PTH
    E. DiGeorge syndrome

83. What is the most accurate definition of acidemia?
    A. pH > 7.44
    B. pH < 7.0
    C. pH > 7.0
    D. decreased serum CO_2
    E. increased serum bicarbonate

84. According to the Henderson-Hasselbalch equation, in order to maintain pH an increase in bicarbonate should be compensated for by this change in CO_2:
    A. increase (retain more)
    B. decrease (retain less)
    C. no change
    D. changes in CO_2 do not compensate for changes in bicarbonate
    E. intracellular shift of CO_2

85. All of the following variables are directly measured by arterial blood gas analyzers, <u>except</u>:
    A. pH
    B. $PaCO_2$
    C. PaO_2
    D. percent oxygen saturation (SaO_2)
    E. all of the above are directly measured

86. Which of the following techniques is superior in detecting carbon monoxide poisoning?
    A. arterial blood gas analyzer
    B. pulse oximeter
    C. co-oximeter
    D. peripheral blood smear
    E. all are equivalent

87. Which of the following equations best estimates the anion gap?
    A. $[HCO_3^-] + [K^+] - [Na^+]$
    B. $([Na^+] - [K^+]) - [HCO_3^-]$
    C. $([Cl^-] - [HCO_3^-]) + [Na^+]$
    D. $[HCO_3^-] - ([Na^+] - [Cl^-])$
    E. $[Na^+] - ([Cl^-] + [HCO_3^-])$

88. In general, in which relative directions do changes in pH and bicarbonate go in metabolic and respiratory disorders, respectively?
    A. same direction, opposite direction
    B. opposite direction, same direction
    C. opposite in both
    D. same in both
    E. it depends on the cause

1: Clinical Chemistry Questions

89. Which two of the following calculations assist in determining the cause of metabolic acidosis?
    A. anion gap
    B. osmolal gap
    C. $[HCO_3^-]$
    D. A & B
    E. A, B, C

90. What relationship exists between creatinine concentration and glomerular filtration rate?
    A. directly related
    B. inversely related
    C. not related
    D. complex interaction - sometimes related, sometimes not
    E. cannot be predicted

91. All of the following criteria are utilized in the calculation of Modification of Diet in Renal Disease (MDRD) study equation eGFR, except:
    A. serum creatinine
    B. gender
    C. patient age
    D. patient race
    E. body mass

92. What type of azotemia is most likely when the BUN/creatinine ratio is maintained but the levels of both are elevated?
    A. prerenal azotemia
    B. renal azotemia
    C. postrenal azotemia
    D. A & B
    E. A, B, C

93. Which of the following is the most standardized definition of proteinuria?
    A. >150mg/day of urinary protein
    B. >300 mg/day of urinary protein
    C. >3mg/day of urinary protein
    D. > or equal to 2+ on spot urine protein testing
    E. none of the above

94. The presence of beta$_2$-microglobulin or lysozyme in the urine is suggestive of dysfunction of this portion of the kidney:
    A. afferent arteriole
    B. juxtaglomerular apparatus
    C. glomerulus
    D. renal tubule
    E. efferent arteriole

95. Which of the following criteria is most critical to defining the stage of chronic kidney disease?
    A. patient age
    B. patient gender
    C. patient race
    D. glomerular filtration rate
    E. hemoglobin

1: Clinical Chemistry Questions

96. Which of the following conditions is an indication for dialysis?
    A.   severe metabolic alkalosis
    B.   volume depletion
    C.   hypokalemia
    D.   uremic pericarditis
    E.   none of the above are indications for dialysis

97. What is the typical result for fractional excretion of sodium (FENa) in pre-renal acute renal failure?
    A.   increased (>2%)
    B.   decreased (<1%)
    C.   no change
    D.   it depends on the cause of prerenal azotemia

98. Pigmented casts are most suspicious for this type of renal pathology:
    A.   prerenal acute renal failure
    B.   glomerulonephritis
    C.   acute tubular necrosis
    D.   tubulointerstitial nephritis
    E.   bladder pathology

99. What's the most common cause of renal failure in cirrhotic patients?
    A.   NSAIDs
    B.   radiocontrast dye
    C.   aminoglycosides
    D.   spontaneous bacterial peritonitis
    E.   volume overload

100. At what wavelength light is bilirubin absorbance maximal?
    A.   150 nm
    B.   260 nm
    C.   320 nm
    D.   450 nm
    E.   620 nm

101. Which two variables are plotted on a Liley curve?
    A.   delta OD_{320} v. hCG
    B.   delta OD_{450} v. EGA
    C.   EGA v. hCG
    D.   hCG v. delta OD_{200}
    E.   none of the above

102. All of the following hormones share a common alpha subunit, except:
    A.   prolactin
    B.   TSH
    C.   FSH
    D.   LH
    E.   hCG

1: Clinical Chemistry Questions

103. Which of the following outcomes in hCG testing is associated most commonly with heterophile antibodies?
    A. true positives
    B. false positives
    C. true negatives
    D. false negatives
    E. it depends

104. At what point in normal gestation does hCG usually reach maximum levels?
    A. within the first two weeks after conception
    B. end of first trimester
    C. end of second trimester
    D. end of third trimester
    E. 2 weeks post-partum

105. What's the most common site for ectopic pregnancies?
    A. ovary
    B. fallopian tube
    C. cornu
    D. uterus
    E. abdomen

106. Beyond hCG levels and ultrasound, which of the following tests has been helpful in distinguishing an intrauterine pregnancy from an abnormal pregnancy?
    A. serum progesterone
    B. serum estrogen
    C. serum inhibin
    D. computerized tomographic (CT) imaging
    E. abdominal plain film radiography

107. Which of the following is not a part of the so-called "quad test"?
    A. hCG
    B. alpha-fetoprotein
    C. dimeric inhibin A
    D. progesterone
    E. unconjugated estriol

108. Which of the following patterns is associated with Edwards' syndrome?
    A. increased AFP, increased hCG, increased estriol
    B. decreased AFP, increased hCG, increased estriol
    C. decreased AFP, decreased hCG, increased estriol
    D. increased AFP, decreased hCG, decreased estriol
    E. decreased AFP, decreased hCG, decreased estriol

109. Which of the following patterns is associated with neural tube defects?
    A. increased AFP, normal hCG, decreased estriol
    B. increased AFP, increased hCG, increased estriol
    C. decreased AFP, normal hCG, decreased estriol
    D. decreased AFP, increased hCG, decreased estriol
    E. normal AFP, increased hCG, increased estriol

1: Clinical Chemistry Questions

110. Which of the following patterns is associated with Down syndrome (trisomy 21)?
    A. decreased AFP, decreased hCG, decreased estriol
    B. decreased AFP, increased hCG, decreased estriol
    C. increased AFP, increased hCG, increased estriol
    D. increased AFP, decreased hCG, increased estriol
    E. decreased AFP, decreased hCG, increased estriol

111. What is the maternal age above which ACOG 2007 guidelines recommend invasive screening?
    A. 27
    B. 32
    C. 35
    D. 37
    E. 42

112. What is the effect typically of increased maternal weight on maternal serum alpha fetoprotein levels?
    A. varies with fetal gender
    B. increased
    C. decreased
    D. no change

113. Which of the following organs synthesizes dimeric inhibin as seen in maternal serum?
    A. fetal gonads
    B. maternal ovaries
    C. fetal kidney
    D. placenta
    E. maternal liver

114. All of the following are part of the definition of pre-term labor, except:
    A. rupture of membranes
    B. regular contractions
    C. prior to 37 weeks
    D. associated cervical changes
    E. all of the above are strictly considered to be part of the definition

115. Type II pneumocytes produce surfactant, which is predominantly composed of a mix of phospholipids called lecithin. What is the primary component of lecithin?
    A. phosphatidylcholine
    B. phosphatidylglycerol
    C. phosphatidylinositol
    D. phosphatidylethanolamine
    E. sphingomyelin

116. During which time frame in gestation is the assessment of fetal lung maturity most necessary?
    A. prior to 30 weeks
    B. 30-34 weeks
    C. 34-37 weeks
    D. 37-39 weeks
    E. after 39 weeks

1: Clinical Chemistry Questions

117. What lecithin:sphingomyelin ratio is considered to be consistent with fetal lung maturity?
    A. 1:1
    B. 2:1
    C. 1:2
    D. 5:1
    E. 1:5

118. Which of the following analytes can be measured as an indication of lung maturity when confounding factors preclude accurate determination of maturity by L:S ratios?
    A. lecithin alone
    B. phosphatidylinositol
    C. phosphatidylinositol phosphate
    D. phosphatidyl glycerol
    E. diacylglycerol

119. Which of the following is typically INCREASED in pregnancy?
    A. GFR (glomerular filtration rate)
    B. BUN (blood urea nitrogen)
    C. creatinine
    D. urate
    E. none of the above are typically increased

120. At which point with all other risks being equal is a mother's risk of thromboembolism the highest?
    A. pre-pregnancy
    B. first trimester
    C. second trimester
    D. third trimester
    E. postpartum

121. Which of the following autoimmune diseases tends to actually decrease in severity during pregnancy?
    A. rheumatoid arthritis
    B. Graves disease
    C. myasthenia gravis
    D. A & B
    E. A, B, C

122. What is the most common cause of death due to lupus in pregnant women?
    A. hypertension
    B. hypercoagulation
    C. lupus pneumonitis
    D. renal failure
    E. Libman-Sacks endocarditis

123. Which of the following cause Sheehan syndrome?
    A. pregnancy-associated pituitary enlargement
    B. severe blood loss during pregnancy
    C. thromboembolic disease
    D. A & B
    E. A, B, C

1: Clinical Chemistry Questions

124. Which of the following is the cause of hyperemesis gravidarum?
    A. hypothyroidism
    B. hyperthyroidism
    C. high levels of hCG
    D. high levels of progesterone
    E. none of the above

125. What is the most commonly associated comorbidity of acute fatty liver of pregnancy?
    A. pulmonary embolism
    B. Budd-Chiari syndrome
    C. hepatic adenoma
    D. disseminated intravascular coagulation
    E. cirrhosis

126. All of the following are common forms of investigation into recurrent pregnancy loss, except:
    A. parental karyotyping
    B. endometrial biopsy
    C. lupus anticoagulant testing
    D. urine drug screen
    E. thyroid function tests

127. What type of kinetics does the elimination of most drugs or foreign agents follow?
    A. zero order
    B. first order
    C. second order
    D. mixed order
    E. higher order

128. How many half-lives (with dosing at the half-life) are typically needed to reach a steady state?
    A. 1
    B. 2
    C. 5
    D. 10
    E. 20

129. Under which condition is a protein-bound drug usually at its most efficacious?
    A. high serum protein levels
    B. low serum protein levels
    C. high hydrostatic pressure
    D. low hydrostatic pressure
    E. none of the above

130. What does a high volume of distribution for a drug imply?
    A. high plasma concentration
    B. strict limitation to the vascular space
    C. lipophilicity and hydrophobicity
    D. wide distribution into vascular, extravascular, and adipose tissue
    E. none of the above

1: Clinical Chemistry Questions

131. What is the most common modality used in urine testing for drugs of abuse?
     A. immunoassay
     B. mass spectrophotometry
     C. electrophoresis
     D. cell culture
     E. tasting

132. Match the drug of abuse with the key metabolite:
     A. cocaine
     B. heroin
     C. amphetamines
     D. PCP
     E. cannibis

     1. norepinephrine and phenylacetone
     2. hydroxylated and glucoronidated drug forms
     3. Δ-9-THC-COOH
     4. N-acetylmorphine
     5. benzoylecgonine

133. What is the physiological basis of acute cocaine-induced chest pain?
     A. hypercoagulability and thrombus development
     B. direct antiplatelet activity
     C. coronary vasoconstriction
     D. increased blood pressure
     E. neurotoxicity

134. Which of the following tests is most significantly affected by cocaine use?
     A. myoglobin
     B. CK-MB
     C. troponin I
     D. A & B
     E. A, B, C

135. Which of the following drugs can provide a therapeutic as well as diagnostic effect in patients with acute opiate intoxication?
     A. nalmefene
     B. naloxone
     C. methadone
     D. A & B
     E. A, B, C

136. What is the mechanism of barbiturate-mediated CNS depression?
     A. opiate receptor agonist
     B. NMDA receptor agonist
     C. potentiation of NMDA-dependent activity
     D. potentiation of GABA-dependent activity
     E. potentiation of glutamate-dependent activity

1: Clinical Chemistry Questions

137. Which of the following conditions is associated with the highest average hCG levels?
    A. normal intrauterine pregnancy
    B. ectopic pregnancy
    C. partial mole
    D. complete mole
    E. choriocarcinoma

138. Which of the following is a potential risk of long-term amphetamine use?
    A. Alzheimer-like syndrome
    B. Parkinsonian syndrome
    C. rhabdomyolysis
    D. cirrhosis
    E. all of the above

139. What is the mechanism of action of phencyclidine?
    A. direct serotonergic activity
    B. inhibition of serotonin reuptake
    C. direct cholinergic activity
    D. inhibition of catecholamine reuptake
    E. a combination of several of the above mechanisms

140. At what blood alcohol level (BAL) does one start worrying about coma and death from alcohol poisoning (in general)?
    A. 0.05%
    B. 0.1%
    C. 0.3%
    D. 0.4%
    E. 0.8%

141. What is the first hepatic metabolite of ethanol?
    A. cocaethylene
    B. acetic acid
    C. methanol
    D. ethylene glycol
    E. acetaldehyde

142. Which sample is preferred for quantitative alcohol testing in a living patient with a suspected overdose?
    A. vitreous humor
    B. breath
    C. whole blood
    D. urine
    E. serum

143. In the legal definition of alcohol level limits for operation of a motor vehicle, what sample is used for standards?
    A. vitreous humor
    B. breath
    C. whole blood
    D. urine
    E. serum

1: Clinical Chemistry Questions

144. Under normal circumstances which test is the most sensitive and specific for chronic alcohol consumption?
    A.   carbohydrate-deficient transferrin (CDT)
    B.   serum alkaline phosphatase (AP)
    C.   gamma-glutamyl transferase (GGT)
    D.   alcohol dehydrogenase (ADH)
    E.   alanine aminotransferase (ALT)

145. Which of the following toxidromes is most likely to be seen in a farm worker who has just been spraying pesticides?
    A.   altered mental status, hypopnea/apnea
    B.   salivation, lacrimation, urination, diarrhea, GI cramps, and emesis
    C.   hyperthermia, dry skin, altered mental status, psychosis
    D.   hypertension, tachycardia, mydriasis, anxiety, hyperthermia
    E.   hallucinations, anxiety, hyperthermia

146. What is the calculated osmolarity for a sodium of 140 mEq/L, blood urea nitrogen of 10 mg/dL, and a glucose of 180 mg/dL?
    A.   340 mOsm/L
    B.   330 mOsm/L
    C.   318 mOsm/L
    D.   312 mOsm/L
    E.   384 mOsm/L

147. Which ingestion would be most suspect in a patient with both and anion and osmolar gap?
    A.   whiskey
    B.   rubbing alcohol
    C.   windshield washer fluid
    D.   nail polish remover
    E.   aspirin

148. Which of the following values is calculated in an arterial blood gas analyzer?
    A.   oxygen saturation of blood
    B.   hemoglobin oxygen affinity
    C.   oxygen tension of blood
    D.   pH of blood
    E.   all of the above are directly measured by an ABG analyzer

149. Which of the following forms of hemoglobin will a pulse oximeter measure?
    A.   oxyhemoglobin
    B.   deoxyhemoglobin
    C.   carboxyhemoglobin
    D.   A & B
    E.   A, B, C

150. Why has ethanol been historically used in the treatment of ethylene glycol or methanol poisoning?
    A.   ethanol prevents the development of an anion gap
    B.   ethanol increases diuresis and elimination
    C.   ethanol directly binds methanol and ethylene glycol, effectively neutralizing them
    D.   ethanol competes with ethylene glycol and methanol for alcohol dehydrogenase
    E.   ethanol makes the patient less anxious

1: Clinical Chemistry Questions

151. Which two body sites are the primary storage sites for lead? (pick two)
   A. vitreous humor
   B. hair
   C. bone
   D. erythrocytes
   E. gingiva

152. What is the preferred screening test for lead toxicity?
   A. blood lead levels
   B. free erythrocyte protoporphyrin (FEP)
   C. zinc protoporphyrin (ZPP)
   D. hair lead levels
   E. urine lead levels

153. Above what level is considered an elevated lead concentration when screening children?
   A. 5 microgram/dL
   B. 10 microgram/dL
   C. 35 microgram/dL
   D. 50 microgram/dL
   E. 100 microgram/dL

154. Which of the following modalities is best for measuring blood carbon monoxide levels?
   A. pulse oximeter
   B. co-oximeter
   C. blood gas analyzer
   D. hemoglobin levels
   E. V/Q scan

155. Which of the following ancillary tools is used to assess the risk of acetaminophen overdose?
   A. Levey-Jennings chart
   B. Rumack-Matthew nomogram
   C. Henderson-Hasselbalch equation
   D. Friedewald equation
   E. Michaelis-Menten equation

156. Which of the following compounds is the toxic metabolite of acetaminophen primarily responsible for hepatotoxicity?
   A. acetaminophen phosphate
   B. N-acetylcysteine
   C. N-acetyl-p-benzoquinoneimine
   D. glutathione
   E. acetaminophen sulfate

157. Which of the following is most consistent with cyanide poisoning?
   A. elevated serum lactate, anion gap metabolic acidosis
   B. elevated serum lactate, metabolic alkalosis
   C. decreased serum lactate, anion gap metabolic acidosis
   D. decreased serum lactate, metabolic alkalosis
   E. normal serum lactate, normal serum pH

1: Clinical Chemistry Questions

158. Which of the following is most consistent with salicylate intoxication?
    A. respiratory alkalosis
    B. metabolic acidosis
    C. respiratory acidosis
    D. A & B
    E. A, B, C

159. Which of the following is the most reliable test for the diagnosis of acute arsenic ingestion?
    A. fingernail arsenic quantitation
    B. quantitative 24-hour urinary arsenic levels
    C. blood arsenic levels
    D. serum arsenic levels
    E. hair arsenic quantitation

160. Which of the following tests can give likelihood information for seizure risk in tricyclic antidepressant overdose?
    A. blood oxygen partial pressure
    B. EKG
    C. urine sediment analysis
    D. renal biopsy
    E. none of the above

161. Which of the following types of poisoning can result in either autonomic instability and a desquamative erythematous rash of the palms and feet OR personality changes with irritability and fine motor disturbances?
    A. lead
    B. mercury
    C. carbamates
    D. organophosphates
    E. arsenic

162. A hat maker is suspected to have mercury poisoning due to his increasingly erratic behavior. What is the preferred method to confirm the diagnosis?
    A. 24-hour urine mercury levels
    B. hair mercury levels
    C. whole blood mercury levels
    D. liver dry mercury weight
    E. vitreous mercury levels

163. Which of the following drugs can substantially alter the risk of digoxin toxicity?
    A. fluoroquinolone
    B. alprazolam
    C. lithium
    D. quinidine
    E. aspirin

164. Which of the following means are used to metabolize procainamide?
    A. hepatic
    B. renal
    C. respiratory
    D. A & B
    E. A, B, C

1: Clinical Chemistry Questions

165. What's the most reliable means of predicting quinidine toxicity?
      A. serum quinidine levels
      B. whole blood quinidine levels
      C. 24-hour urinary quinidine levels
      D. liver function tests
      E. EKG

166. Which of the following agents causes fetal hydantoin syndrome?
      A. procainamide
      B. lithium
      C. quinidine
      D. amiodarone
      E. none of the above

167. What is the recommended monitoring interval for lithium levels in patients stable on therapy?
      A. 1-3 days
      B. 1-3 weeks
      C. 1-3 months
      D. 6-12 months
      E. every other year

168. All of the following organs potentially have a significant risk of amiodarone toxicity, except:
      A. thyroid
      B. kidney
      C. liver
      D. peripheral nerves
      E. lungs

169. Which of the following fatty acids have several double bonds along their hydrocarbon chains?
      A. saturated fatty acids
      B. monosaturated fatty acids
      C. monounsaturated fatty acids
      D. polysaturated fatty acids
      E. polyunsaturated fatty acids

170. All of the following are components of lipoprotein particles, except:
      A. chylomicrons
      B. cholesterol
      C. triglyceride
      D. phospholipids
      E. apolipoproteins

1: Clinical Chemistry Questions

171. Match the lipoprotein with its role:
    A.   chylomicron
    B.   VLDL
    C.   LDL
    D.   HDL

    1.   scavenge peripheral cholesterol to return to the liver
    2.   transport cholesterol to somatic cells
    3.   transport ingested lipid from enterocytes to somatic cells and liver
    4.   transport triglycerides to somatic cells

172. Which of the following variables are usually measured in a standard lipid quantitation?
    A.   total cholesterol
    B.   HDL
    C.   LDL
    D.   A & B
    E.   A, B, C

173. Match the type of lipid disorder by the lipoproteins increased in each:
    A.   I
    B.   II
    C.   III
    D.   IV
    E.   V

    1.   IDL
    2.   LDL
    3.   VLDL
    4.   chylomicrons
    5.   VLDL & chylomicrons

174. All of the following are common manifestations of elevated triglycerides, except:
    A.   eruptive xanthomas
    B.   premature atherosclerosis
    C.   tuberous xanthomas
    D.   xanthelasmas
    E.   acute pancreatitis

175. Tangier disease, smoking, obesity, and a sedentary lifestyle all have this in common:
    A.   increased apolipoprotein A-1
    B.   decreased triglycerides
    C.   increased cholesterol
    D.   decreased HDL
    E.   increased cholesterol

1: Clinical Chemistry Questions

176. Which of the following most accurately represents the cholesterol and LDL target values (in mg/dL) as recommended by the National Cholesterol Education Program (NCEP), Third Adult Treatment Panel (ATIII)?
    A.   <100, <200
    B.   <100, <100
    C.   <200, <200
    D.   <100, <50
    E.   <200, <100

177. Which of the following hormones is primarily responsible for the glucose intolerance associated with pregnancy?
    A.   human placental lactogen
    B.   progesterone
    C.   human chorionic gonadotropin
    D.   estrogen
    E.   alpha fetoprotein

178. How does laboratory glucose measurement compare to non-calibrated point of care (POC) glucose testing (in general)?
    A.   lab levels run higher that POC levels
    B.   lab levels run lower than POC levels
    C.   lab levels and POC levels are effectively the same
    D.   POC levels run higher than lab levels
    E.   none of the above

179. In patients with a normal RBC survival, what time span of glucose control is represented by hemoglobin A1c levels?
    A.   3 weeks
    B.   3 months
    C.   6 months
    D.   1 year
    E.   1-3 years

180. In addition to hypoglycemic symptoms and plasma glucose less than 45 mg/dL, what other symptom/sign completes the Whipple triad of the clinical presentation of insulinoma?
    A.   gastric pain
    B.   increased serum C peptide
    C.   diarrhea
    D.   relief of symptoms with glucose administration
    E.   oliguria

181. Why is the measured C peptide concentration usually several-fold higher than that of insulin in an individual without renal failure?
    A.   insulin is produced at half the rate of C peptide
    B.   insulin is metabolized faster than C peptide
    C.   C peptide is made in more islet cells than insulin
    D.   measured C peptide concentration is artifactually high in standard assays
    E.   all of the above contribute to higher C peptide than insulin ratios

1: Clinical Chemistry Questions

182. Which of the following is a cause of hyperinsulinemic hypoglycemia?
    A. autoimmune hypoglycemia
    B. liver failure
    C. starvation
    D. alcohol
    E. insulinoma

183. Which of the following autoantibodies are associated with type I diabetes?
    A. anti-GAD65
    B. anti-ICA512
    C. anti-IAA
    D. none of the above
    E. all of the above

184. Which of the following statements about diabetes diagnosis is true?
    A. a fasting plasma glucose greater than or equal to 120 mg/dL
    B. classical symptoms of diabetes and casual plasma glucose greater than 200 mg/dL
    C. oral glucose tolerance test with 75 g glucose load and two hour glucose greater than 200 mg/dL
    D. 24-28wks gestation oral glucose tolerance test with 100 g glucose and 1 hour plasma glucose greater than 150 mg/dL
    E. all of the above are true

185. All of the following are typically required for the diagnosis of diabetic ketoacidosis, except:
    A. hyperglycemia
    B. ketosis
    C. monocytosis
    D. metabolic acidosis
    E. all of the above are required

186. The nitroprusside technique to measure ketones can be used to directly measure which of the following compounds?
    A. acetone
    B. acetoacetic acid
    C. beta-hydroxybutyrate
    D. A & B
    E. A, B, C

187. Administration of which of the following is critical in the treatment of diabetic ketoacidosis?
    A. magnesium
    B. potassium
    C. sodium
    D. bicarbonate
    E. urea nitrogen

188. In a patient with mental status changes and hyperglycemia, which of the following is helpful in distinguishing diabetic ketoacidosis from hyperglycemic hyperosmolar nonketotic coma (HHNC)?
    A. level of hyperglycemia
    B. venous pH
    C. type of diabetes mellitus
    D. all of the above
    E. none of the above

1: Clinical Chemistry Questions

189. All of the following are components of the metabolic syndrome, <u>except</u>:
    A. obesity
    B. tachycardia
    C. insulin resistance
    D. hyperlipidemia
    E. hypertension

190. All of the following are characteristics of a good tumor marker screening test, <u>except</u>:
    A. high prevalence of disease
    B. cost-effective outcomes
    C. high pretest probability of disease
    D. dependence on heterophile antibodies
    E. low analytic sensitivity

191. Approximately what percentage of men with PSA elevated in the range of 4-10 ng/mL will be found to have prostate cancer?
    A. 0.1-0.5%
    B. 1-2%
    C. 10-20%
    D. 30-40%
    E. 85-90%

192. Which of the following statements regarding PSA testing best correlates with the presence of prostate cancer?
    A. free PSA less than 10%
    B. decreased bound PSA fraction
    C. PSA velocity greater than 0.25 ng/mL/yr
    D. PSA density greater than 0.05
    E. decreased pro-PSA

193. Which form of recurrence is most consistent with a rising post-treatment PSA?
    A. local recurrence
    B. distant metastatic recurrence
    C. micrometastatic lymph node disease
    D. angioinvasive disease
    E. cannot be determined

194. Which of the following colon cancer scenarios about higher CEA levels is true?
    A. poorly differentiated tumors produce more CEA than well-differentiated tumors
    B. confined tumors produce more CEA than metastatic tumors
    C. left-sided tumors produce more CEA than right-sided tumors
    D. diploid tumors produce more CEA than aneuploid tumors
    E. smokers on average have lower CEA than non-smokers

195. Which of the following thyroid tumors is associated with increased serum thyroglobulin?
    A. follicular carcinoma
    B. papillary carcinoma
    C. medullary carcinoma
    D. A & B
    E. A, B, C

1: Clinical Chemistry Questions

196. Which of the following conditions is associated with increased tumor-associated trypsin inhibitor (TATI)?
    A.   mucinous ovarian carcinoma
    B.   pancreatitis
    C.   urothelial carcinoma
    D.   pancreatic adenocarcinoma
    E.   all of the above

197. Which of the following conditions is most commonly associated with elevated CA-125?
    A.   sarcoidosis
    B.   non-mucinous epithelial ovarian neoplasm
    C.   mucinous epithelial ovarian neoplasm
    D.   gastric carcinoma
    E.   cirrhosis

198. Which of the following antibodies are directed against MUC1?
    A.   CA27-29
    B.   BR27-29
    C.   CA15-3
    D.   A & B
    E.   A, B, C

199. The combination of a weight loss of greater than 20 pounds, bilirubin greater than 3 mg/dL, and a CA19-9 greater than 37 units/L has an almost 100% positive predictive value for this type of carcinoma:
    A.   hepatocellular
    B.   biliary
    C.   splenic
    D.   pancreatic adenocarcinoma
    E.   chronic adenocarcinoma

200. Which of the following RBC antigens is the same as the CA19-9 antigen?
    A.   A
    B.   B
    C.   M
    D.   D (Rh)
    E.   Lewis

201. Which of the following tumors is associated with elevated alpha-fetoprotein?
    A.   hepatocellular carcinoma
    B.   yolk sac tumor
    C.   hepatoid gastric carcinoma
    D.   A & B
    E.   A, B, C

202. In which of the following conditions has beta 2 microglobulin been shown to represent an independent prognostic factor?
    A.   hepatocellular carcinoma
    B.   NK/T-cell lymphoma
    C.   extranodal marginal zone lymphoma
    D.   invasive ductal carcinoma of the breast
    E.   multiple myeloma

1: Clinical Chemistry Questions

203. Which of the following types of carcinoid tumors is most commonly associated with high levels of serotonin production?
     A. foregut
     B. midgut
     C. hindgut
     D. atypical carcinoids
     E. no specific type is associated with high serotonin

204. Which of the following tumors is associated with elevated plasma chromogranin A levels?
     A. pheochromocytoma
     B. carcinoid tumor
     C. pancreatic islet cell tumor
     D. small cell neuroendocrine tumor
     E. all of the above

205. Which immunohistochemical pattern is most consistent with medullary thyroid carcinoma?
     A. calcitonin (-), CEA (-), thyroglobulin (+)
     B. calcitonin (+), CEA (-), thyroglobulin (+)
     C. calcitonin (+), CEA (+), thyroglobulin (+)
     D. calcitonin (+), CEA (+), thyroglobulin (-)
     E. calcitonin (-), CEA (+), thyroglobulin (+)

206. Which of the following patterns is most consistent with a paraganglioma?
     A. elevation of predominantly norepinephrine and normetanephrine
     B. elevation of predominantly norepinephrine, metanephrine, and normetanephrine
     C. elevation of predominantly norepinephrine, epinephrine, metanephrine, and normetanephrine
     D. elevation of predominantly norepinephrine, epinephrine, and normetanephrine
     E. elevation of predominantly epinephrine and normetanephrine

207. For which of the following conditions are the NMP22 (nuclear matrix protein 22) and BTA (bladder tumor antigen) tests best suited?
     A. ruling out recurrent low-grade disease
     B. ruling in recurrent low-grade disease
     C. ruling out recurrent high-grade disease
     D. ruling in recurrent high-grade disease
     E. initial diagnosis of high-grade disease

208. Which of the following tests has been shown to be a potential useful screening tool for prostatic adenocarcinoma?
     A. prostate volume determination
     B. urine DD3 levels
     C. serum HVA and VMA levels
     D. NMP22 levels
     E. serum calcitonin

209. Which of the following patterns is most consistent with hyperthyroidism?
     A. decreased TSH, increased total T4, increased T3 resin uptake
     B. increased TSH, decreased total T4, decreased T3 resin uptake
     C. normal TSH, decreased to normal total T4, normal T3 resin uptake
     D. normal TSH, increased total T4, decreased T3 resin uptake
     E. decreased TSH, decreased total T4, increased T3 resin uptake

1: Clinical Chemistry Questions

210. All of the following are causes of hyperthyroidism, <u>except</u>:
    A. Graves disease
    B. pituitary adenoma
    C. toxic adenoma Plummer syndrome
    D. Hashimoto thyroiditis
    E. toxic multinodular goiter

211. Which of the following antibodies is/are associated with Hashimoto thyroiditis?
    A. anti-microsomal
    B. anti-thyroglobulin
    C. LATS
    D. A & B
    E. A, B, C

212. Which of the following descriptions best fits Refetoff syndrome?
    A. autosomal dominant peripheral resistance to thyroid hormone
    B. autosomal recessive congenital thyroiditis
    C. autosomal recessive thyroid agenesis
    D. autosomal dominant TSH gene deletion
    E. X-linked recessive absence of thyroid-binding globulin

213. What is the most common cause of sick euthyroid syndrome?
    A. medication effect
    B. critical illness
    C. increased thyroid binding globulin
    D. autoimmune destruction of thyroid
    E. radiation

214. What is the typical effect of amiodarone on thyroid function in the developed world?
    A. hyperthyroidism
    B. euthyroidism
    C. hypothyroidism
    D. increased anti-TSH antibodies
    E. none of the above

215. At what time of the day are cortisol levels typically highest and lowest, respectively?
    A. midnight, 8 a.m.
    B. 8 a.m., midnight
    C. 6 a.m., 6 p.m.
    D. 6 p.m., 6 a.m.
    E. there are no usual peaks or troughs

216. Which of the following is the best test for confirming Cushing disease?
    A. serum TSH
    B. 24-hour urine cortisol
    C. low dose dexamethasone suppression test
    D. high dose dexamethasone suppression test
    E. metyrapone stimulation test

1: Clinical Chemistry Questions

217. What is the best time to collect samples of salivary cortisol to be used as a screening tool for Cushing syndrome?
    A. early morning
    B. mid day
    C. early evening
    D. late-night
    E. the collection time is immaterial

218. What's the most common non-iatrogenic cause of Cushing syndrome?
    A. Cushing disease
    B. ectopic ACTH production by tumor
    C. iatrogenic steroid administration
    D. hypothalamic dysfunction
    E. adrenocortical carcinoma

219. Which of the following signs/symptoms is associated with Addison disease?
    A. hypokalemia
    B. hypernatremia
    C. hyperglycemia
    D. hyperpigmentation
    E. osteoporosis

220. What's the most common cause of Conn syndrome?
    A. pituitary adenoma
    B. adrenal adenoma
    C. juxtaglomerular cell tumor of the kidney
    D. renal artery stenosis
    E. ectopic hormone production by tumor

221. What is the most common cause of congenital adrenal hyperplasia?
    A. 11-hydroxylase deficiency
    B. 17-hydroxylase deficiency
    C. 21-hydroxylase deficiency
    D. growth hormone deficiency
    E. 17-hydroxyprogesterone deficiency

222. What is the most common cause of salt-wasting congenital adrenal hyperplasia?
    A. 11-hydroxylase deficiency
    B. 17-hydroxylase deficiency
    C. 21-hydroxylase deficiency
    D. growth hormone deficiency
    E. 17-hydroxyprogesterone deficiency

223. All of the following pituitary hormones are produced by basophilic cells, except:
    A. FSH
    B. TSH
    C. LH
    D. GH
    E. ACTH

1: Clinical Chemistry Questions

224. What's the most commonly secreted hormone due to a pituitary tumor?
     A. ACTH
     B. prolactin
     C. GH
     D. LSH
     E. TSH

225. How is an insulin tolerance test used to measure growth hormone?
     A. insulin-like growth factor is measured after insulin administration as a growth hormone surrogate
     B. insulin creates hypoglycemia, stimulating GH production
     C. insulin causes ion shifts which are sensed in the pituitary and lead to GH release
     D. insulin inhibits growth hormone uptake leading to increased serum GH levels
     E. insulin directly stimulates the release of GHRH from the hypothalamus

226. How does administration of a GnRH agonist inhibit FSH and LH?
     A. by acting as a synthetic nonstimulatory FSH/LH mimic
     B. by downregulating FSH or LH receptors
     C. by disrupting FSH/LH-mediated cell signaling
     D. by inhibiting production of FSH and LH
     E. by increasing synthesis of an inhibitory substance

227. Which of the following profiles is most consistent with diabetes insipidus?
     A. hypernatremia with a low urine osmolarity
     B. hypernatremia with a high urine osmolarity
     C. hyponatremia with a low urine osmolarity
     D. hyponatremia with a high urine osmolarity
     E. hyperkalemia with unchanged urine osmolarity

228. Which of the following samples is the most useful in diagnosing hyperglycemia in a postmortem situation?
     A. arterial serum
     B. whole arterial blood
     C. venous blood
     D. intravesicle urine
     E. vitreous humor

229. Which one of the following vitreous chemistry patterns is most consistent with decomposition?
     A. increased sodium, increased chloride, increased potassium
     B. decreased sodium, decreased chloride, increased potassium
     C. decreased sodium, increased chloride, increased potassium
     D. increased sodium, increased chloride, decreased potassium
     E. decreased sodium, decreased chloride, decreased potassium

230. Which of the following tests provides the most accurate evidence for death caused by anaphylaxis?
     A. total serum immunoglobulin
     B. total serum IgE
     C. serum alpha-tryptase
     D. serum beta-tryptase
     E. peripheral eosinophil count

1: Clinical Chemistry Questions

231. Which of the following is the best advantage of the Clinitest method v. the dipstick method for detecting glucose in the urine?
    A. ability to detect other "reducing substances"
    B. superior glucose detection sensitivity
    C. increased specificity
    D. increased positive predictive value
    E. cost

232. Which of the following unique patterns is most consistent with free light chains (Bence-Jones proteins) in urine?
    A. precipitate at 40°, then redissolve at 60°
    B. precipitate at 100°, then cool to redissolve at 60°
    C. heat to precipitate at 40°, redissolve at 100°, then cool to reprecipitate at 60° and redissolve at 40°
    D. heat to precipitate at 100°, redissolve with cooling to 60°, reprecipitate at 40°
    E. none of the above are accurate

233. Which of the following can be distinguished from hemoglobinuria on a urine dipstick via urine microscopy?
    A. myoglobinuria
    B. hematuria
    C. proteinuria
    D. bilirubinemia
    E. cholesterol

234. Which of the following common causes of urinary tract infections will give a positive nitrite test?
    A. *Enterococcus faecalis*
    B. *Neisseria gonorrheae*
    C. *Escherichia coli*
    D. *Mycobacterium tuberculosis*
    E. *Candida albicans*

235. All of the following are causes of increased urine specific gravity, <u>except</u>:
    A. diabetes mellitus
    B. diabetes insipidus
    C. congestive heart failure
    D. proteinuria
    E. syndrome of inappropriate antidiuretic hormone

236. What's the composition of the most common kidney stone?
    A. calcium oxalate
    B. calcium phosphate
    C. magnesium ammonium phosphate
    D. urate
    E. cystine

237. Which of the following urine microscopy findings is most consistent with glomerular bleeding?
    A. uniform RBC morphology
    B. red blood cell casts
    C. uniform hemoglobin concentration
    D. lack of erythrophagocytosis
    E. none of the above

1: Clinical Chemistry Questions

238. Which of the following types of casts is most specific for glomerulonephritis?
    A. hyaline casts
    B. red blood cell casts
    C. white blood cell casts
    D. tubular casts
    E. waxy casts

239. All of the following modalities can be used to diagnose cerebrospinal fluid leak in cases of rhinorrhea or otorrhea of unknown etiology, <u>except</u>:
    A. glucose measurement
    B. fluid protein electrophoresis
    C. specific gravity
    D. asialated transferrin measurement
    E. protein measurement

240. In addition to the presence of oligoclonal bands, which of the following findings is most supportive of a diagnosis of multiple sclerosis?
    A. increased serum albumin
    B. intrathecal IgG synthesis
    C. increased CSF albumin
    D. intrathecal IgA synthesis
    E. CSF glutamine

241. Which of the following cell types is seen more often in normal neonatal CSF compared to adult CSF?
    A. lymphocytes
    B. monocytes
    C. neutrophils
    D. ependymal cells
    E. eosinophils

242. Which of the following causes of meningitis is associated with a normal CSF glucose?
    A. *Neisseria meningitidis*
    B. *Mycobacterium tuberculosis*
    C. JC virus
    D. *Escherichia coli*
    E. herpes simplex virus

243. Which of the following pleural fluid test results confirms your clinical suspicion of an exudate?
    A. pleural fluid to serum protein ratio >0.3
    B. pleural fluid to serum LDH ratio >0.3
    C. pleural fluid LDH >200, or 2/3 the upper limit of serum LDH
    D. specific gravity >1.006
    E. pleural fluid protein >1 g/L

244. Which feature most specifically distinguishes a parapneumonic pleural effusion from an empyema?
    A. the presence of neutrophils
    B. specific gravity >1.010
    C. LDH levels
    D. the absence of bacteria
    E. acidic pH

1: Clinical Chemistry Questions

245. Which of the following tests are characteristically elevated in a pleural effusion associated with rheumatoid arthritis?
    A.   pH
    B.   glucose
    C.   LDH
    D.   A & B
    E.   A, B, C

246. Which of the following criteria is considered positive for a diagnostic peritoneal lavage?
    A.   >1 mL gross blood
    B.   RBCs >1000/mL
    C.   WBCs >5/mL
    D.   DPL fluid in Foley catheter
    E.   mesothelial cells >100/mL

247. Which of the following crystals is most strongly birefringent?
    A.   calcium pyrophosphate
    B.   monosodium urate
    C.   hydroxyapatite
    D.   corticosteroid
    E.   cholesterol

1: Clinical Chemistry Answers

1.   B.   **RATE OF ENZYME ACTIVITY VARIES LINEARLY WITH SUBSTRATE CONCENTRATION WHEN ENZYME IS FULLY SATURATED.**

The enzyme is working at its maximum rate (V_{max}); it cannot go any faster. Therefore, with all other things being equal, the only thing that alters reaction rate is the enzyme concentration. Because of this in the presence of substrate excess, enzyme concentration can be determined.
QCCP2, **Methods**, p 2

2.   D.   **NADH ABSORBS LIGHT AT 340NM; NAD DOES NOT.**

The formation or disappearance of NADH can be measured by light absorption at 340nm. Reaction products can be measured by coupling the reaction to the utilization of NAD or NADH, or indirectly by coupling a subsequent "measuring" reaction to NAD or NADH. The concentration of reaction products are calculated from the NAD/NADH ratio.
QCCP2, **Methods**, p 2

3.   A.   **ALKALINE PHOSPHATASE, PH10; ACID PHOSPHATASE, PH5.**

At pH10 (alkaline pH), alkaline phosphatase can be assayed; at pH5 (acidic pH), acid phosphatase can be assayed. While nitrophenyl phosphatase is a real enzyme, nitrophenyl kinase doesn't exist (as far as I know).
QCCP2, **Methods**, p 2

4.   E.   **ACTIVITY UNDERESTIMATES IMMUNOASSAY.**

There are multiple potential causes for enzyme activity to be lower than enzyme concentration: inhibitors, macroenzymes, lack of cofactors, proteolytically-inactive enzymes, among others.
QCCP2, **Methods**, p 2

5.   C.   **AN ENZYME BOUND TO AN ANTIBODY, INHIBITING THE ENZYME AND PREVENTING IT FROM BEING CLEARED.**

Macroenzymes are enzymes bound to antibodies, which inhibit enzyme function and block enzyme clearance. The other choices are somewhat plausible, but none of them describe a macroenzyme.
QCCP2, **Methods**, p 2

6.   D.   **1/[S] v. 1/v.**

Strictly speaking, a Lineweaver-Burk is a means to express a non-linear asymptotic concept (how the rate of the reaction varies with the substrate concentration) in a linear fashion by using the reciprocals of reaction rate and substrate concentration.
QCCP2, **Types of enzyme inhibition**, p 2

7.   D.   **-1/KM v. 1/VMAX.**

The Lineweaver-Burk equation is the reciprocal of the Michaelis-Menten equation. The terms can be shuffled around to yield the equation that describes a straight line ($y = mx + b$), where y is the y-coordinate, m is the slope of the line, x is the x-coordinate and b is the y-intercept (the point at which the line crosses the y axis or where $x = 0$). The resultant equation of the line in a Lineweaver-Burk plot is $1/v = Km/V_{MAX}(1[S]) + 1/V_{MAX}$. Get it? $y = 1/v$, $m = Km/V_{MAX}$, $x = 1/[S]$, and $b = 1/V_{MAX}$.
QCCP2, **Types of enzyme inhibition**, p 2

1: Clinical Chemistry Answers

8. A. **COMPETITIVE INHIBITION.**

    It is necessary to know the mechanisms of inhibition to determine which type can be overcome by increasing substrate. Competitive inhibitors bind reversibly to the enzyme and prevent substrate binding. Therefore, by increasing substrate one can "compete" for binding enzyme and shift the steady state toward the binding of substrate rather than inhibitor (and vice-versa of course). Noncompetitive inhibitors bind the enzyme at a different site than the substrate binding site, effectively decreasing the amount of useful enzyme without affecting the binding of substrate to enzyme. This is why the Km, a function of binding, is unaffected, but the reaction rate decreases. Uncompetitive inhibitors bind and stabilize the enzyme-substrate complex. This results in decreasing the Km (can't bind enzyme if it's wrapped up in a stable intermediate complex) and decreasing the V_{MAX} (same concept - product can't be formed if the substrate is stuck to the enzyme).
    QCCP2, **Types of enzyme inhibition,** p 2-3

9. B. **AMOUNT OF ENZYME THAT CATALYZES THE CONVERSION OF 1 MICROMOLE OF SUBSTRATE PER MINUTE.**

    Choice A is the definition of a katal (1 IU = 16.7 nanokatals). C is the definition of INR. D is the definition of molar concentration. E is the definition of a mole.
    QCCP2, **Units for expressing enzyme activity,** p 3

10. B. **ALT.**

    ALT is mainly confined to the mitochondria (80%) of liver and kidney. ALT has an "L" in it, like "liver." AST is at its highest concentration in the heart and has been used as a marker, although non-specific, of cardiac injury.
    QCCP2, **Hepatic enzymes and other liver function tests,** p 3

11. D. **HIGHER, LOWER.**

    Heparin elevates the AST/ALT while renal failure results in a lower ALT/AST.
    QCCP2, **AST and ALT,** p 3

12. B. **LD2, ACUTE MI, HEMOLYSIS, OR RENAL INFARCTION.**

    Tricky question, I'll give you that. Actually, two separate questions, but you weren't fooled. LD2 is highest in serum, except when LD1 levels rise higher than LD2 - the so-called "flipped ratio," when the LD1>LD2 that can occur with acute MI, hemolysis or renal infarction.
    QCCP2, **Lactate dehydrogenase,** p 4

13. E. **LD6.**

    Usually seen in the setting of cardiovascular collapse, an elevated LD6 portends a poor outcome.
    QCCP2, **Lactate dehydrogenase,** p 4

14. A. **PLACENTA.**

    Prostatic acid phosphatase has been used as a serum and immunohistochemical marker of prostatic adenocarcinoma; tartrate-resistant acid phosphatase is found in red blood cells and is a marker for hairy cell leukemia. While placenta is one of the major sources of alkaline phosphatase, it is not a major source of acid phosphatase.
    QCCP2, **Alkaline phosphatase,** p 4

1: Clinical Chemistry Answers

15. D. **BONE.**

"Bone burns" - heat inactivates the bone isoenzyme.
QCCP2, **Alkaline phosphatase**, p 4

16. B. **OSTEOBLASTS.**

Osteoblasts make bone, which also explains why bone alkaline phosphatase is particularly high in Paget disease of the bone.
QCCP2, **Alkaline phosphatase**, p 4

17. E. **ALL OF THE ABOVE ARE ASSOCIATED WITH MILD INCREASES IN ALKALINE PHOSPHATASE.**

Also hyperthyroidism and some drugs, such as ibuprofen and acetaminophen.
QCCP2, **Alkaline phosphatase**, p 5

18. B. **GGT.**

E. **5' NUCLEOTIDASE.**

GGT is primarily found in the biliary epithelial cells that line the small interlobular bile ducts and ductules as well as the smooth endoplasmic reticulum of the hepatocytes. 5' NT is also found in biliary epithelium.
QCCP2, **GGT, 5' NT**, p 5

19. A. **LIVER.**

While the skeletal muscle and gut are the main sources of ammonia, the liver is responsible for clearing it.
QCCP2, **Ammonia**, p 5

20. D. **GLUCURONIDATION.**

Unconjugated bilirubin is a heme breakdown product; it is tightly bound to albumin in the bloodstream when it comes to the liver for glucuronidation. The now water-soluble conjugated bilirubin can be excreted in bile, which intestinal bacteria convert to urobilinogen for excretion in feces and urine.
QCCP2, **Bilirubin**, p 6

21. B. **DIRECT IS MEASURED IN THE DIAZO-COLORIMETRIC ASSAY, WHILE INDIRECT IS CALCULATED.**

While many of the answers are somewhat correct, the single <u>best</u> answer is that the direct bilirubin is measured in the reaction with the diazo compound in the absence of an accelerator. Addition of an accelerator, such as alcohol) results in a measurement of total bilirubin. Indirect is calculated as total minus direct.
QCCP2, **Bilirubin**, p 6

22. E. **DUBIN-JOHNSON.**

The black liver of Dubin-Johnson syndrome is due to a defect in the transmembrane secretion of conjugated bilirubin into the canaliculis, while all the other selections are various causes of unconjugated hyperbilirubinemia.
QCCP2, **Bilirubin, T1.2**, p 6

1: Clinical Chemistry Answers

23. C. **FACTOR VII, PT.**

Factor VII's half life is 12 hours and the protime (PT) is a sensitive marker of impaired hepatic synthetic function. Note that bile salts are required for the absorption of vitamin K. Since vitamin K is required for the function of many of the coagulation factors, administration of parenteral vitamin K can be used to distinguish a PT elevated due to cholestasis/impaired vitamin K absorption from decreased hepatic synthetic function.

QCCP2, **Additional tests of hepatic function,** p 7

24. A. **PHYSIOLOGICAL JAUNDICE DUE TO HEPATIC ENZYMES NOT BEING UP TO CAPACITY.**

All of the other choices are potential causes of neonatal jaundice, but physiological jaundice is the most common cause. An infant's liver many not be up to full capacity and therefore unable to conjugate bilirubin for excretion. This can be exacerbated by peripartum hemolysis, which leads to an increased bilirubin load, or breast milk jaundice, where the breast milk contains inhibitors of bilirubin conjugation.

QCCP2, **Neonatal jaundice,** p 7

25. A. **JAUNDICE THAT APPEARS WITHIN 24 HOURS OF BIRTH.**

Signs that warn a physician that an infant may not just have physiological jaundice include jaundice within 24 hours of birth, rising bilirubin after 1 week, persistence past 10 days, a total bilirubin >12 mg/dL, a single day increase in bilirubin >5 mg/dL, or a direct bilirubin >2 mg/dL.

QCCP2, **Neonatal jaundice,** p 8

26. E. **20 MG/DL AT ANY TIME.**

The first three choices are indications for phototherapy, which converts unconjugated bilirubin into a water-soluble form. Phototherapy is not useful for a conjugated bilirubinemia.

QCCP2, **Neonatal jaundice,** p 8

27. A. **TRANSCUTANEOUS BILIRUBIN LEVELS.**

Transcutaneous bilirubin measurements can detect hyperbilirubinemia before the onset of clinically apparent jaundice and can be used to screen otherwise healthy infants while sparing a venipuncture. Blood velocity can be used *in utero* to assess the risk of hyperbilirubinemia.

QCCP2, **Neonatal jaundice,** p 8

28. C. **HCV.**

Approximately 80% of acute HCV infections lead to chronic disease. HAV does not lead to chronic disease and only a small proportion of HBV infections lead to chronic disease. Drug-induced acute hepatitis occurs within the first four months of drug administration.

QCCP2, **Laboratory evaluation of acute hepatic injury,** p 8

29. D. **A & B.**

Both HAV and HBV can be detected with serological testing (IgM anti-HAV, IgM anti-HBc, HBsAg). Serological testing for HCV, however, is only 60% sensitive in acute infections. RNA testing for HCV is 90-95% sensitive.

QCCP2, **Laboratory evaluation of acute hepatic injury,** p 8

1: Clinical Chemistry Answers

30. D. ISCHEMIA.

Ischemic and toxic injuries lead to the most profound elevations in transaminases, sometimes >100 times the upper limit of normal. So if AST is >3000 U/L, 90% of the time, the cause is a toxin.
QCCP2, **Transaminases,** p 9)

31. E. A & D.

An AST:ALT ratio >2 is present in over 80% of patients with toxic, ischemic, and alcoholic hepatitis.
QCCP2, **Transaminases,** p 9

32. G. A & D.

HAV and alcoholic hepatitis are the most common causes of jaundice (~70%), and 20-30% of acute HBV and HAV.
QCCP2, **Bilirubin,** p 9

33. D. PROTIME (PT).

The protime is the most consistent indicator of prognosis in acute hepatic injury. A PT prolongation >4.0 seconds indicates severe injury and an unfavorable prognosis. The other selections are tests of injury, while the PT is a test of loss of function.
QCCP2, **Laboratory evaluation of acute hepatic injury,** p 9

34. A. SALIVARY, INHIBITED, D. PANCREATIC, UNINHIBITED.

There are 6 isoenzymes of serum amylase as analyzed by serum electrophoresis. The fastest migrating are pancreatic; the slowest are salivary. While the salivary types are inhibited by wheat germ lectin, the pancreatic ones typically are not inhibited. I remember that the only place wheat germ lectin would come in contact with amylase would be in the mouth, so the salivary types are the ones affected.
QCCP2, **Amylase,** p 9

35. C. PSEUDOCYST.

Serum amylase rises 2-24 hours after the onset of acute hepatitis, with a resolution of values within 2-3 days. Persistent elevations should be a cause for concern of complications.
QCCP2, **Amylase,** p 9

36. A. HYPERTRIGLYCERIDEMIA.

Interestingly enough and depending on the assay, triglycerides competitively interfere with the amylase assay.
QCCP2, **Amylase,** p 9

37. C. ANTIBODY BOUND TO AMYLASE, LEADING TO DECREASED RENAL CLEARANCE.

Ig-amylase is referred to as macroamylase. Macroamylase cannot be cleared by the kidney due to its large size (like a bowling ball trying to pass through a sieve), which leads to increased serum amylase and decreased urinary amylase.
QCCP2, **Amylase,** p 10

1: Clinical Chemistry Answers

38.   D.   **ALL OF THE ABOVE ARE ADVANTAGES OF LIPASE.**

     All are true, which is why lipase is a better test for acute pancreatitis - "Lipase Lasts Longer and Lies Less."
     QCCP2, **Lipase,** p 10

39.   B.   **HEMATOCRIT.**

     In addition to the criteria presented in the question choices, WBC count, rather than hematocrit, is used at admission to calculate the prognosis of a patient presenting with acute pancreatitis. The hematocrit is assessed at 48 hours post-admission.
     QCCP2, **Laboratory evaluation of acute pancreatitis,** p 10

40.   D.   **AT LEAST 48 HOURS.**

     5 criteria are assessed at admission. 5 more are assessed 48 hours later.
     QCCP2, **Laboratory evaluation of acute pancreatitis,** p 10

41.   A.   **TSC1.**

     Cationic trypsinogen (PRSS-1), pancreatic secretory trypsin inhibitor (PSTI), and cystic fibrosis transmembrane conductance regulator (CFTR) have all been implicated as causes of recurrent pancreatitis.
     QCCP2, **Laboratory evaluation of acute pancreatitis,** p 10

42.   C.   **ELASTASE-1.**

     Fecal fat, chymotrypsin, and elastase-1 are all sensitive and specific, with elastase being the most so. D-xylose is a measure of small bowel mucosal absorptive capacity, not pancreatic exocrine function.
     QCCP2, **Tests of pancreatic exocrine function,** p 11

43.   1-E, 2-D, 3-C, 4-B, 5-A.

     CEA is elevated in the mucinous neoplasms, while serous cystadenoma and solid-pseudopapillary tumors have decreased levels of all three.
     QCCP2, **T1.6, Pancreatic Cyst Evaluation,** p 11

44.   C.   **CK-BB.**

     BB is the fastest migrating and is present in nearly all tissues of the body, though found primarily in the brain. (A BB would migrate faster than an M&M, with a MB in between).
     QCCP2, **Creatine kinase (CK),** p 11

45.   C.   **CK-MM.**

     MM is present in the serum, due mostly to contributions from skeletal muscle (which is the source of most MB).
     QCCP2, **Creatine kinase,** p 12

46.   D.   **MITOCHONDRIAL CK.**

     Mitochondrial CK, if seen on electrophoresis, appears as a faint band migrating slightly slower than CK-MM. Macro-CK is another abnormal CK that is composed of a complex of antibody-bound CK.
     QCCP2, **Creatine kinase,** p 12

1: Clinical Chemistry Answers

47.   D.   **A & B.**

The gene that encodes TnC is expressed in both cardiac and skeletal muscle, whereas TnI and TnT have separate cardiac and skeletal muscle genes. These two immunoassays can distinguish between the skeletal and cardiac forms.
QCCP2, **Troponin I,** p 12

48.   B.   **cTnI.**

cTnI is marginally more cardiac-specific than cTnT, while there is no cardiac-specific TnC isoform. Troponins for the most part are much more specific than either CK-MB or myoglobin, both of which are often elevated following vigorous exercise or skeletal muscle injury.
QCCP2, **Troponin I,** p 12

49.   D.   **A & C.**

Usually within moments of an acute MI, there is an elevation of the myoglobin. Unfortunately, very sensitive myoglobin is very nonspecific and can be elevated due to a number of causes.
QCCP2, **Myoglobin,** p 12

50.   B.   **COBALT.**

The amino terminus of albumin is modified with exposure to a number of conditions, such as acidosis, hypoxemia, and free radicals. The modification decreased the ability of albumin to bind cobalt. The amount of unbound cobalt reflects the level of ischemia-modified albumin.
QCCP2, **Ischemia-modified albumin,** p 13

51.   D.   **N-TERM-PRO-BNP**

A-type natriuretic peptide is released in response to increased ventricular as well as increased atrial filling pressures. For that reason, it's not as specific as BNP, which is only released in response to increased ventricular filling pressure (stretch). It is released as an inactive pro-BNP peptide which when cleaved releases an active BNP as well as the regulatory N-term-pro-BNP, a very stable molecule. Little is known about C-type natriuretic peptide.
QCCP2, **B-type natriuretic peptide,** p 13

52.   C.   **CONGESTIVE HEART FAILURE.**

All are considered to be in a spectrum of disease. Stable angina is reproducible and most likely due to progressive stenosis of coronary arteries. Unstable angina may represent further stenosis, but with a little less predictable event as well, such as a transient clot or vasospasm, causing transient ischemia. Acute MI is the best characterized and is the condition that we can most readily identify.
QCCP2, **Acute coronary syndrome,** p 13

53.   A.   **INCREASED SENSITIVITY.**

The specificity of a single elevated troponin is very high; serial measurements don't change that. However, a mildly elevated troponin many not be sensitive enough to detect AMI. Serial measurements of troponin increase the sensitivity, but don't change the ability of the test to change its negative predictive value.
QCCP2, **Acute myocardial infarction,** p 14

1: Clinical Chemistry Answers

54. C. **TROPONIN IS NOT HELPFUL IN DETERMINING THE TIME COURSE OF** AMI.

Troponin rises more slowly and stays elevated longer than CK-MB. If CK-MB continues to rise, it may indicate an acute event or an extension of an existing infarction, while a downward trend of CK-MB may indicate resolution of an infarction.
QCCP2, **Acute myocardial infarction,** p 14

55. D. **AMMONIUM NITROGEN RELEASED BY ACID DIGESTION.**

All of the techniques presented are used to measure protein. The Kjedahl technique is cumbersome and makes assumptions about average nitrogen content. Colorimetric assays are preferred for the measurement of protein, and all involve formation of a colored precipitate under alkaline or acidic conditions and then measuring the absorbance at the appropriate wavelength. Refractometry is used but has many interferences. Dye-binding is limited by uneven dye uptake by proteins.
QCCP2, **Protein quantitation,** p 14-15

56. A. **NEGATIVE, ANODE.**

Most proteins bear a net negative charge at physiologic pH and as such migrate toward the anode or positive pole when subject to an electromotive force. Remember, anions have negative charges and are attracted to the positive pole or anode. Cations bear positive charges and are attracted to the negative pole or cathode.
QCCP2, **Protein separation,** p 15

57. A. **ALBUMIN.**

Albumin accounts for the majority of normal serum protein and is the fastest migrating major protein followed by the alpha, beta, then gamma region proteins.
QCCP2, **Protein separation,** p 15

58. D. **IMMUNOPRECIPITATION.**

While immunoprecipitation can be used to characterize proteins, it is not commonly used to characterize monoclonal proteins. All the other techniques, especially immunofixation, are commonly used to identify and classify monoclonal proteins identified by serum electrophoresis.
QCCP2, **Immunofixation and immunotyping,** p 16

59. D. **A & B.**

Protein-losing conditions are responsible for the greatest decrements in serum albumin. The ability of the liver to synthesize albumin is preserved with decreases only being apparent with severe end-stage liver disease.
QCCP2, **Major Serum Proteins,** p 17

60. D. **MAINTENANCE OF SERUM OSMOTIC PRESSURE.**

Pre-albumin does function in the capacity to bind thyroid hormone, vitamin A, and is the precursor in cardiac amyloidosis and familial amyloid polyneuropathy. Albumin, rather than pre-albumin, is responsible for maintenance of serum osmotic pressure. Pre-albumin is prominent in the CSF.
QCCP2, **Pre-albumin,** p 17-18

1: Clinical Chemistry Answers

61. E. **BETA-1.**

Transferrin is the predominant beta-1 protein. On standard serum electrophoresis, beta does not resolve into beta-1 and beta-2, but can on high-resolution electrophoresis. (In the beta-2 region migrates IgA, C-reactive protein can be in beta-2 or gamma-2). The predominant alpha-1 band is alpha-1-antitrypsin; alpha-2 has haptoglobin and ceruloplasmin.
QCCP2, **T1.7,** p 18

62. B. **ALPHA-2-MACROGLOBULIN.**

Due to its large size, alpha-2-macroglobulin is typically not lost with nephrotic syndrome. As a result of the loss of other smaller proteins and fluid, the alpha-2-macroglobulin concentration increases.
QCCP2, **alpha-2-macroglobulin,** p 19

63. C. **TRANSFERRIN.**

Both the unmodified and asialated forms of transferrin can cross the blood-brain barrier through active transport. This accounts for the double transferrin peak typically seen in CSF electrophoresis.
QCCP2, **Transferrin,** p 19

64. B. **FIBRINOGEN.**

Normally blood clots to make serum, and fibrinogen is consumed. In the event of incomplete clotting (such as in heparinized patients), fibrinogen may appear at the beta-gamma interface.
QCCP2, **Fibrinogen,** p 19-20

65. B. **NORMAL VARIANT.**

Bisalbuminemia is a normal variant seen in heterozygotes for different albumin allotypes. There is no clinical significance.
QCCP2, **Bisalbuminemia,** p 20

66. C. **ALPHA-2.**

Albumin is usually the most commonly affected protein. Due to its small size, it is lost in both selective and non-selective proteinuria. Other proteins also start to decrease in the serum in non-selective proteinuria, except alpha-2-macroglobulin, due to its large size.
QCCP2, **Nephrotic syndrome,** p 20

67. B. **CIRRHOSIS.**

Predominantly due to increased IgA, beta-gamma bridging is seen with cirrhosis. Cirrhosis can also show hypoalbuminemia with blunted alpha-1 and alpha-2 peaks.
QCCP2, **Beta-gamma bridging,** p 20

68. E. **ALL OF THE ABOVE ARE POTENTIAL CAUSES OF HYPOGAMMAGLOBULINEMIA.**

It may be counter-intuitive, but a significant portion of cases of myeloma can exhibit hypogammaglobulinemia, especially when there is a concomitant Bence-Jones protein seen on urine protein electrophoresis.
QCCP2, **Monoclonal gammopathy,** p 22

1: Clinical Chemistry Answers

69. A. **OLIGOCLONAL GAMMA BANDS.**

Oligoclonal bands, though they can be present in CSF protein electrophoresis, are distinctly NOT normal. Oligoclonal bands in CSF but not in a concurrent SPEP support a diagnosis of multiple sclerosis.

QCCP2, **CSF protein electrophoresis,** p 22

70. B. **GLOMERULAR PROTEINURIA.**

Glomerular proteinuria occurs due to a loss of the selective filtration of the glomerulus - large proteins, such as alpha-2 macroglobulin are retained while very small proteins are resorbed in the tubules, leaving medium-sized proteins, such as albumin in the urine. Tubular proteinuria is due to the loss of small protein resorption, while overflow proteinuria is due to very high serum levels of a protein overwhelming the kidney's filtration and resorption capacity.

QCCP2, **Urine protein electrophoresis,** p 23

71. A. **TYPE I.**

Type I cryoglobulins are monoclonal, associated with monoclonal gammopathies, such as myeloma or Waldenstrom macroglobulinemia. Type II is a mixture of polyclonal IgG and monoclonal IgM, while Type III is a mixture of two or more polyclonal antibodies.

QCCP2, **Cryoglobulinemia,** p 23

72. C. **HEPATITIS C VIRUS.**

Prior to the advent of HCV testing, approximately 1/2 of all cases of mixed cryoglobulinemia had no apparent cause. With testing, the majority of these cases were found to be due to HCV.

QCCP2, **Mixed cryoglobulinemia (types II and III),** p 24

73. A. **MEMBRANOPROLIFERATIVE GLOMERULONEPHRITIS, TYPE II.**

Cryoglobulinemia is a deposition disease leaving dense immune complex deposits within the mesangium and subendothelium, often with the characteristic tubuloreticular inclusions or "interferon fingerprints." There is often an associated vasculitis.

QCCP2, **Mixed cryoglobulinemia,** p 24

74. B. **CEREBRAL EDEMA.**

Carefully read the question if you chose central pontine myelinolysis. That most often occurs when hyponatremia is corrected too <u>rapidly</u>. Hyponatremia is usually described as a serum sodium level of less than 135mM.

QCCP2, **Hyponatremia,** p 24

75. D. **RENAL TUBULAR ACIDOSIS, TYPE I.**

The causes of true hyponatremia (relatively low sodium compared to water) can be subdivided according to the patient's volume status (assessed clinically). Hypovolemic patients tend to be hyponatremic due to water loss either through the kidneys or GI tract. Euvolemic patients are often hyponatremic due to drugs and similar conditions. Hypervolemic patients are hyponatremic due to the "oses" - cardiosis, nephrosis, and cirrhosis, better known as congestive heart failure, nephrotic syndrome, and cirrhosis.

QCCP2, **Hyponatremia,** p 24

1: Clinical Chemistry Answers

76. D. **ALL OF THE ABOVE.**

   Measurement of urinary potassium helps to distinguish renal potassium losses from other causes. Transcellular shifts come into play most often with correction of diabetic ketoacidosis. As the hyperglycemia of ketoacidosis is corrected, the concomitant hyperkalemia is often overcorrected as potassium moves back into cells. For that reason, it is important to include supplemental potassium when correcting the hyperglycemia of diabetic ketoacidosis.
   QCCP2, **Hypokalemia,** p 25

77. D. **A & B.**

   Type I, or distal renal tubular acidosis, is due to the inability to produce an acid urine. Type II, or proximal renal tubular acidosis, is due to bicarbonate wasting. Both are associated with hypokalemia. There is no Type III RTA. Type IV renal tubular acidosis is due to aldosterone deficiency and is associated with hyperkalemia.
   QCCP2, **Hyperkalemia,** p 25

78. A. **EXCESS PARATHYROID HORMONE.**

   Straightforward question - too much PTH. The most common cause is a parathyroid adenoma, followed by parathyroid hyperplasia and carcinoma,
   QCCP2, **Hypercalcemia,** p 25

79. C. **PRIMARY HYPERPARATHYROIDISM.**

   Most causes of hypercalcemia also cause hyperphosphatemia. The combination of high calcium and high phosphate leads to increased calcium phosphate crystal formation and deposition. Crystals are often deposited in the kidney, leading to stones or in vessels with severe end-stage renal disease (calciphylaxis).
   QCCP2, **Hypercalcemia,** p 25-26

80. D. **A & B.**

   80-90% of hypercalcemia is due to hyperparathyroidism or malignancy (often with the paraneoplastic expression of PTHrp). PTH is synthesized as an intact protein then digested into three fragments. Intact and N-terminal PTH have biological activity and, as a result, short half-lives.
   QCCP2, **Hypercalcemia,** p 26-27

81. C. **12.0 MG/DL.**

   Since a significant portion of serum calcium is bound to albumin and the fraction that is unbound is biochemically active, it may be necessary to adjust the measured calcium to get an estimate of what the true calcium level is. For each 1 g/dL the albumin drops below the "normal" level of 4 g/dL, add 0.8 mg/dL to the total calcium. In this case, albumin drops 2 g/dL below 4, so you would add 1.6 mg/dL to the measured calcium of 10.4 mg/dl to get 12 mg/dL. This is significant because, while 10.4 mg/dL is not commonly thought of as hypercalcemia, 12 mg/dL is.
   QCCP2, **Hypercalcemia, laboratory evaluation,** p 27

1: Clinical Chemistry Answers

82. D. **PERIPHERAL RESISTANCE TO PTH.**

The first three choices are causes of primary hyperparathyroidism (PTH overproduction). Secondary hyperparathyroidism is due to increased physiological PTH as a response to increased resistance to PTH activity, most commonly in end-stage renal disease. diGeorge syndrome is a cause of hypoparathyroidism.
QCCP2, **Differential diagnosis,** p 28

83. B. **pH < 7.0.**

Physiological pH is generally accepted to be 7.0 to 7.44. pH above 7.44 is considered alkalemia, while below 7.0 is considered acidemia. Decreased serum CO_2 and increased bicarbonate would tend to increase the pH, thus causing alkalemia.
QCCP2, **Acid-base disorders,** p 28

84. A. **INCREASE (RETAIN MORE).**

The Henderson-Hasselbalch equation describes the action of a weak acid and its conjugate base in response to changes in pH. Conversely, changes in this ratio of acid to base have predictable changes on the $[H^+]$, which is represented by pH. According to the equation $pH = pKa + \log([base]/[acid])$. If base concentration (bicarbonate in this case) were to increase, in order for pH to remain constant (remember, the pKa is a constant), then the acid concentration would also have to increase. This is accomplished by retaining more CO_2 by a compensatory decrease in respiration.
QCCP2, **Acid-base disorders,** p 28

85. D. **PERCENT OXYGEN SATURATION (SaO_2).**

SaO_2 is calculated from the hematocrit and the PaO_2 plotted on a standard hemoglobin oxygen dissociation curve.
QCCP2, **Acid-base disorders,** p 29

86. C. **CO-OXIMETER.**

The co-oximeter has the ability to directly measure the proportions of several hemoglobin subtypes. The other techniques, if they possess the ability to do so, calculate the proportions rather than measure them. In addition, multiple potential confounding elements are present in some of the techniques, such as poor peripheral perfusion or recent transfusion.
QCCP2, **Acid-base disorders,** p 29

87. E. $[Na^+] - ([Cl^-] + [HCO_3^-])$.

Sodium is the major plasma cation (with only a minor contribution from potassium, which is mostly an intracellular cation), while chloride and bicarbonate are the major anions. Since electrical neutrality must be maintained, the overall number of positive charges must equal the overall number of negative charges. Therefore, the difference between the major measured cations and anions must be due to unmeasured anions, the so-called anion gap. Increases in unmeasured anions, such as lactate, cause a decrease in the measured anions in order to maintain electrical neutrality. This is the basis of the increased anion gap.
QCCP2, **Acid-base disorder,** p 29

1: Clinical Chemistry Answers

88. A. **SAME DIRECTION, OPPOSITE DIRECTION.**

For the most part in metabolic disorders, a change in pH with a change in bicarbonate go in the same direction. That is, as pH increases so does bicarbonate. The opposite holds true for simple respiratory disorders - as pH increases, bicarb decreases, and vice-versa.
QCCP2, **Acid-base disorders,** p 30

89. D. **A & B.**

Increased anion gap acidoses usually fall into discrete categories by the most common unmeasured anions, most commonly lactate, urea, or ketones. These can be further characterized by whether there is an osmolal gap - that is, the presence of unmeasured osmolytes, such as methanol or propylene glycol.
QCCP2, **T1.13, Increased osmolal gap,** p 30

90. B. **INVERSELY RELATED.**

Creatinine is freely filtered and constantly produced, making it an excellent marker of glomerular filtration function. Because a small amount of the creatinine is resorbed in the tubules, creatinine tends to overestimate the GFR. As creatinine rises, it indicates a decrease in the filtration rate.
QCCP2, **Creatinine and GFR calculations,** p 31

91. E. **BODY MASS.**

The MDRD equation is an improvement of the calculation of GFR from creatinine in a 24-hour urine. Its use has been validated on adults with impaired kidney function. Caution should be exercised when using it with other groups as there are several different formulae, dependent on whether or not the lab uses a creatinine assay calibrated to isotope dilution spectroscopy or not.
QCCP2, **Creatinine and GFR calculations,** p 31-32

92. B. **RENAL AZOTEMIA.**

A maintained ratio with elevated BUN (azotemia) is suggestive of an intrinsic renal defect, most commonly glomerulonephritis or tubulointerstitial nephritis. Deranged ratios, such as when BUN increases more than creatinine, is suggestive of impaired renal perfusion, such as prerenal (insufficient volume to the kidney) and postrenal (insufficient volume out of the kidney).
QCCP2, **BUN/creatinine ratio,** p 32

93. B. **>300MG/DAY URINARY PROTEIN.**

24-hour urine collection and protein determination are the standard for measuring proteinuria. Normally, less than 150 mg/day of protein is excreted in the urine, predominantly Tamm-Horsfall protein. The lower limit of detection of the urine protein assay is 3 mg/day. Spot urine protein readings can be misleading.
QCCP2, **Urine protein and urine albumin,** p 32

94. D. **RENAL TUBULE.**

Both are freely filtered by the glomerulus but then resorbed in the proximal convoluted tubule. Dysfunction in the tubule leads to an inability to resorb the proteins, and hence, their presence in the urine.
QCCP2, **Urine protein and urine albumin,** p 33

1: Clinical Chemistry Answers

95.   D.   **GLOMERULAR FILTRATION RATE.**

Chronic renal disease is defined as a GFR <60 mL/min or 3+ months of albuminuria. Stage is defined by albuminuria with either no decrease in GFR (Stage 1), mild decrease in GRF (Stage 2), moderate decrease in GFR (Stage 3), severe decrease (Stage 4), or finally, end-stage (Stage 5) renal failure.
QCCP2, **Laboratory screening for chronic kidney disease,** p 33

96.   D.   **UREMIC PERICARDITIS.**

A number of conditions are indications for dialysis, but of the choices presented, end-organ damage due to uremia is the only cause for which dialysis is indicated. Metabolic acidosis, volume overload, and certain drug overdoses are indications.
QCCP2, **Laboratory screening for chronic kidney disease,** p 34

97.   B.   **DECREASED (<1%).**

The fractional excretion of sodium is a useful calculation to help distinguish pre-renal causes of acute renal failure. Diuresis or high glucose levels can confound using FENa.
QCCP2, **Laboratory screening for chronic kidney disease,** p 34

98.   C.   **ACUTE TUBULAR NECROSIS.**

Hyaline casts are suggestive of prerenal disease, red cell casts are suggestive of glomerulonephritis, and white blood cell casts are seen most commonly with tubulointerstitial nephritis. Acute tubular necrosis is most commonly associated with pigmented casts. Rhabomyolysis is the prototypical cause of ATN that can present with the myoglobin-pigmented casts.
QCCP2, **Laboratory screening for chronic kidney disease,** p 34

99.   D.   **SPONTANEOUS BACTERIAL PERITONITIS.**

All of the presentations are potential causes of renal failure in patients with cirrhosis, but SBP is the most common and must be excluded.
QCCP2, **Hepatorenal syndrome,** p 34

100.   D.   **450NM.**

The spectrum of visible light goes from approximately 400-700 nm. Colors appear as their distinct entities due to the fact that colored objects absorb the wavelengths of light that do not pertain and reflects those that do. For example, a red object reflects light at the "red" wavelength (~650nm) and absorbs other wavelengths. The yellow-green bilirubin optimally absorbs at 450 nm (roughly the reflectance of indigo).
QCCP2, **Amniotic fluid bilirubin,** p 34

101.   B.   **DELTA OD_{450} VERSUS EGA.**

The absorbance wavelength is plotted on a semilog plot and a straight line drawn from OD_{550} to OD_{350}. The difference between the actual absorbance of amniotic fluid at OD_{450}nm and the theoretical line is the delta OD_{450}. The value represents the difference in the amniotic fluid between the background and any bilirubin present. The delta OD_{450} is then plotted against the estimated gestational age (EGA) on a Liley chart. Bilirubin is a surrogate for hemolysis. Plotting values on the chart assists with clinical decision making for either delivery or intrauterine transfusion.
QCCP2, **Amniotic fluid bilirubin,** p 35

1: Clinical Chemistry Answers

102.   A.   **PROLACTIN.**

The common alpha subunit is paired with a unique beta subunit. For this reason, most specific assays are directed against the beta subunit. Prolactin is a single chain polypeptide, similar to growth hormone or placental lactogen. *QCCP2,* **Maternal serum human chorionic gonadotropin,** p 35

103.   B.   **FALSE POSITIVES.**

The most common cause of false positive hCG is said to be heterophile antibodies. There are a number of ways to deal with false positive results due to heterophile antibodies. Basically, either get rid of the antibodies or run the assay on a machine that is not affected by heterophile antibodies. False negatives in hCG testing may occur with urine tests due to low sensitivity; false negatives are very rare in these kinds of serum tests. *QCCP2,* **hCG,** p 35

104.   B.   **END OF FIRST TRIMESTER.**

The hCG doubles every 2 days up to 1200 mIU/mL, every 3 days up to ~6000 mIU/mL and every 4 days until the peak at the end of the first trimester where it can reach 100,000 mIU/mL. It decays within a few weeks to a plateau of ~10,000 mIU/mL. *QCCP2,* **hCG,** p 35

105.   B.   **FALLOPIAN TUBE.**

All of the choices are possible sites of fetal implantation, with the vast majority of ectopic pregnancies occurring in the fallopian tube as most fertilization occurs there. Any dysfunction of the tubal ciliary apparatus could lead to implantation. An implantation within the uterus is normal. I hope that you already knew that. *QCCP2,* **hCG in ectopic pregnancy,** p 36

106.   A.   **SERUM PROGESTERONE.**

Serum progesterone levels above 25 ng/mL are almost diagnostic of a normal intrauterine conception, less than 5 ng/mL is consistent with an abnormal pregnancy. *QCCP2,* **hCG in ectopic pregnancy,** p 36

107.   D.   **PROGESTERONE.**

The triple test consists of the hCG, maternal serum alpha fetoprotein (MSAFP), and unconjugated estriol. The addition of dimeric inhibin A to the triple test makes it the quad test. Because inhibin levels are stable throughout the second trimester, it helps to "standardize" the levels of the other tests and improve the sensitivity. *QCCP2,* **Prenatal screening for trisomy and neural tube defects,** p 37

108.   E.   **DECREASED AFP, DECREASED hCG, DECREASED ESTRIOL.**

Somewhat sensitive, but not very specific for trisomy 18, the triple test is a fairly effective screening tool, but not a good diagnostic test. Amniotic karyotypic analysis can confirm the diagnosis. *QCCP2,* **Prenatal screening for trisomy and neural tube defects,** p 37

1: Clinical Chemistry Answers

109. A. INCREASED AFP, NORMAL hCG, DECREASED ESTRIOL.

Increased AFP (>2 multiples of the mean) should suggest neural tube defect. An elevated AFP should be repeated if done early, otherwise ultrasound is indicated to further workup the patient. Gestational age, multiple gestations, anatomic abnormalities, or fetal demise must be excluded. After that, amniocentesis should be performed to further workup the case.
QCCP2, **Prenatal screening for trisomy and neural tube defects,** p 38

110. B. DECREASED AFP, INCREASED hCG, DECREASED ESTRIOL.

In addition, inhibin is usually increased in Down syndrome. The mnemonic "It gets <u>ME Down</u>" helps me to remember that both MSAFP and estriol are down in Down syndrome. Like any abnormality in the triple test screening exam, it should be followed up. In this case, high-resolution ultrasound and amniocentesis with karyotyping have been used.
QCCP2, **Prenatal screening for trisomy and neural tube defects,** p 38

111. C. 35.

The same guidelines mandate that all pregnant women are to be offered non-invasive testing. After age 35, which is considered "advanced maternal age," or in the event of a positive triple test at any age, the option for invasive screening such as amniocentesis, should be offered.
QCCP2, **Prenatal screening for trisomy and neural tube defects,** p 38

112. C. DECREASED.

Increased maternal weight can have a dilutional effect on the serum levels of a number of analytes, MSAFP included. As a result, MSAFP levels may be artifactually lower.
QCCP2, **Prenatal screening for trisomy and neural tube defects,** p 38

113. D. PLACENTA.

Elevated in Down syndrome, DIA is produced by the placenta. DIA levels, unlike unconjugated estriol, MSAFP, and hCG remain relatively constant during pregnancy.
QCCP2, **Prenatal screening for trisomy and neural tube defects,** p 38

114. A. RUPTURE OF MEMBRANES.

Premature labor is defined as regular contractions with associated cervical changes prior to 37 weeks of gestation. PPROM-premature labor with premature rupture of membranes is a separate entity.

115. A. PHOSPHATIDYLCHOLINE.

Lecithin is composed of multiple types of phospholipids, predominant among these is disaturated phosphatidylcholine (DSPC). DSPC levels can be directly measured to assess for fetal lung maturity.
QCCP2, **Determination of Fetal Lung Maturity,** p 39-40

116. C. 34-37 WEEKS.

Prior to 34 weeks, the fetal lung is almost certainly immature, therefore obviating the need for assessment of lung maturity at that age. Similarly, after 37 weeks, lung maturity is very likely, also eliminating the need for testing.
QCCP2, **Determination of Fetal Lung Maturity,** p 39

1: Clinical Chemistry Answers

117. B. **2:1.**

2:1 is considered a reliable cutoff for most pregnancies. Typically the lecithin levels rise until the ratio reaches 2:1, which usually occurs around 35 weeks. The chances of developing respiratory distress syndrome are very low, with a ratio of 2:1 or higher. It is important to remember that a number of conditions, such as maternal diabetes, blood, and meconium can affect the interpretation of the L:S ratio.

QCCP2, **Determination of Fetal Lung Maturity,** p 39

118. D. **PHOSPHATIDYLGLYCEROL.**

Since the presence of blood or meconium doesn't inhibit the measurement of phosphatidyl glycerol, which first appears around 36 weeks, it is an excellent surrogate for the lecithin:sphingomyelin ratio. Alternatively, disaturated phosphatidyl choline can also be measured.

QCCP2, **Determination of Fetal Lung Maturity,** p 39-40

119. A. **GLOMERULAR FILTRATION RATE (GFR).**

Perhaps due to an increased plasma volume, the GFR usually increases in pregnancy. As a result the BUN, creatinine, and urate usually decrease.

QCCP2, **Laboratory Evaluation of Diseases in Pregnancy,** p 40

120. E. **POSTPARTUM.**

The incidence of thromboembolism such as DVT rises from 1/2000 antepartum to up to 1/700 postpartum. The risk during pregnancy (and immediately postpartum) is much greater than pre-pregnancy.

QCCP2, **Medical conditions of importance in pregnancy,** p 40

121. D. **A & B.**

Pregnancy tends to ameliorate the effects of rheumatoid arthritis and, less reliably, Graves disease. SLE and myasthenia tend to become worse during pregnancy.

QCCP2, **Medical conditions of importance in pregnancy,** p 40

122. C. **LUPUS PNEUMONITIS.**

Pulmonary hemorrhage secondary to lupus pneumonitis is the most common cause of death in pregnant women with SLE. Pregnancy-induced hypertension must be distinguished from a lupus cause of hypertension because the treatments are very different. Thromboembolism and pulmonary embolism are causes of morbidity and mortality in SLE patients, but at a lower rate than pneumonitis. The renal failure associated with lupus is usually irreversible.

QCCP2, **Medical conditions of importance in pregnancy,** p 41

123. D. **A & B.**

The vast majority (~90%) of patients have a history of severe postpartum bleeding. In addition to the physiological enlargement of the pituitary during pregnancy, pituitary apoplexy can occur. This is the cause of Sheehan syndrome, which is manifested as lethargy, weakness, amenorrhea, and the inability to lactate.

QCCP2, **Medical conditions of importance in pregnancy,** p 41

1: Clinical Chemistry Answers

124.   C.   HIGH LEVELS OF hCG.

Hyperemesis gravidarum is the most common <u>cause</u> of hyperthyroidism in pregnancy. It is thought that very high levels of hCG cause hyperemesis gravidarum.
QCCP2, **Medical conditions of importance in pregnancy**, p 41

125.   D.   DISSEMINATED INTRAVASCULAR COAGULATION (DIC).

Because DIC is commonly seen with acute fatty liver of pregnancy it is a medical emergency, although somewhat rare it is associated with very high mortality. Acute fatty liver presents late in pregnancy and can be associated with multiple metabolic defects.
QCCP2, **Medical conditions of importance in pregnancy**, p 42

126.   D.   URINE DRUG SCREEN.

Recurrent pregnancy loss is defined as two or more spontaneous abortions. A number of clinical and laboratory investigations are done in the case of recurrent loss, but urine drug screen is usually not one of them.
QCCP2, **Recurrent pregnancy loss**, p 42

127.   B.   FIRST ORDER.

Most drugs are eliminated by first-order kinetics, where the rate is proportional to the concentration of the drug. An exponential decrease in drug concentration occurs with time as the body eliminates a constant proportion of the drug. Zero-order reactions occur at a constant rate, irrespective of drug concentration. The concentration of the drug is much greater than the Km of the enzyme. Notable drugs eliminated by zero-order kinetics are alcohol and high dose phenytoin or salicylates. A second-order reaction is more complex and the rate is dependent on the product of the concentration of two reactants, while mixed or higher order reactions have a fractional rate constant.
QCCP2, **Toxicology**, p 42

128.   C.   5.

After 5 half-lives, a drug dosed at every half-life will reach steady state. It is important to realize that steady state is a fluctuating condition with trough levels prior to dosing and peaks shortly after.
QCCP2, **Half-life**, p 43

129.   B.   LOW SERUM PROTEIN LEVELS.

Active drug is most commonly the unbound or free form. Any condition that increases the amount of unbound drug, such as decreased protein, a change in pH, etc., can potentially increase the efficacy.
QCCP2, **Half-life**, p 43

130.   D.   WIDE DISTRIBUTION INTO VASCULAR, EXTRAVASCULAR, AND ADIPOSE TISSUE.

Simply stated, the volume of distribution is how many places in the body a drug can inhabit. A large V_D implies that the drug can be in many of these places, while a small one implies the drug is more limited. To express the V_D mathematically, divide the dose of the drug by the plasma concentration.
QCCP2, **Volume of distribution**, p 43

1: Clinical Chemistry Answers

131. A. **IMMUNOASSAY.**

Because immunoassay is most commonly used, there is a risk of cross-reaction and false positive results. A positive screen can then be confirmed with a more specific testing modality, such as gas chromatography/mass spectrometry.
QCCP2, **Drugs of abuse screening,** p 43

132. A-5, B-4, C-1, D-2, E-3.

Cocaine, or benzoylmethyl ecgonine, is very rapidly metabolized to the stable urine-excreted compound, benzoylecgonine. Heroin, or diacetylmorphine, is deacetylated in a stepwise fashion, yielding first a monoacetylated metabolite, N-acetylmorphine, more commonly known as 6-monoacetylated morphine (6-MAM). This is important because it allows the distinction of heroin from morphine or other prescribed opiates. Phencyclidine (PCP) is metabolized by cytochrome P_{450} oxidase in the liver into glucoronidated and hydroxylated water-soluble forms. Finally, the active ingredient in cannibis, tetrahydrocannibinol (THC), is modified to a water-soluble form, delta-9-THC-COOH.
QCCP2, **T1.18, Selected Drugs of Abuse,** p 43

133. C. **CORONARY VASOCONSTRICTION.**

While increased heart rate and blood pressure often accompany cocaine ingestion, it is the ability of the drug to cause coronary vasoconstriction that leads to the chest pain. Prolonged cocaine use can also be atherogenic and cause left ventricular hypertrophy. Usually the end result of vasoconstriction is myocardial infarction.
QCCP2, **Cocaine,** p 44

134. B. **CK-MB.**

Both myoglobin and CK-MB are less cardiospecific than troponin in the first place. Secondly, cocaine has an effect on skeletal muscle, which non-specifically elevates myoglobin and CK-MB. Therefore, those two tests (and likely, LDH as well) become even less cardiospecific in patients who use cocaine.
QCCP2, **Cocaine,** p 44

135. D. **A & B.**

Both nalmefene and naloxone are opiate antagonists. When given to cases of suspected opiate overdose, they can suddenly reverse the effects of opiates. Patients who do not respond to opiate antagonists can presumably be excluded from opiate intoxication. Methadone is an opiate agonist used in the treatment of opiate addiction.
QCCP2, **Opiates,** p 44

136. D. **POTENTIATION OF GABA-DEPENDENT ACTIVITY.**

Gamma aminobutyric acid (GABA) is a CNS inhibitor with an unclear mechanism of action. It is known that barbiturates can work through the GABA receptor and stimulate its activity, but not through the same mechanism as benzodiazepines.
QCCP2, **Barbiturates,** p 45

137. D. **COMPLETE MOLE.**

On average, gestational trophoblastic disease presents with hCG levels higher than those of a normal pregnancy. Complete moles have a much higher risk that any other pre-existing condition to develop choriocarcinoma.
QCCP2, **hCG in gestational trophoblastic disease,** p 37

1: Clinical Chemistry Answers

138.   B.   **PARKINSONIAN SYNDROME.**

Amphetamines work by stimulating the release of dopamine and in doing so can cause the death of the dopamine-secreting cells in the CNS. Lack of dopamine can result in a Parkinsonian condition, often where patients experience a locked-in phenomenon.
QCCP2, **Amphetamines,** p 45

139.   D.   **INHIBITION OF CATECHOLAMINE REUPTAKE.**

PCP functions as an inhibitor of catecholamine reuptake. Beyond the hallucinatory activities of PCP, patients with active intoxication exhibit symptoms of dopamine toxicity - bradycardia, hypotension, hypoglycemia, and hypopnea.
QCCP2, **PCP,** p 45

140.   D.   **0.4%.**

Of course, if somebody survived a BAL of 0.8%, one would worry about coma and death, but the question asked at what BAL does one <u>start</u> to worry, and 0.4% is the level at which there is first a very real risk of coma and death.
QCCP2, **T1.19, Clinical Effects of Blood Alcohol,** p 45

141.   E.   **ACETYLALDEHYDE.**

Both gastric and hepatic alcohol dehydrogenase facilitate the oxidation of ethanol to acetylaldehyde. When the alcohol dehydrogenase system is overwhelmed by excess ethanol, the microsomal ethanol oxidizing system contributes to the oxidation of ethanol. Acetylaldehyde is then further oxidized to acetate in the liver by aldehyde dehydrogenase. Many of the unpleasant side effects of alcohol - flushing, nausea, etc - are due to a buildup of acetaldehyde. The drug disulfram inhibits aldehyde dehydrogenase, perpetuating the unpleasant effects and helping to promote teetotalling.
QCCP2, **Ethanol,** p 46

142.   E.   **SERUM.**

Vitreous, breath alcohol, and whole blood are more commonly used in the post-mortem investigation of blood alcohol levels (just try to collect vitreous humor from a living patient!). Either serum or plasma are preferred samples when evaluating alcohol levels in living patients. Urine can be used, but usually only for qualitative testing.
QCCP2, **Ethanol,** 46

143.   C.   **WHOLE BLOOD.**

Even though the previous question stated that plasma or serum is the preferred sample, one must carefully read the question. For <u>overdose</u>, the preferred sample is plasma or serum, but to define what level is safe to operate a motor vehicle, whole blood is used. This is important because whole blood ethanol levels are usually lower than serum levels. The legal limits vary by state but are typically in the range of 0.8-1.0%.
QCCP2, **Ethanol,** p 46

1: Clinical Chemistry Answers

144.   A.   **CARBOHYDRATE-DEFICIENT TRANSFERRIN.**

For the most part, CDT is the most sensitive and specific of the choices, though all of them can be altered with chronic alcohol consumption. CDT levels rise faster than GGT in response to ethanol. There are a few caveats with CDT, however. Heavy female drinkers have lower average levels than their male counterparts and certain liver diseases can cause CDT elevations in the absence of alcohol consumption.
QCCP2, **Ethanol,** p 43

145.   B.   **SALIVATION, LACRIMATION, URINATION, DIARRHEA, GI CRAMPS, AND EMESIS.**

Certain insecticides, such as malathion and parathion, are converted to organophosphates after ingestion. Organophosphates are cholinesterase inhibitors with potent cholinergic activity. The mnemonic "SLUDGES" is helpful in remembering the cardinal features of cholinergic toxicity - <u>s</u>alivation, <u>l</u>acrimation, <u>u</u>rination, <u>d</u>iarrhea, <u>G</u>I cramps, <u>e</u>mesis. Imagine a farm worker trudging through a field of SLUDGE.
QCCP2, **T1.20, Common toxidromes,** p 47

146.   E.   **384 mOsm/L.**

Sodium is the major serum osmolyte, but BUN and glucose both provide a significant amount of osmolytes, too. To calculate the serum osmolarity, multiply the sodium concentration by two, add BUN/2.5 and glucose/18. In this case, a sodium of 140 multiplied by two is 280, added to 10/2.5 plus 180/1.8 is 384 mOsm/L.
QCCP2, **Calculation of osmolar gap,** p 47

147.   C.   **WINDSHIELD WASHER FLUID.**

Ethanol, isopropanol, and acetone (as in whiskey, rubbing alcohol, and nail polish remover, respectively) all can cause an osmolar gap, but usually without a concomitant anion gap. Conversely, salicylates can cause an anion gap but no osmolar gap. Windshield wiper fluid contains methanol, which like the ethylene glycol in antifreeze can cause both an anion and osmolar gap.
QCCP2, **Tables 1.21 and 1.22,** p 47-49

148.   A.   **OXYGEN SATURATION OF BLOOD.**

ABG analyzers measure oxygen tension and pH. From those values and a standard hemoglobin oxygen affinity graph, the oxygen saturation is calculated. Because the calculation is based on a standard curve, anything that affects the ability of hemoglobin to bind oxygen can cause inaccurate oxygen saturation readings.
QCCP2, **Measurement of blood gases,** p 47

149.   D.   **A & B.**

Pulse oximetry uses transdermal illumination to measure the absorption of light by oxyhemoglobin and deoxyhemoglobin. Alternate forms of hemoglobin, such as methemoglobin and carboxyhemoglobin can interfere with these results.
QCCP2, **Measurement of blood gases,** p 48

1: Clinical Chemistry Answers

150. D. **ETHANOL COMPETES WITH ETHYLENE GLYCOL AND METHANOL FOR ALCOHOL DEHYDROGENASE.**

While ethylene glycol and methanol have little direct toxicity, the metabolites glycolic acid/oxalate and formaldehyde/formic acid are both extremely toxic. The enzyme alcohol dehydrogenase is responsible for the metabolism of ethanol, methanol, and ethylene glycol. Supplying the patient with excess ethanol allows for competitive inhibition of alcohol dehydrogenase and therefore decreased production of toxic metabolites. In doing so, ethanol <u>delays</u> the development of an anion gap in patients with methanol and ethylene glyngestion - it does not prevent it.

QCCP2, **Toxic alcohol poisoning,** p 49

151. C. **BONE.**

D. **ERYTHROCYTES.**

In addition to bone and erythrocytes, a significant portion of lead is stored in the kidneys.

QCCP2, **Lead poisoning,** p 49

152. A. **BLOOD LEAD LEVELS.**

Previously, FEP and ZPP were used as screening tools. Lead inhibits delta-ALA-dehydratase, an enzyme involved in heme synthesis. As a result, a precursor, free erythrocyte protoporphyrin (EP) accumulates. Furthermore, FEP can bind zinc and produce zinc protoporphyrin (ZPP). The problem with using ZPP and FEP as screening tools is that they are both non-specific and insufficiently sensitive.

QCCP2, **Lead poisoning,** p 49-50

153. B. **10 MICROGRAMS/DL.**

The CDC recommendations stipulate blood levels should be less than 10 micrograms/dL. For this only, blood lead levels by atomic absorption spectrophotometry are sufficiently sensitive. FEP and ZPP are only detectable at lead levels greater than 35 micrograms/dL, which is not sensitive enough for screening.

QCCP2, **Lead poisoning,** p 50

154. B. **CO-OXIMETER.**

Co-oximeter analysis from either arterial or venous blood directly measures carbon monoxide-bound hemoglobin. Pulse oximeters and blood gas analyzers don't measure variant hemoglobins, such as hemoglobin-CO, and may actually provide falsely normal readings. Hemoglobin levels give no indication of carbon monoxide levels and a V/Q scan is to look for oxygenation/perfusion mismatch.

QCCP2, **Carbon monoxide (CO) poisoning,** p 51

155. B. **RUMACK-MATTHEW NOMOGRAM.**

The Rumack-Matthew nomogram is a plot of acetaminophen levels (in micrograms/mL or micromoles/L) on the y axis v. time after ingestion on the x axis. Two straight lines of equal linear regressive slope are drawn to delimit those below as low risk and those above as high risk. Importantly, the nomogram is used with the assumption that the patient has taken a single ingestion of acetaminophen at a defined time at least four hours prior.

QCCP2, **Acetaminophen poisoning,** p 51

1: Clinical Chemistry Answers

156.   C.   N-ACETYL-P-BENZOQUINONEIMINE.

The cytochrome P_{450} system converts acetaminophen to the toxic metabolite, N-acetyl-p-benzoquinoneimine (NAPQI), which is responsible for the majority of the hepatic toxicity. Glutathione-S-transferase then converts NAPQI to a less toxic metabolite. However, in the process glutathione is depleted and excess NAPQI can cause direct zone 3 hepatic toxicity. Treatment is by providing excess glutathione equivalents in the form of N-acetylcysteine.
QCCP2, **Acetaminophen poisoning,** p 52

157.   A.   ELEVATED SERUM LACTATE, ANION GAP METABOLIC ACIDOSIS.

The causes of anion gap metabolic acidosis can be divided into two categories - conditions that cause elevated serum lactate, such as cyanide, and those that are due to unmeasured organic anions. Lactate elevation in cyanide poisoning is fairly universal, so a normal serum lactate can eliminate cyanide as a cause of patient symptoms.
QCCP2, **Cyanide poisoning,** p 52

158.   E.   A, B, C.

It all depends on when you check. Initially, aspirin triggers a tachypnea resulting in respiratory alkalosis. Then it facilitates anaerobic metabolism, the production of lactate (just like cyanide) and the development of an anion gap metabolic acidosis. Remember, "MUDPILES"? This is the mnemonic to help recall the causes of anion gap metabolic acidosis - methanol, uremia, diabetic ketoacidosis, paraldehyde, isoniazid, lactate, ethanol, salicylates. Eventually, this can be followed by CNS depression and a respiratory acidosis.
QCCP2, **Salicylates,** p 53

159.   B.   QUANTITATIVE 24-HOUR URINARY ARSENIC LEVELS.

Another "go-with-the-longest-answer-if-you-don't-know" question. Blood arsenic is unreliable due to rapid clearance and distribution. Fingernails and hair can be used but elevated levels are more consistent with chronic prolonged ingestion or exposure.
QCCP2, **Arsenic,** p 53

160.   B.   EKG.

Actually, a widened QRS, in addition to an increased risk of arrhythmia, is predictive of a likelihood of seizures, especially if the QRS is greater than 0.1.
QCCP2, **Tricyclic antidepressants,** p 54

161.   B.   MERCURY.

The chronic exposure to mercury usually occurs through occupational inhalation or ingestion of contaminated FISH. The manifestations of mercury usually take the form of one of two syndromes. Feer syndrome (acrodynia) has autonomic signs - sweating and hemodynamic instability in addition to the characteristic desquamation of the palms and soles. Erethism is more central nervous system-centered, with personality changes and fine motor difficulties.
QCCP2, **Mercury,** p 54

1: Clinical Chemistry Answers

162. A. **24-HOUR URINE MERCURY LEVELS.**

Elemental mercury is typically inhaled during occupational exposure. It is readily excreted in the urine. Organic mercury, however, is absorbed through the GI tract in contaminated food and not excreted in the urine. Therefore, hair or blood levels are used for diagnosis. Just try to collect vitreous humor from a living patient.
QCCP2, **Mercury,** p 54

163. D. **QUINIDINE.**

Quinidine has multiple roles in enhancing the function of digoxin. It has a direct role in increasing the drug's effects on the heart, but also inhibits the elimination of digoxin by competing for the common P-glycoprotein binding site. As a result, both quinidine and digoxin toxicity is increased when simultaneously administered.
QCCP2, **Digoxin,** p 54

164. D. **A & B.**

Procainamide is acetylated in the liver to an active metabolite, N-acetyl procainamide, which in turn is renally excreted. Therefore, both renal and liver dysfunction can affect procainamide levels.
QCCP2, **Procainamide,** p 55

165. E. **EKG.**

Levels - serum, urinary, or otherwise - are unreliable. The only reliable means of assessing quinidine toxicity is by EKG. As the drug blocks ion channels, toxicity usually manifests with cardiac symptoms, such as a prolonged QT, widened QRS, and arrhythmias.
QCCP2, **Quinidine,** p 55

166. E. **NONE OF THE ABOVE.**

The causative agent of fetal hydantoin syndrome is *in utero* exposure of a fetus to phenytoin. The typical manifestations include characteristic facial anomalies, as well as growth and mental retardation.
QCCP2, **phenytoin,** p 55

167. C. **1-3 MONTHS.**

Because of the very narrow therapeutic range and the proximity of therapeutic and toxic levels, it is of paramount importance to monitor levels for initial dosing. The half-life of lithium ranges from 8-40 hours, so steady levels will be achieved after 5 half-lives or 1.5 days to 1 week. Initially, it is recommended to check levels after the initial interval. Samples should be collected 12 hours after last dose.
QCCP2, **Lithium,** p 55-56

168. B. **KIDNEY.**

The thyroid and lungs have the highest incidence of toxic reactions to amiodarone. It is also important to remember that amiodarone effects on the liver can affect warfarin and digoxin levels.
QCCP2, **Amiodarone,** p 56

1: Clinical Chemistry Answers

169. E. **POLYUNSATURATED FATTY ACIDS.**

Whether a fatty acid is fully saturated with hydrogen groups (saturated) or has a single double bond (monounsaturated) with less hydrogen or even less hydrogen with multiple double bonds (polyunsaturated) affects its chemical properties. Saturated fatty acids are less fluid in the cell membrane due to their rigid structure. Unsaturated fatty acids have bends in their chains due to the double bonds and therefore pack less tightly into a membrane which leads to greater membrane fluidity.
QCCP2, **Lipids,** p 56

170. A. **CHYLOMICRONS.**

All the different classes of lipoproteins are composed of varying amounts of common building blocks - cholesterol, triglyceride, phospholipid, and apolipoproteins. Chylomicrons are a class of lipoproteins that contain a large amount of triglyceride and as a result are very dense.
QCCP2, **Lipids,** p 56

171. A-3, B-4, C-2, D-1.

If you can visualize the function of each lipoprotein, you can guess the amount of lipid and protein in each. There are four basic rules:

1. In general, the ratio of triglycerides/lipid and protein are inversely proportional - the more lipid, the less protein and vice-versa.

2. The lipoproteins migrate depending on the amount the protein - more protein migrates further.

3. Protein is denser than lipid.

4. The name of the lipoprotein tells you the density!

As far as the main function of each of the lipoproteins - chylomicrons take dietary triglycerides to the liver. The liver repackages the triglycerides into VLDL to deliver triglycerides to tissue. Once the triglyceride is dropped off, the lipoprotein becomes IDL and then LDL. To monitor the amount of the peripheral lipid, the liver makes HDL, whose role is to take back triglyceride from the periphery and return it to the liver.
QCCP2, **Lipid,** p 57

172. D. **A & B.**

Total cholesterol, triglycerides, and HDL are directly measured using a series of enzymatic reactions. Because it is difficult to separate LDL from other lipoproteins, its levels are calculated rather than directly measured. The cholesterol in LDL is basically what's left over when the measurable sources of cholesterol are subtracted from total cholesterol. The Friedewald equation is this calculation. (LDL cholesterol = total cholesterol - HDL cholesterol - VLDL.) Since the VLDL is not usually measured, an equivalent substitute is the triglycerides divided by 5. Under certain conditions, such as triglycerides above 400, the Friedewald equation is not applicable.
QCCP2, **Methods,** p 57

1: Clinical Chemistry Answers

173.   A-4, B-2, C-1, D-3, E-5.

There are several ways to classify lipid disorders. When classified by which lipoprotein is elevated, they can be subsequently categorized by electrophoretic mobility. Since charged molecules move through an electric field and protein determines the charge of a lipoprotein, the different lipoproteins can be sorted by electrophoresis. The molecules with the most charged protein move the furthest. The bands are then numbered from the least mobile to the most - I = chylomicrons, II = LDL, III = IDL, IV = VLDL. V is tricky, but the mnemonic I + IV = V helps (I = chylomicrons, IV = VLDL, V = chylomicrons + VLDL).
QCCP2, **Lipids,** T1.25 p 58

174.   B.   PREMATURE ATHEROSCLEROSIS.

Atherosclerosis is most commonly seen with elevated cholesterol. While there is a significant amount of cholesterol in LDL and IDL, chylomicrons don't contain much cholesterol. In addition to chylomicrons, VLDL also contains a considerable amount of triglyceride and therefore both are associated with xanthomas, xanthelasmas, and pancreatitis.
QCCP2, **Lipids,** p 59

175.   D.   DECREASED HDL.

Tangier disease is an autosomal recessive condition named for the small Chesapeake Bay island where the predominance of cases of the disease have been described. A mutation in the ABC1 cholesterol transporter prevents intracellular cholesterol from being excreted to be packaged with apolipoprotein-A1 to make HDL. As a result, HDL and apolipoprotein A1 levels are decreased to absent and serum cholesterol is greatly reduced. Intracellular cholesterol deposits are commonly seen as the characteristic orange tonsils.
QCCP2, **Lipid disorders,** p 60

176.   E.   <200, <100.

The target ranges are specified especially for those with a history of coronary artery disease with a target IDL <100 mg/dL. More liberal guidelines are proposed for those with fewer risk factors. Cholesterol >240 and LDL >160 are considered to be elevated and medication is indicated. Values between optimal and elevated are considered borderline and can be treated with lifestyle changes.
QCCP2, **Lipids in the assessment of CAD risk,** T1.27, p 60

177.   A.   HUMAN PLACENTAL LACTOGEN.

HPL or somatomammotropin is functionally similar to growth hormone. HPL's main function is to modify maternal metabolism to provide more fuel in the form of glucose or ketones to the fetus. This is accomplished through the utilization of maternal free fatty acids and increasing maternal insulin resistance.
QCCP2, **Carbohydrates,** p 60

178.   A.   LAB LEVELS RUN HIGHER THAN POC LEVELS.

Laboratory glucose measurement is typically performed on plasma, while POC testing is done on whole blood. Unless the POC instrument is calibrated, its levels will routinely be lower than the laboratory plasma glucose levels. Hematocrit also affects the correlation between plasma and whole blood levels.
QCCP2, **Carbohydrates,** p 61

1: Clinical Chemistry Answers

179. B. **3 MONTHS.**

For all intents and purposes, a red blood cell lifespan is 4 months, but a majority of cells in circulation have been around for less than half of that time. As a result, it is generally accepted that HbA1c gives an indication of glucose control for the previous 1-3 weeks.
QCCP2, **Carbohydrates**, p 61

180. D. **RELIEF OF SYMPTOMS WITH GLUCOSE ADMINISTRATION.**

Another "choose-the-longest-answer" question! While several of the choices listed above may be associated with insulinoma, the classical Whipple triad is hypoglycemia, symptoms, glucose <45 mg/dL and relief of symptoms by administration of glucose.
QCCP2, **Hypoglycemia**, p 62

181. B. **INSULIN IS METABOLIZED FASTER THAN C-PEPTIDE.**

Initially, insulin is secreted by pancreatic islet cells as a prohormone of disulfide-bonded A & B chains linked by a C chain. Therefore, they are secreted in equimolar amounts. After secretion, the relatively stable C peptide is cleaved, leaving its active A-B peptide, which is rapidly metabolized, leading to the skewed C-peptide:insulin ratio of 5-15:1.
QCCP2, **Carbohydrate**, p 61

182. E. **INSULINOMA.**

The causes of hypoglycemia can be divided into those that result from excess insulin and those that don't. Furthermore, the hypoinsulinemic causes of hypoglycemia can be divided into ketotic and non-ketotic, while most causes of hypoinsulinemic hypoglycemia are associated with ketosis. It should be noted that causes of non-ketotic hypoglycemia are usually due to an insulin-like activity, such as in starvation, liver failure, and autoimmune hypoglycemia.
QCCP2, **Hypoglycemia**, p 63

183. E. **ALL OF THE ABOVE.**

Almost all cases of type I diabetes are associated with at least one of those autoantibodies that cause islet B cell destruction.
QCCP2, **Diabetes mellitus**, p 63

184. C. **ORAL GLUCOSE TOLERANCE TEST WITH 75 G GLUCOSE LOAD AND TWO HOUR GLUCOSE GREATER THAN 200 MG/DL.**

There are many diagnostic modalities used for diabetes. In the case of "non-gestational diabetes," three major tests are used: fasting plasma glucose, casual plasma glucose, and oral glucose tolerance test. A positive test should be repeated on a different day. A combination of tests can be used. For the fasting plasma, a level of 126 mg/dL or above is considered diagnostic of diabetes. A random plasma glucose of 200 mg/dL, in addition to symptoms of diabetes, is considered diagnostic. Finally, a 75 g oral glucose tolerance test with a 2 hour plasma glucose of 200 mg/dL or higher is positive. In pregnancy, a 100 g oral glucose tolerance test is used and glucose levels are checked before dosage and for 3 hours afterward at 1-hour intervals. Two abnormal values during the test are considered positive for gestational diabetes. The cutoff values for gestational diabetes are a fasting glucose of 95 mg/dL or more, a 1 hour of 180+, 2 hour of 155+, 3 hour of 140+.
QCCP2, **Diabetes mellitus**, p 63-64

1: Clinical Chemistry Answers

185.   C.   **MONOCYTOSIS.**

Hyperglycemia, ketosis, and anion gap metabolic acidosis support a diagnosis of diabetic ketoacidosis. The diagnosis can be made on clinical presentation with the presence of urine glucose and ketones, as well. A plasma glucose level of 200 mg/dL or more with a venous pH <7.3 or bicarbonate <15 mmole/L is consistent with diabetic ketoacidosis.
QCCP2, **Diabetic ketoacidosis,** p 64

186.   D.   **A & B.**

The measured ketones, acetone, and acetoacetic acid comprise only a minority of the ketones in diabetic ketacidosis. However, there is inter-conversion of each type, which accounts for the appearance of an increased ketone level with initial treatment as beta-hydroxybutyrate is converted to the other ketones, which in turn are measured.
QCCP2, **Diabetic ketoacidosis,** p 65

187.   B.   **POTASSIUM.**

Transcellular shifts of potassium in diabetic ketoacidosis in response to elevated glucose lead to high serum levels and subsequent urinary loss, but low cellular levels when insulin is initiated. There is a shift of potassium into the cell, further lowering the levels and potentially causing a severe hypokalemia.
QCCP2, **Diabetic ketoacidosis,** p 65

188.   D.   **ALL OF THE ABOVE.**

DKA and HHNC vary in several ways. DKA is more common in type I DM, and presents with an acidic pH and a low level hyperglycemia. HHNC is more common in type 2 DM and presents with extremely high hyperglycemia and normal pH. The prognosis for HHNC is typically also more dire with a 10% mortality rate (it has COMA in the name!).
QCCP2, **HHNC,** p 65

189.   B.   **TACHYCARDIA.**

The constellation can also include increased PAI-1 and CRP. The dyslipidemia usually manifests as increased VLDL/LDL/triglycerides with decreased HDL. Patients with metabolic syndrome have a significantly increased risk of accelerated atherosclerosis.
QCCP2, **The Metabolic Syndrome,** p 65

190.   D.   **DEPENDENCE ON HETEROPHILE ANTIBODIES.**

In order for a screening test to be cost-effective - that is, the cost of detection is less than the cost of sorting out false results - the test should have a high positive predictive value (PPV). The PPV is increased when there is a high prevalence of disease and when pretest probability is high. Low analytic sensitivity means the test is able to detect low amounts of analyte or more specifically the lowest analyte concentration that registers above zero.
QCCP2, **Tumor markers,** p 66

1: Clinical Chemistry Answers

191. D. **30-40%.**

A little less than half of men with mildly elevated PSA will have prostate cancer on biopsy. Very high levels of PSA (>10ng/dL) are associated with a very high incidence of prostate cancer, but intermediate levels of 4-10 ng/dL are less likely to be associated with cancer. More importantly, the trajectory of PSA elevation is more indicative of cancer than isolated elevated values.
QCCP2, **PSA,** p 66

192. A. **FREE PSA LESS THAN 10%.**

While PSA levels are a somewhat useful tool in screening for prostate cancer, substantial improvement is needed. Multiple techniques have been used to in order to improve the use of PSA: setting age-specific ranges, calculating PSA density, velocity of PSA changes, measuring unbound/bound PSA ratios, and measuring the levels of PSA isoforms. Two of the most useful techniques have been measuring the percent of PSA bound (free PSA <10% correlates well with prostate cancer) and levels of pro-PSA (high pro-PSA correlates with CA).
QCCP2, **PSA,** p 67

193. E. **CANNOT BE DETERMINED.**

Biochemical failure, or rising post-treatment PSA, is indicated as either 3 consecutive increases or 1 increase so large that hormone therapy is indicated. While post-treatment PSA is useful in the determination of recurrence, it cannot help to distinguish where the recurrence arises.
QCCP2, **PSA,** p 69

194. C. **LEFT-SIDED TUMORS PRODUCE MORE CEA THAN RIGHT-SIDED TUMORS.**

With the exception of choice C, all the choices presented are inverted. Other things associated with high CEA are bowel obstruction, peptic ulcer disease, inflammatory bowel disease, pancreatitis, and cirrhosis.
QCCP2, **CEA,** p 68

195. D. **A & B.**

Both follicular cancer and papillary thyroid cancer are associated with elevated thyroglobulin. The precursor of medullary carcinoma is the C-cell and is associated with elevated calcitonin rather than thyroglobulin.
QCCP2, **Thyroglobulin,** p 68-69

196. E. **ALL OF THE ABOVE.**

The expression of TATI is a poor prognostic sign. In addition to all the conditions listed above, elevated TATI is associated with renal failure (due to decreased clearance), renal cell carcinoma, and gastric carcinoma. The elevation seen in pancreatic adenocarcinoma is fairly consistent. However, because it is elevated in pancreatitis, it is of limited use.
QCCP2, **TATI,** p 69

197. B. **NON-MUCINOUS EPITHELIAL OVARIAN NEOPLASM.**

The most used aspect of CA-125 is the monitoring of patients with non-mucinous epithelial ovarian neoplasm. It is a poor tool to be used for screening as it is only elevated in 1/2 of early stage disease, but also because it is has a low positive predictive value.
QCCP2, **CA-125,** p 69

1: Clinical Chemistry Answers

198.   E.   **A, B, C.**

All of the antibodies are directed against different epitopes of the MUC1 gene product, which is most commonly associated with breast cancer. Like many other tumor markers, it is a poor tool for screening due to the very nonspecific elevations seen in conditions such as cysts, cirrhosis, sarcoidosis, and lupus. In addition, a number of other carcinomas are associated with elevated CA27-29, such as colon, stomach, pancreas, prostate, and lung. *QCCP2,* **CA27-29,** p 70

199.   D.   **PANCREATIC ADENOCARCINOMA.**

If only 2 of the 3 signs are present, the PPV drops to 90%. CA19-9 is also elevated in some non-neoplastic diseases, such as cirrhosis and pancreatitis, and some intestinal and esophageal adenocarcinomas. Like most of the other relatively tumor-specific markers mentioned previously, CA19-9 is not a very useful as a screening tool, but it mostly utilized to monitor disease recurrence or response to treatment. *QCCP2,* **CA19-9,** p 70

200.   E.   **LEWIS.**

It is important to note that patients negative for both Lewis A and B antigens are unable to produce CA19-9. In their case, CA19-9 is not useful as a tool to monitor disease recurrence or response to treatment. *QCCP2,* **CA19-9,** p 70

201.   E.   **A, B, C.**

AFP is not tumor-specific. In fetal serum, it provides the function of albumin, the major intravascular oncotic protein. In addition, non-neoplastic conditions, such as pregnancy and cirrhosis, may show elevations in AFP. *QCCP2,* **AFP,** p 71

202.   E.   **MULTIPLE MYELOMA.**

Any cell rapidly turning over, with the exception of red blood cells, has the capacity to shed beta-2-microglobulin. MHC Class I proteins along with beta-2-microglobulin are on the surface of nearly all nucleated cells, providing an important recognition receptor for cytotoxic T cells. Therefore, there is the potential for elevated beta-2-microglobulin in almost any tumor. Hematological malignancies are the best studied and increased beta-2-microglobulin has been shown in CLL, non-Hodgkin lymphoma, and multiple myeloma. Of these, only multiple myeloma has beta-2-microglobulin been shown to be an independent prognostic factor. *QCCP2,* **Beta-2-microglobulin,** p 71

203.   B.   **MIDGUT.**

All carcinoids are capable of producing serotonin, but only ones of midgut (duodenum to hepatic flexure of colon) are associated with very high serotonin. Foregut carcinoids also produce serotonin, albeit in small amounts, and hindgut carcinoids typically are not associated with serotonin expression. *QCCP2,* **Carcinoid tumors,** p 72

204.   E.   **ALL OF THE ABOVE.**

There are number of peptides produced by carcinoid-type tumors. Of these, plasma chromogranin A levels have been used to track response to treatment and help diagnose carcinoid tumors. *QCCP2,* **Carcinoid tumors,** p 72

1: Clinical Chemistry Answers

205. D. CALCITONIN (+), CEA (+), THYROGLOBULIN (-).

While elevated calcitonin is associated with medullary thyroid carcinoma (MTC), it is not specific and can be seen elevated in other neoplastic (breast cancer) and non-neoplastic (Hashimoto thyroiditis) conditions. However, when combined with elevated CEA and a lack of thyroglobulin expression, the specificity becomes very high.
QCCP2, **Calcitonin,** p 73

206. A. ELEVATION OF PREDOMINANTLY NOREPINEPHRINE AND NORMETANEPHRINE.

Normetanephrine is metabolized to normetanephrine, while epinephrine is metabolized to metanephrine. While adrenal tumors (pheochromocytoma) can secrete both norepinephrine and epinephrine (and normetanephrine, metanephrine), extra-adrenal chromaffin tumors (paragangliomas) secrete predominantly norepinephrine and normetanephrine.
QCCP2, **Markers of paragangliomas and pheochromocytoma,** p 73

207. A. RULING OUT RECURRENT LOW GRADE DISEASE.

Again, most tumor-specific antigens have a greater role in the detection of recurrent disease instead of the initial diagnosis. In the case of NMP22, >70% of patients will have elevated levels and recurrent disease, while even more (>80%) of patients with normal levels will not have recurrence, making it most effective in ruling out recurrent disease. In addition, while there is a moderate increase in sensitivity of detecting low-grade disease, there is no such benefit in the detection of high-grade disease.
QCCP2, **Urine markers for urothelial carcinoma,** p 73

208. B. URINE DD3 LEVELS.

The DD3 mRNA is encoded by the gene PCA3. It has been shown to be significantly upregulated in prostatic adenocarcinoma from post-prostate massage urine specimens. The DD3 transcript can be detected from extracted RNA via RT-PCR.
QCCP2, **Urine PCA3/DD3 for prostatic carcinoma,** p 74

209. B. INCREASED TSH, DECREASED TOTAL T4, DECREASED T3 RESIN UPTAKE.

First of all, it's hypothyroidism, so there must be decreased T4. That narrows it down to choices B and E. The normal response to decreased circulating thyroid hormone is increased thyroid stimulating hormone from the anterior pituitary, which leaves choice B. Choice A describes hyperthyroidism; C sick euthyroid syndrome; D excess thyroid-binding globulin. T3 resin uptake is a complex test designed to get around the protein-binding confounder in measuring total T3 and T4. T3 resin uptake levels parallel T3 and T4 levels.
QCCP2, **Thyroid chemistry,** p 75

210. D. HASHIMOTO THYROIDITIS.

If it has toxic in the name, you can almost guarantee that it's hyperfunctioning. Most adenomas are also hyperfunctioning. Graves is the leading cause of hyperthyroidism, while Hashimoto thyroiditis is one of the leading causes of hypothyroidism.
QCCP2, **Hyper-hypothyroidism,** p 75-76

1: Clinical Chemistry Answers

211.   D.   **A & B.**

Both anti-microsomal and anti-thyroglobulin are present in Hashimoto thyroiditis. As a matter of fact, a case of histologic lymphocytic thyroiditis should not be called Hashimoto thyroiditis without serum confirmation of antibodies.
QCCP2, **Hypothyroidism,** p 76

212.   A.   AUTOSOMAL DOMINANT PERIPHERAL RESISTANCE TO THYROID HORMONE.

Refetoff syndrome is one of myriad causes of congenital neonatal hypothyroidism. It is an extremely rare autosomal dominant condition where there is peripheral unresponsiveness to thyroid hormone. As a result, thyroid hormone is made but not utilized.
QCCP2, **Neonatal hypothyroidism,** p 76

213.   B.   CRITICAL ILLNESS.

The sick euthyroid syndrome refers to the decreased thyroid hormone secondary to a critical illness. Usually it occurs in elderly sick patients. TSH is usually normal despite the mildly decreased T3. Since the first line test for dyshormonogenic conditions is TSH, it is often overlooked.
QCCP2, **Euthyroid sick syndrome,** p 76-77

214.   C.   HYPOTHYROIDISM.

For the most part, the effect of amiodarone is unpredictable. However, there is the general trend of it causing hypothyroidism in iodine-replete conditions, such as in the developed world, and hyperthyroidism in iodine-poor regions.
QCCP2, **Amiodarone,** p 77

215.   B.   8 A.M., MIDNIGHT.

The easiest way to remember when peaks and troughs occur is to think about when babies are usually born (or at least when labor begins). Usually in the small hours of the morning, corresponding to the a.m. cortisol spike. And like most people, at the end of the day, you are tired and so is your pituitary, where there is a significant trough at midnight. This is also why an elevated midnight serum cortisol is suggestive of Cushing syndrome. This also explains why the 24-hour urine cortisol is a superior test of overall cortisol levels - it negates diurnal variation.
QCCP2, **Adrenal cortex tests,** p 77

216.   D.   HIGH DOSE DEXAMETHASONE SUPPRESSION TEST.

While urine cortisol and low dose DST would be positive in cases of Cushing disease, they cannot distinguish Cushing syndrome (elevated serum cortisol) from Cushing disease (elevated serum cortisol due to a pituitary adenoma). The DST suppresses ACTH in the pituitary and CRH in the hypothalamus, and therefore will discover if the patient has hypercortisolism due to upstream causes.
QCCP2, **Adrenal cortex,** p 77

1: Clinical Chemistry Answers

217. D. LATE-NIGHT.

Remember that typically, the most significant trough of cortisol occurs around midnight ("you and your pituitary are tired"). It would make sense that the best time to assay elevated cortisol is when the cortisol should be at its lowest. The salivary cortisol is an excellent screening tool with very high sensitivity and specificity for elevated free cortisol.

QCCP2, **Adrenal cortex,** p 78

218. A. CUSHING DISEASE.

To be honest, iatrogenic Cushing syndrome should be in a separate category of what the "non-iatrogenic causes." Administration of steroids is probably the most common cause of Cushing syndrome. Outside of those cases, the most common organic cause of Cushing syndrome is cortisol overproduction due to pituitary adenoma and increased ACTH.

QCCP2, **Cushing syndrome,** p 78

219. D. HYPERPIGMENTATION.

Like with hypercortisolism, hypocortisolism can be divided into an eponymous general "syndrome" and specific cause of the syndrome, "disease." Addison syndrome is defined as hypocortisolism, while Addison disease is defined as hypocortisolism due to primary adrenal insufficiency. When cortisol drops, the pituitary produces more ACTH, but it is stimulated by the CRH from the hypothalamus. CRH is secreted in a prohormone (POMC) that also encodes an opiate and melanocyte-stimulating hormone (MSH), which accounts for the hyperpigmentation.

QCCP2, **Addison syndrome,** p 78, **and ACTH,** p 80

220. B. ADRENAL ADENOMA.

Conn syndrome refers to the constellation of symptoms secondary to hyperaldosteronism (hypernatremia, hypokalemia, hypertension). While renal artery stenosis (bilateral, usually) and juxtaglomerular tumors can cause reactive (secondary) hyperaldosteronism, the most common cause of hyperaldosteronism is primary overproduction from an adrenal adenoma. Extra credit - which layer of the adrenal cortex is responsible for the production of aldosterone? The answer is zona glomerulosa.

QCCP2, **Conn syndrome,** p 79

221. C. 21-HYDROXYLASE DEFICIENCY.

Deficiency of the enzyme 21-hydroxylase accounts for the majority of cases of CAH. The gene encoding 21-hydroxylase is in the MHC complex on 6p21.3 and mutations are typically due to gene conversion by recombination between an active gene and a colocated pseudogene.

QCCP2, **Congenital adrenal hyperplasia,** p 79

222. C. 21-HYDROXYLASE DEFICIENCY.

As detailed above, 21-hydroxylase is the overall most common cause of CAH, but also the most common cause of the salt-wasting form. Typically, patients with salt-wasting have more severe disease and hence earlier presentation overall, with girls presenting earlier than boys due to the high incidence of ambiguous genitalia. Salt-losing is due to the decreased aldosterone, which results in decreased reabsorption of sodium from the urine and hence hyponatremia.

QCCP2, **Congenital adrenal hyperplasia,** p 79

1: Clinical Chemistry Answers

223. **D. GH.**

The majority of hormones in the anterior pituitary are produced by basophilic cells. Remember, the differentiation of acidophils from basophils is made with a supravital stain, such as acridine orange. The only anterior pituitary hormones produced by acidophils are prolactin and growth hormone. The remaining hormones, luteinizing hormone, follicle-stimulating hormone, thyroid-stimulating hormone, and adrenocorticotrophic hormone are produced by basophils. The mnemonic "TOGA FLAP" helps with recall of the hormones of the pituitary: TSH, oxytocin, GH, ACTH, FSH, LH, ADH, prolactin. Oxytocin and ADH are produced by the posterior pituitary.
QCCP2, **Pituitary,** p 80

224. **B. PROLACTIN.**

The most common pituitary secretory tumor is the prolactinoma and it is usually very small. Interestingly, due to its unique means of control (dopamine-mediated repression), prolactin is unlikely to be hyposecreted like the other pituitary hormones with a stalk-compressive lesion.
QCCP2, **Pituitary,** p 80

225. **B. INSULIN CREATES HYPOGLYCEMIA, STIMULATING GH PRODUCTION.**

The insulin intolerance test is used in cases of suspected growth hormone deficiency. Similarly, clonidine, arginine, or exercise can be used to provoke growth hormone expression. Insulin administration results in hypoglycemia, which causes a reflexive stimulation of growth hormone secretion. Insufficient growth hormone levels are indicative of deficiency. In cases of growth hormone excess, IGF-1 can be measured - increased levels are indicative of excess.
QCCP2, **Growth hormone,** p 80

226. **D. BY INHIBITING PRODUCTION OF FSH AND LH.**

Leuprolide and goserelin are both GnRH agonists used as therapy against hormone-sensitive malignancies, such as prostate cancer. A GnRH agonist works as an initial stimulant of FSH/LH production, but then it begins to be inhibitory, decreasing the amounts of FSH and LH. LH normally functions to increase androgen production; therefore inhibition of LH leads to inhibition of testosterone.
QCCP2, **FSH and LH,** p 81

227. **A. HYPERNATREMIA WITH LOW URINE OSMOLARITY.**

A simple way to think of hypernatremia and hyponatremia is as derangements in body water rather than sodium. That is, hypernatremia is having too little water; hyponatremia is having too much. Then remember that diabetes insipidus is the result of inadequate anti-diuretic hormone - either because there in not enough made (central DI) or because the kidneys don't respond (nephrogenic DI). Anti-diuretic hormone helps us to conserve water by activating water channels (aquaporins) in the collecting duct and "taking back" water from urine. Without ADH, we would get rid of excess water in the urine, leading to the characteristic hypernatremia with low urine osmolarity. SIADH would be expected to have the opposite presentation.
QCCP2, **ADH,** p 81

1: Clinical Chemistry Answers

228.   E.   **VITREOUS HUMOR.**

Okay, this is one of those times that you can collect vitreous humor. Blood levels of glucose tend to rise post-mortem; vitreous levels tend to drop. Therefore, an elevated post-mortem vitreous glucose is suggestive of hyperglycemia. However, since vitreous glucose levels drop post-mortem it would be inappropriate to diagnose hypoglycemia from a vitreous sample.
QCCP2, **Glucose**, p 82

229.   B.   **DECREASED SODIUM, DECREASED CHLORIDE, INCREASED POTASSIUM.**

If you remember one thing about vitreous chemistry, remember that elevated potassium (>15 mEq/L) is indicative of decomposition. The vitreous potassium level rises in a consistent linear fashion after death and provides a fairly standard indication of the proximate interval post-mortem. If you want to remember two things about vitreous humor chemistry, see the previous question.
QCCP2, **Sodium and chloride, potassium**, p 82

230.   D.   **SERUM BETA-TRYPTASE.**

I know that the answer to this question is not in the text, but it is an important issue. Serum tryptase is one of the most reliable means of diagnosing anaphylaxis, specifically, beta-tryptase, which is released during mast cell and eosinophil activation. Alpha-tryptase is present in the serum and its levels don't change much with anaphylaxis.
QCCP2, **Tryptase and post-mortem diagnosis of anaphylaxis**, p 83

231.   A.   **ABILITY TO DETECT OTHER "REDUCING SUBSTANCES."**

Some of the above choices may or may not be true, depending on the circumstances. However, the ability to measure other reducing substances, such as galactose, is the clear advantage of Clinitest.
QCCP2, **Urine glucose**, p 83

232.   C.   **HEAT TO PRECIPITATE AT 40°, REDISSOLVE AT 100°, THEN COOL TO REPRECIPITATE AT 60° AND REDISSOLVE AT 40°.**

We have another "longest-answer-is-correct" question. Bence-Jones proteins have the unique property that, when heated, they will precipitate when the temperature reaches 40-60°C. Continued heating to 100°C will make the proteins redissolve. If then allowed to cool, the proteins will reprecipitate when the temperature reaches 60°C and, finally, again redissolve at 40°C. Nowadays, a urine protein electrophoresis is done more often to answer the same question.
QCCP2, **Urine protein**, p 83

233.   B.   **HEMATURIA.**

The most common hemoglobin confounder on urine dipstick is myoglobin. However, myoglobinuria and hemoglobinuria cannot be differentiated by microscopy. Red blood cells will also give a positive result on urine dipstick and can be differentiated on urine microscopy.
QCCP2, **Urine hemoglobin**, p 83

1: Clinical Chemistry Answers

234. C. *ESCHERICHIA COLI.*

While nitrate may be present in normal urine, nitrite is usually only due to presence of bacteria that are capable of reducing nitrate to nitrite. Also, urine must be incubated with the organism for a sufficient length of time in order for the nitrite to form. In addition, the patient's diet must include sufficient nitrate precursors.
QCCP2, **Urine nitrite,** p 84

235. B. DIABETES INSIPIDUS.

Increased specific gravity is consistent with increased urine concentration either due to less solvent (water) or more solute (protein, glucose, etc). In the case of diabetes insipidus there is a lack of water conservation leading to profound diuresis of very dilute urine.
QCCP2, **Urine specific gravity,** p 84

236. A. CALCIUM OXALATE.

The order of choices is roughly the incidence from most common to less common causes of nephrolithiasis. Increased urine calcium and oxalate, along with decreased urine volume and citrate, promote the production of calcium oxalate stones. Calcium phosphate stones are also promoted by hypercalciuria, frequently in the face of hypercalcemia. MAP stones are promoted by urea-splitting organisms such as *Proteus mirabilis.* Increased uric acid promotes urate stones, and cystine stones are almost exclusively seen in the setting of cystinuria, an autosomal recessive defect in amino acid transport.
QCCP2, **Nephrolithiasis,** p 84-85

237. B. RED BLOOD CELL CASTS.

Damage to the glomerulus usually results in bad-looking sediment including polymorphous red blood cells, red cell casts, and erythrophagocytosis. Non-glomerular bleeding results in a more refined sediment with uniform red blood cells, no casts nor erythrophagocytosis.
QCCP2, **Casts,** p 86

238. B. RED BLOOD CELL CASTS.

Both hyaline and waxy casts are relatively non-specific and can be seen with almost any type of renal injury, RBC/WBC and tubular casts are more specific. RBC casts are usually indicative of renal glomerular damage, such as that due to glomerulonephritis. WBC casts are seen most often with tubulointerstitial disease, such as pyelonephritis. Tubular casts are made of shed necrotic renal tubular cells and are indicative of acute tubular necrosis.
QCCP2, **Casts,** p 86

239. C. SPECIFIC GRAVITY.

Measuring the protein or glucose concentration of the fluid is a very nonspecific test. One is looking for the characteristic concentrations of each analyte (~60% of serum levels). Protein electrophoresis and measurement of asialated transferrin are more specific. CSF has a characteristic "twin transferrin" peak due to the presence of asialated transferring that is not seen in serum. In addition, CSF has a prominent pre-albumin band.
QCCP2, **CSF,** p 87

1: Clinical Chemistry Answers

240.   B.   INTRATHECAL IgG SYNTHESIS.

Oligoclonal bands are one of the most sensitive tests for detecting MS (in concert with clinical and radiological findings). In addition to the presence of oligoclonal bands, intrathecal IgG synthesis demonstrates activity and is suggestive of MS. Intrathecal IgA synthesis is seen most commonly with cerebral adrenoleukodystrophy, while glutamine in the CSF is associated with hepatic encephalopathy.

QCCP2, **CSF,** p 87

241.   B.   MONOCYTES.

Overall there should be very few cells present in the CSF. Neonates tend to have more monocytes and fewer lymphocytes than adults. When WBCs are present in the CSF, the differential for a normal neonate is different than that of a normal adult. Higher numbers of leukocytes are tolerated in the neonatal CSF.

QCCP2, **IVL CSF differential counts, T1.38,** p 87

242.   C.   JC VIRUS.

Most bacterial, mycobacterial, and fungal causes of meningitis are associated with decreased CSF glucose, while most viral meningitides are associated with normal CSF glucose. However, HSV causes of meningoencephalitis are actually also associated with decreased CSF glucose.

QCCP2, **CSF differential counts in meningitis, T1.39,** p 88

243.   C.   PLEURAL FLUID LDH >200, OR 2/3 THE UPPER LIMIT OF SERUM LDH.

The Light criteria are the most commonly used guidelines for the determination of whether an effusion is an exudate or transudate. Once the fluid is categorized, then potential etiologies can be explored. A protein ratio >0.5, an LDH ratio >0.6, and LDH >200 are all suggestive of an exudate. Some other ancillary tests can also be performed to help with determination, such as specific gravity (>1.01 implies exudate, also protein >3g/dL, cholesterol >45 mg/dL, and a bilirubin ratio >0.6).

QCCP2, **Pleural fluid,** p 88

244.   D.   THE ABSENCE OF BACTERIA.

An empyema is usually the result of a secondarily-infected parapneumonic effusion. Neutrophils can be present in a parapneumonic effusion, but not to the levels seen in an empyema. The pH of an empyema tends to be acidic. The most important differentiation factor is the presence or absence of bacteria.

QCCP2, **Parapneumonic effusion,** p 88

245.   C.   LDH.

Typically, the pH and glucose are decreased, while the LDH and rheumatoid factor levels are elevated.

QCCP2, **Collagen vascular diseases,** p 89

246.   D.   DPL FLUID IN FOLEY CATHETER.

More than 15mL of blood, 100,000 red blood cells/mL, 500 white blood cells/mL are considered positive findings. Finding lavage fluid in the places other than the peritoneum, such as in the bladder or pleural space, is also considered a positive finding. Finally, if any bacteria is present on gram stain, that is considered a positive finding.

QCCP2, **Peritoneal fluid microscopy,** p 89

1: Clinical Chemistry Answers

247.   B.   **MONOSODIUM URATE.**

Monosodium urate is the most strongly birefringent crystal seen in synovial fluids. Urate crystals are needle-shaped with negative birefringence and rapid extinction (goes away quickly with a small change in the angle of the compensator) under polarization. Negatively birefringent crystals are yellow when parallel to the long axis of the compensator and blue when perpendicular. Positive birefringence is the opposite. Urate crystals are needle-shaped and a needle looks like a minus sign (negative birefringence). Also, ye__ll__ow and para__ll__el have double "l's." See the text for an additional helpful mnemonic.

QCCP2, **Synovial fluid microscopy,** p 90

Chapter 2

Blood Banking and Transfusion

1. What is the most common minimum age for blood donation?
    A. 14 years old
    B. 16 years old
    C. 18 years old
    D. 21 years old
    E. 24 years old

2. What is the minimum acceptable hemoglobin (g/dL)/hematocrit (%) for allogeneic blood donation?
    A. 9/27
    B. 10/30
    C. 12.5/38
    D. 15/45
    E. 17/50

3. Which of the following statements regarding whole blood collections of volumes less than 300 mL is true?
    A. the sample can only be used for non-transfusion (ie, research) purposes
    B. the remaining 150 mL of volume must be made up with saline
    C. the sample should be set aside for pediatric use only
    D. the sample can only be used for component therapy
    E. the amount of anticoagulant must be proportionally decreased

4. Which of the following best separates a vasovagal reaction from a hypovolemic reaction?
    A. respiration rate
    B. skin temperature
    C. peripheral capillary refill rate
    D. pulse
    E. SaO_2

5. For which of the following conditions is the deferral for whole blood donation the longest?
    A. viral hepatitis after 11th birthday
    B. positive syphilis screening test
    C. recent blood donation
    D. being incarcerated for >72 hours
    E. paying for sex

6. The following patients arrive at your blood drive. Which one cannot donate today?
    A. a 72-year-old man who had West Nile Virus encephalitis 2 months ago
    B. a 39-year-old woman who took Soritane for acne as a teenager, but has not taken it since then
    C. a 42-year-old man who spent 2 days in jail last month after getting drunk, fighting, and getting a tattoo in Mexico
    D. a 21-year-old man who had the anthrax vaccine 6 months ago
    E. a 56-year-old man who had an accidental needle stick a year and a half ago

2: Blood Banking and Transfusion Questions

7. What should be the next step in typing donor blood that tests negative with anti-D?
    A. nothing, it's negative!
    B. test for other Rh antigens, such as C and E
    C. repeat test to confirm
    D. test for weak D
    E. only recipient blood needs to be retested in this scenario

8. What is the blood type (ABO and Rh) of a patient that tests 4+ with anti-A, 0 with anti-B, 3+ with anti-D on forward type, and 0 with A cells and 3+ with B cells on reverse testing?
    A. A positive
    B. B positive
    C. A negative
    D. B negative
    E. AB positive

9. All of the following are required infectious disease screening tests for donor blood, except:
    A. anti-HCV
    B. anti-HTLV-I
    C. HIV RNA
    D. serological testing for babesiosis
    E. serological testing for West Nile virus

10. Which of the following is the most common cause of fatal acute hemolytic transfusion reactions?
    A. manufacturing flaws
    B. clerical errors
    C. emergency release of unmatched blood
    D. failure to premedicate
    E. infusion mistakes

11. All of the following are required for the labeling of blood samples for recipients, except:
    A. 2 unique patient identifiers
    B. patient's stated blood type
    C. phlebotomist ID
    D. date of collection
    E. all of the above are required

12. What's the most common cause of alloantibodies that appear as a positive antibody screen?
    A. solid tumor
    B. atopy
    C. concomitant viral infection
    D. hematolymphoid malignancy
    E. previous transfusion or pregnancy

13. In an indirect antiglobulin test all of the following may be performed, except:
    A. addition of patient serum to the test blood cells
    B. addition of patient serum to patient blood cells
    C. incubation at 37°C for 10 minutes
    D. addition of antihuman globulin
    E. addition of high ionic strength buffer

2: Blood Banking and Transfusion Questions

14. Besides reviewing ABO and Rh types, what is the main purpose of reviewing previous transfusion records prior to initiation of transfusion?
    A. look for history of high-risk behavior
    B. look for previous allergic transfusion reactions
    C. look for previous febrile nonhemolytic transfusion reactions
    D. look for previously documented alloantibodies
    E. look for patterns of blood usage

15. All of the following are required prior to the release of all red blood cells, <u>except</u>:
    A. forward typing
    B. reverse typing
    C. antibody screen
    D. antibody panel
    E. cross match

16. Red blood cells of which of the following blood types are acceptable to give to patients with Bombay phenotype?
    A. A negative
    B. O negative
    C. O positive
    D. A positive
    E. none of the above

17. What is the most common ABO blood type in African-Americans?
    A. A
    B. B
    C. O
    D. AB
    E. there is no single dominant blood type

18. What is the most common Rh phenotype in African-Americans?
    A. R^1
    B. DCe
    C. R°
    D. dcE
    E. dCE

19. Which of the following statements concerning the reactions of the weak D phenotype is correct?
    A. negative with immediate spin with anti-D reagent
    B. negative after 37°C incubation with anti-D reagent
    C. positive at AHG phase with anti-D reagent
    D. A & B
    E. A, B, C

20. Which of the following genotypes or phenotypes accounts for the majority of cases of the weak D phenotype?
    A. R°/r'
    B. R^1/R°
    C. r"/r'
    D. r^y/r^y
    E. R^1/R^2

2: Blood Banking and Transfusion Questions

21. Which of the following antigens is affected most by the Rh_{null} phenotype?
    A. Jk^a
    B. Fy^a
    C. Lw
    D. M
    E. N

22. What percentage of D-negative recipients will develop anti-D antibodies after a single exposure to a unit of D-positive red cells?
    A. 1%
    B. 10%
    C. 50%
    D. 80%
    E. 100%

23. An antibody detected in a patient's serum turns out to anti-E. What additional antibody should be suspected?
    A. anti-e
    B. anti-D
    C. anti-C
    D. anti-c
    E. anti-G

24. All of the following antigens are enhanced by enzyme treatment, except:
    A. Rh antigens
    B. Kidd
    C. Duffy
    D. Lewis
    E. all of the above are enhanced by enzyme

25. Which of the following phenotypes is most common in African-Americans?
    A. Jk (a+b-)
    B. Jk (a+b+)
    C. Jk (a-b+)
    D. Jk (a-b-)
    E. it depends on ancestry

26. Which of the following features explains why different Jk+ cell lines may give different results in an antibody panel?
    A. anergy
    B. dosage
    C. antigen enhancement
    D. antigen destruction
    E. cross-reactivity

27. In which of the following patients is one most likely to encounter the i antigen?
    A. 36-year-old African-American woman
    B. 78-year-old Asian man
    C. 24-year-old Hispanic woman
    D. 2-month-old Caucasian boy
    E. 17-year-old African-American boy

2: Blood Banking and Transfusion Questions

28. Which of the following descriptions best fits the function of the Le gene?
    A. fucosyltransferase that adds fucose to type 1 oligosaccharides
    B. fucosyltransferase that adds fucose to type 2 oligosaccharides
    C. N-acetylgalactosamine transferase that adds N-acetylgalactosamine to type 1 oligosaccharides
    D. N-acetylgalactosamine transferase that adds N-acetylgalactosamine to type 2 oligosaccharides
    E. oligosaccharide branching enzyme that converts i antigen to I antigen

29. What is the most common Lewis phenotype?
    A. Le (a-b-)
    B. Le (a+b-)
    C. Le (a-b+)
    D. Le (a+b+)
    E. it depends on race of the individual

30. Which Duffy phenotype confers resistance to malaria?
    A. Fy (a+b+)
    B. Fy (a+b-)
    C. Fy (a-b+)
    D. Fy (a-b-)
    E. there is no Duffy phenotype that confers resistance to malaria

31. Which of the following MNS antibodies is clinically insignificant?
    A. anti-M
    B. anti-S
    C. anti-s
    D. anti-U
    E. all MNS antibodies are clinically significant

32. Which blood group antigen is associated with the McLeod phenotype?
    A. Kidd
    B. Duffy
    C. Kell
    D. MNS
    E. Lutheran

33. The P antigen is significant for a number of varied properties. Which of the following is not one of them?
    A. the cause of acquired B phenotype
    B. the target of antibodies in paroxysmal cold hemoglobinuria
    C. agglutinated by hydatid cyst fluid
    D. the receptor for parvovirus B19
    E. agglutinated by pigeon egg fluid

34. All of the following genes are encoded within the major histocompatibility complex, except:
    A. HFE
    B. TNF
    C. PKHD1
    D. complement proteins
    E. 21-hydroxylase

2: Blood Banking and Transfusion Questions

35. Class II HLA genes encode proteins found on all the following cell types, except:
    A. macrophages
    B. megakaryocytes
    C. activated T-cells
    D. B-cells
    E. all of the above express Class II HLA antigens

36. Which of the following reactions is considered positive in terms of an antibody panel?
    A. agglutination
    B. hemolysis
    C. coagulation
    D. A & B
    E. A, B, C

37. Which of the following is added to blood in a direct antiglobulin test?
    A. nothing (just incubate at 37°C)
    B. antihuman globulin
    C. patient serum
    D. patient RBCs
    E. antibodies of known specificity

38. Which of the following is considered "clinically significant"?
    A. an antibody that causes hemolytic disease of the newborn
    B. a warm-reacting IgG antibody
    C. a cold-reacting P antigen
    D. IgM anti-ABO
    E. all of the above

39. Which of the following criteria is most commonly used to establish the identity of a particular alloantibody in a routine antibody panel?
    A. positivity with 1 cell, negativity with 1 cell
    B. positivity with 5 cells, negativity with 1 cell
    C. positivity with 1 cell, negativity with 5 cells
    D. positivity with 1 cell, negativity with 3 cells
    E. positivity with 3 cells, negativity with 3 cells

40. All of the following techniques are useful in the evaluation of the nonroutine antibody panel, except:
    A. adsorption
    B. high ionic strength saline
    C. enzyme incubation
    D. neutralization
    E. all of the above are commonly used in evaluating nonroutine panels

41. Which of the following antibodies usually displays dosage?
    A. Duffy
    B. Kidd
    C. MNS
    D. C/c
    E. all of the above

2: Blood Banking and Transfusion Questions

42. All of the following are properties of high-titer low-avidity antibodies (HTLA), except:
    A. they are directed against high incidence antigens
    B. they exhibit irreversible binding to test cells
    C. they are usually weakly-reactive to all cells in panel
    D. they are still reactive when highly diluted
    E. all of the above are features of HTLA

43. Which of the following antigens is only made when bacterial neuraminidase activates it?
    A. Cad
    B. Tn
    C. Wr^a
    D. Kp^a
    E. Gy

44. Which of the following neutralizing substance and antigens are correctly matched?
    A. hydatid cyst fluid; H
    B. breast milk; I
    C. saliva; P_1
    D. pigeon eggs; Le^a
    E. guinea pig urine; Chido

45. Which of the following lectins and binding substrates are incorrectly matched?
    A. *Dolichos biflorus*, B
    B. *Ulex europaeus*, H
    C. *Vicea graminea*, N
    D. *Lotus tetragonolobus*, H
    E. *Bandeiraea simplicifolia*, B

46. All of the following antigens are enhanced by enzyme digestion, except:
    A. Lewis
    B. P
    C. Rh
    D. I/i
    E. Fy^a

47. Which of the following is among the most common cause of a positive crossmatch with a negative antibody screen?
    A. anti-C
    B. anti-ABO
    C. anti-Le^a
    D. anti-Kell
    E. antibodies to reagents

48. Which of the following conditions explains why an A-negative patient with colon cancer can forward type as AB, but have anti-B antibodies on reverse typing?
    A. acquired B phenotype
    B. anti-Lw antibody
    C. AZB phenotype
    D. high titer, low-avidity antibodies
    E. antibodies to reagents

2: Blood Banking and Transfusion Questions

49. Which of the following questions is the <u>most</u> important one to ask in a patient with a positive DAT?
    A. has the patient been recently transfused?
    B. has the patient has a recent bone marrow transplant?
    C. what medications is the patient taking?
    D. is the patient hemolyzing RBCs?
    E. is the result a false positive?

50. Which of the following grades of RBC agglutination during the AHG phase is most correlated with the chance that hemolysis will occur?
    A. m+
    B. 1+
    C. 3+
    D. 4+
    E. the risk of hemolysis is not correlated with the grade of agglutination

51. What are the most common autoantibodies?
    A. warm autoantibodies
    B. antibodies that cause warm autoimmune hemolytic anemia
    C. benign cold autoagglutinins
    D. cold antibodies that cause autoimmune hemolytic anemia
    E. antibodies that cause cold agglutinin syndrome

52. At what temperature does hemolysis occur with paroxysmal cold hemoglobinuria?
    A. <0°C
    B. 4°C
    C. 10°C
    D. 20°C
    E. 37°C

53. Which of the following techniques is suitable for helping to detect potential alloantibody in the presence of a cold autoantibody?
    A. perform all tests at 37°C
    B. use monospecific anti-IgG AHG reagent instead of polyspecific
    C. adsorption of cold autoantibody with autologous red cells
    D. A & B
    E. A, B, C

54. All of the following are potential mechanisms for a drug-induced positive DAT, <u>except</u>:
    A. immune complex
    B. nonimmune protein adsorption
    C. true autoimmune hemolytic anemia
    D. cold autoantibody
    E. drug-hapten mechanism

55. Which of the following antigens is most commonly associated with maternal immune thrombocytopenic purpura?
    A. red blood cell glycophorin A
    B. platelet GPIIb/IIIa
    C. platelet PLA1
    D. red blood cell CD59
    E. red blood cell GPIIb/IIIa

2: Blood Banking and Transfusion Questions

56. What is the approximate risk of a serious *in utero* hemorrhage in a fetus affected by neonatal alloimmune thrombocytopenic purpura (NATP)?
    A. 0%
    B. 1%
    C. 10%
    D. 50%
    E. >90%

57. All of the following antibody classes are capable of causing hemolytic disease of the newborn (HDN), <u>except</u>:
    A. IgG1
    B. IgG2
    C. IgG3
    D. IgG4
    E. all of the above can cause HDN

58. What is the most common antigen involved in HDN?
    A. Rh
    B. ABO
    C. Kell
    D. c
    E. Duffy

59. What is the prime titer decision point for the presence of a clinically-significant anti-D antibody in pregnancy?
    A. 1:1000
    B. 1:100
    C. 1:50
    D. 1:16
    E. 1:4

60. What is the range of risk reduction for the development of anti-D with the use of prophylactic RhIg?
    A. 100% decreased to 50%
    B. 100% decreased to 10%
    C. 80% decreased to 10%
    D. 8% decreased to 0.1%
    E. 1% decreased to 0.5%

61. How much whole blood is one complete dose (300 micrograms) of RhIg capable of protecting against the development of anti-D antibody?
    A. 300 mL
    B. 100 mL
    C. 30 mL
    D. 10 mL
    E. 1 mL

62. All of the following are potential risks in chronic transfusion of sickle cell disease patients, <u>except</u>:
    A. iron accumulation
    B. infectious disease
    C. autoantibody development
    D. volume overload
    E. stroke

2: Blood Banking and Transfusion Questions

63. All of the following are associated with massive transfusion, <u>except</u>:
    A. anti-D development
    B. decreased oxygen-carrying capacity
    C. dilutional coagulopathy
    D. raised body temperature
    E. raised serum potassium

64. What percentage of viable RBCs present in the circulation 24 hours after transfusion is considered in the determination of allowable storage time?
    A. 100%
    B. 90%
    C. 75%
    D. 50%
    E. 25%

65. Which of the following blood products has the shortest allowable storage time?
    A. whole blood
    B. fresh frozen plasma
    C. apheresis platelets
    D. cryoprecipitate
    E. granulocyte concentrate

66. Which of the following additive solutions extends the shelf life of blood the most?
    A. citrate
    B. heparin
    C. CPD
    D. AS-1
    E. CPDA-1

67. Which of the following clotting factors is/are most labile in <u>stored</u> blood?
    A. Factor V
    B. Factor VIII
    C. Factor VII
    D. A & B
    E. A, B, C

68. The final hematocrit of packed red cells must be no more than:
    A. 50%
    B. 75%
    C. 80%
    D. 90%
    E. 95%

69. In order to qualify as "leukocyte-reduced" for the purpose of avoiding CMV transmission, what must the final white blood cell count not exceed?
    A. $<5 \times 10^6$
    B. $<5 \times 10^7$
    C. $<5 \times 10^8$
    D. $<5 \times 10^9$
    E. $<5 \times 10^{10}$

2: Blood Banking and Transfusion Questions

70. What is the shelf life of washed red blood cells?
    A. 4 hours
    B. 24 hours
    C. 48 hours
    D. 1 week
    E. 28 days

71. What is the approximate amount of iron in a single red blood cell unit?
    A. 200 mg
    B. 100 mg
    C. 200 mg
    D. 100 mg
    E. 10 mg

72. Which of the following fluids may be transfused simultaneously through an infusion line with red blood cells?
    A. antibiotics
    B. 0.45% (1/2 normal) saline
    C. 0.9% (isotonic) saline
    D. lactated Ringer's solution
    E. heparin

73. What is the minimum amount of platelets required in an apheresis platelet unit?
    A. 3×10^{11}
    B. 3×10^{10}
    C. 1×10^{11}
    D. 1×10^{10}
    E. 1×10^{8}

74. What is the appropriate storage temperature for granulocyte concentrates?
    A. 37°C
    B. 20-24°C
    C. 1-6°C
    D. -20°C
    E. -80°C

75. After thawing, what is the time frame within which fresh frozen plasma must be used?
    A. 8 hours
    B. 24 hours
    C. 2 days
    D. 7 days
    E. 30 days

76. All of the following are preferred uses of fresh frozen plasma, except:
    A. multiple factor deficiencies in disseminated intravascular coagulation
    B. reversal of warfarin therapy
    C. massive transfusion
    D. replacement solution in plasmapheresis for thrombotic thrombocytopenic purpura
    E. hemophilia A

2: Blood Banking and Transfusion Questions

77. Cryoprecipitated plasma contains appreciable amounts of all of the following factors, <u>except</u>:
    A. Factor VIII
    B. von Willebrand factor
    C. Factor XIII
    D. Factor V
    E. fibrinogen

78. What is the minimum dose of irradiation that must be delivered to <u>any</u> portion of a product for it to be considered adequately irradiated?
    A. 5 Gy
    B. 25 Gy
    C. 100 Gy
    D. 50 Gy
    E. 15 Gy

79. Which of the following indications is an appropriate usage of irradiated products?
    A. cellular products to immunocompromised hosts
    B. granulocyte concentrates for neutropenic sepsis
    C. prevention of alloimmunization in platelets
    D. red blood cells to prevent CMV transmission
    E. red blood cells to prevent recurrent febrile nonhemolytic transfusion reactions

80. All of the following products would be useful in the treatment of symptomatic anemia in a patient that you wish to remain CMV negative, <u>except</u>:
    A. red blood cells, CMV(-) by serology
    B. frozen, thawed, and deglycerolized red blood cells
    C. washed red blood cells
    D. red blood cells leukoreduced to $<5 \times 10^8$ white blood cells
    E. all of the above are acceptable

81. Which is the first step in the workup of a suspected transfusion reaction?
    A. call the blood bank
    B. stop the transfusion
    C. infuse a bolus of normal saline
    D. paperwork and bag check
    E. check urine for hemoglobin

82. Which of the following is the most common cause of hemolytic transfusion reactions?
    A. ABO incompatibility
    B. Rh incompatibility
    C. paperwork errors
    D. anti-Kidd alloantibodies
    E. mechanical hemolysis due to faulty packaging

83. Which of the following is the most common type of transfusion reaction?
    A. febrile nonhemolytic transfusion reaction
    B. acute hemolytic transfusion reaction
    C. delayed hemolytic transfusion reaction
    D. transfusion-associated graft v. host disease
    E. transfusion-related acute lung injury

2: Blood Banking and Transfusion Questions

84.　What is the most common antibody associated with acute hemolytic transfusion reactions?
　　A.　anti-D
　　B.　anti-Kidd
　　C.　anti-A/anti-B
　　D.　anti-Kell
　　E.　anti-Duffy

85.　All of the following are illness-causing bacteria most commonly associated with red blood cell transfusions, <u>except</u>:
　　A.　*Yersinia enterocolitica*
　　B.　*Serratia liquifaciens*
　　C.　*Citrobacter* spp.
　　D.　*Staphylococcus aureus*
　　E.　*Pseudomonas* spp.

86.　Why are most cases of transfusion-associated graft v. host disease seen in transfusions between related individuals?
　　A.　common disease exposures
　　B.　HLA similarity, not identity
　　C.　shared non-genetic environmental exposures
　　D.　less compatibility
　　E.　less stringent donor requirements

87.　All of the following are associated with transfusion-related acute lung injury, <u>except</u>:
　　A.　patients on induction chemotherapy for lymphoma
　　B.　bypass patients
　　C.　blood stored for long periods of time
　　D.　multiparous female donors
　　E.　patients post-op from lung surgery

88.　What feature of allergic transfusion reactions makes them <u>unique</u>?
　　A.　the patient does not have to be treated; continue transfusion
　　B.　patient serum does not exhibit a positive DAT
　　C.　the reaction does not need to be reported
　　D.　the transfusion can be restarted after treating the patient
　　E.　they cause hemolysis

89.　Which of the following factors involved with the degree of platelet refractoriness is the most important?
　　A.　gender
　　B.　spleen status (present or absent)
　　C.　age
　　D.　height and weight
　　E.　active bleeding

90.　Which of the following viruses is a patient at the <u>highest</u> risk of acquiring through a blood transfusion?
　　A.　hepatitis B virus
　　B.　hepatitis C virus
　　C.　hepatitis A virus
　　D.　human immunodeficiency virus
　　E.　West Nile virus

2: Blood Banking and Transfusion Questions

91. What is the purpose of rapid plasmin reagent testing on donated whole blood?
     A.   detection of *N. gonorrheae* infection
     B.   detection of syphilis infection
     C.   marker of Chagas disease
     D.   detection of past CMV infection
     E.   surrogate marker of high-risk behavior

92. Which of the following red blood cell units would be the most difficult to find in donated blood?
     A.   type B
     B.   c (-)
     C.   Jk (a-b-)
     D.   E (-)
     E.   K (-)

2: Blood Banking and Transfusion Answers

1.   B.   **16 YEARS OLD.**

     The minimum age for whole blood donation is 16 or 17 years old, depending on the state.
     QCCP2, **History and physical exam,** p 104

2.   C.   **12.5/38.**

     Most allogeneic donors must have a minimum hemoglobin concentration of 12.5 g/dL and/or a minimum
     hematocrit of 38%. The regulations for donation of autologous blood are less stringent with a minimum
     hemoglobin of 11 g/dL and a hematocrit of 33%
     QCCP2, **Physical,** p 104

3.   E.   **AMOUNT OF ANTICOAGULANT MUST BE PROPORTIONALLY DECREASED.**

     While many of the choices seem plausible, only choice E is correct. The volume of the average whole blood unit
     should be 450 +/- 50 mL. Anything less than that but more than 300 mL should be labeled as low-volume and
     <u>cannot</u> be used for component therapy. Volume less than 300 mL requires that the amount of anticoagulant be
     proportionally decreased.
     QCCP2, **Volume drawn,** p 104

4.   D.   **PULSE.**

     The manifestations of both of the reactions are overlapping - hypotension, nausea, and syncope. However, a
     vasovagal reaction characteristically manifests with bradycardia while hypovolemia usually has tachycardia. The
     treatment differs primarily in the fact that the hypovolemic patients need volume replacement, while vasovagal
     reactions are treated with supportive therapy.
     QCCP2, **Donor adverse reactions,** p 104

5.   A.   **VIRAL HEPATITIS AFTER 11TH BIRTHDAY.**

     While all the other choices do have stipulated deferral lengths, any viral hepatitis after the 11th birthday is the
     only permanent deferral choice. A positive syphilis screening test is a 12-month post-treatment deferral. The
     interval between whole blood donations should be at least one red blood cell life (8 weeks, 56 days). Being
     incarcerated for more than 72 hours and paying for sex have a 1-year deferral, presumably for the same reasons.
     QCCP2, **Donor deferrals, T2.1,** p 105

6.   C.   **A 42-YEAR-OLD MAN WHO SPENT 2 DAYS IN JAIL LAST MONTH AFTER GETTING DRUNK, FIGHTING,
     AND GETTING A TATTOO IN MEXICO.**

     There is a "must know" list of deferrals that can be divided into three broad categories: permanent or indefinite
     deferral, 12-month deferral, and miscellaneous deferrals. In addition, a donor center may adopt more strict
     criteria than those required. For the most part, permanent deferrals are for someone with a history of viral
     hepatitis after the 11th birthday or other indications of current viral hepatitis (positive anti-HBc, etc), anyone
     with Creutzfeldt-Jakob risk (travel to endemic area, family relative with CJD, bovine insulin in the UK, or a dura
     mater graft) or very high risk of HIV (money for sex or IV drug use).
     QCCP2, **T2.1,** p 105

2: Blood Banking and Transfusion Answers

7.   D.   **TEST FOR WEAK D.**

Weak D refers to D+ donors who do not react at immediate spin or even after incubation at 37°C. Only after addition of AHG is there a reaction. There are several causes of weak D- either due to low amounts of the D antigen or poorly-reactive antigen variants. It is important to label weak D as D (+) because previously sensitized D (-) patients can experience a potential hemolytic transfusion reaction when given weak D cells.
QCCP2, **Laboratory testing of donor blood,** p 106; **and weak D phenotype,** p 111

8.   A.   **A POSITIVE.**

Forward typing tests the patient's red cells for the presence of an antigen (A and Rh in this case). Reverse typing confirms it by testing the patient's serum for the presence of antibodies. In a type A patient, there is an expected naturally-occurring anti-B antibody.
QCCP2, **ABO and Rh,** p 106

9.   D.   **SEROLOGICAL TESTING FOR BABESIOSIS.**

A panel of serological and nucleic acid tests is required to screen donor blood. Among the serological are HBsAg, anti-HBc, anti-HCV, anti-HTLV-I, anti-HTLV-II, anti-HIV1 and 2, RPR, and West Nile virus. Nucleic acid testing for HCV and HIV is also performed. There is no good serological test for babesiosis at this time and screening history questions are used.
QCCP2, **ID screening,** p 106

10.   B.   **CLERICAL ERRORS.**

Of the choices presented, clerical errors account for the largest number of fatal transfusion reactions. For that reason, there must be very strict rules for the labeling of specimens and specimen identification. In 2004, however, the FDA reported that the most common cause of fatal hemolytic transfusion reactions was TRALI (transfusion-related acute lung injury), perhaps due to better controls of clerical issues and increased awareness of TRALI.
QCCP2, **Pretransfusion laboratory testing,** p 106

11.   B.   **PATIENT'S STATED BLOOD TYPE.**

The most common patient identifiers are the patient's name and social security number or hospital medical record number. There must also be a way to identify who the phlebotomist is and when the specimen was collected. Samples that are not clearly labeled with this information should not be accepted by the blood bank. Many blood banks will take the sample from the submitter, so that it cannot be relabeled and resubmitted.
QCCP2, **Proper paperwork and properly identified blood samples,** p 106

12.   E.   **PREVIOUS TRANSFUSION OR PREGNANCY.**

Patients that may have been exposed to foreign blood, such as those previously transfused and pregnant, are the most likely to develop alloantibodies. For this reason, patients with a previous transfusion or pregnancy history must have a sample drawn within three days of testing.
QCCP2, **Antibody screen,** p 107

2: Blood Banking and Transfusion Answers

13.   E.   **ADDITION OF HIGH IONIC STRENGTH BUFFER.**

The indirect antiglobulin test (IAT) is used for the identification of antibodies in the patient's serum. Typically, an antibody screen utilizes patient serum incubated at 37°C. For control purposes, an additional tube utilizing patient blood cells instead of test cells is included.
QCCP2, **Antibody screen,** p 107

14.   D.   **LOOK FOR PREVIOUSLY DOCUMENTED ALLOANTIBODIES.**

While it could be important to review the record for a past history of transfusion reactions, the <u>most</u> important reason to review the previous records is to identify an alloantibody. Several antibodies are known for their evanescent nature, virtually disappearing but then reappearing with an antigen-positive transfusion and causing a hemolytic transfusion reaction.
QCCP2, **Comparison with prior transfusion records,** p 108

15.   D.   **ANTIBODY PANEL.**

Only in case of a positive antibody screen is a panel indicated. All the other choices are required for each and every transfusion. In addition, a visual inspection of the unit and a review of the transfusion history should be performed.
QCCP2, **Pretransfusion Laboratory Testing,** p 106-108

16.   E.   **NONE OF THE ABOVE.**

Because patients with the Bombay phenotype do not make H antigen, they are unable to make ABO antigen. As a result, they have the potential to make an anti-H antibody that could react with any ABO blood type other than Bombay. Also, as H antigen is converted to A or B antigen, less H antigen is present. As a result, type O blood has the most H antigen and would therefore be the <u>worst</u> choice for a Bombay phenotype patient.
QCCP2, **ABO,** p 109

17.   D.   **O.**

In all Americans, white and black, O type blood is the most common, followed by A, B, and AB, respectively.
QCCP2, **T2.4,** p 110

2: Blood Banking and Transfusion Answers

18.   C.   **R°.**

The Weiner classification system (R, r, etc) and the Fisher-Race system (DCE) are both often used. When discussing blood cell phenotypes, the Weiner system is often used, while the Fisher-Race classification is most commonly used for discussing patient phenotypes. It is very easy to convert from one system to the other if one remembers a few principles:

    1.   Organize the Fisher-Race in order of D, C, E. I know that it's not alphabetical, but it makes it easier later.

    2.   In Fisher-Race, capital "D" means the presence of the D antigen, while "d" means the absence of D. Sometimes "d" is omitted. For C and E, the capital and lower case representations are of different alleles.

    3.   In the Weiner system, a capital "R" implies the presence of D (Rh positive), while a lower case "r" implies the absence of D (Rh negative).

    4.   The numbers in the Weiner system after the "R" or "r" represent the position of capitalized antigen after the "D" - for example - R^2 is DcE and R^1 is DCe. Don't be fooled - after "r," hash marks (' or ") are used instead of numbers.

    5.   A naught after the "R" or "r" means that neither of the following antigens are capitalized, eg, R° is Dce.

    6.   Finally, a letter after "R" or "r" means that both of the following antigens are capitalized, eg, r^y is dCE.

Now to answer the question, the R° (quick, what's the Fisher-Race nomenclature?) phenotype is the most common in African-Americans, while R^1 is the most common in whites.
QCCP2, **T2.5,** p 110

19.   E.   **A, B, C.**

The weak D phenotype is of particular concern with donor blood. The possibility exists that the blood could be labeled as Rh negative and transfused to Rh-negative patients who may have been previously sensitized to D antigen. In that case, the transfusion may trigger a hemolytic transfusion reaction. For that reason, all donor blood that tests on forward typing as negative (choice A) must undergo the next two tests to either prove or disprove the presence of weak D.
QCCP2, **Weak D phenotype,** p 111

20.   A.   **R°/ʀ,**

or Dce/Ce, is a common phenotype in the African-American population and results in quantitatively decreased D expression due to the *trans* effect of the C antigen on the other chromosome, the so-called Cepelli effect. The other means of expressing the weak D phenotype is partial D, where certain epitopes of the D antigen are absent. The most significant issue for partial D is in a pregnant woman who could produce anti-D antibodies if exposed to a D+ fetus.
QCCP2, **Weak D phenotype,** p 111

2: Blood Banking and Transfusion Answers

21.　C.　**Lw.**

Certain epitopes are most affected by the Rh$_{null}$ phenotype, where individuals lack the Rh antigens. These include Fy^5, Lw, S, s, and U. Rh$_{null}$ individuals have structural red blood cell abnormalities that result in stomatocytosis and mild chronic anemia.
QCCP2, **Rh$_{null}$,** p 111

22.　D.　**80%.**

Estimates range from 75% to 80% of D-negative individuals exposed to a unit of D positive red cells that subsequently develop anti-D. The antibodies are clinically significant, warm-reactive, non-natural IgG.
QCCP2, **Rh antibodies,** p 111

23.　D.　**ANTI-C.**

The setup is an individual with R^{1}R^1 phenotype (DCe/DCe) being transfused with R^2 (DcE) blood. There is a high likelihood that the patient will develop a detectable anti-E. However, in addition to the anti-E, patients often develop a very weak anti-c - a frequent cause of delayed hemolytic transfusion reactions. For this reason, patients with an anti-E should be given E-negative, c-negative red blood cells.
QCCP2, **Rh antibodies,** p 111

24.　C.　**DUFFY.**

Treatment of red blood cells with enzymes such as papain or ficin leads to predictable changes in the reactivity of the red cells to specific antibodies. Some antigens are enhanced, some destroyed, some unchanged. It's useful to remember them, as they are easily testable. Those that are enhanced include Lewis, I/i, ABO, Rh, P, and Kidd. I use the mnemonic "Lewis Is A Rhotten Peeing Kidd". Among the ones that are destroyed are Duffy, Lutheran, MNS, and Chido. I use the mnemonic "Daffy MeNS Lutheran Choir" and I imagine the church crumbling down on top of them to signify that they are destroyed.
QCCP2, **Assorted Blood Bank Take Home Points,** p 141-142

25.　A.　**JK (A+B-).**

For the most part, the most common phenotype among both whites and blacks is Jk (a+). The major difference phenotypically comes with Jk^b, which is more often positive in whites and negative in blacks.
QCCP2, **T2.6, Kidd phenotypes,** p 112

26.　B.　**DOSAGE.**

Antibodies against Kidd exhibit dosage - that is, homozygotes for Kidd antigens express more antigen than heterozygotes. In antibody panels, there may be red blood cells that are heterozygous or homozygous for the Kidd antigens. Since Kidd antibodies are usually weak, it would not be unusual to get a positive reaction from a homozygous panel red blood cell, but negative from a heterozygote. Also remember that Kidd can be enhanced by enzyme treatment.
QCCP2, **Kidd antibodies,** p 112

ASCP Quick Compendium Companion for Clinical Pathology

2: Blood Banking and Transfusion Answers

27. D. **2-month-old Caucasian boy.**

More important than race or gender for the levels of i antigen is age. The little i antigen is made up of the unbranched type 1 and type 2 precursor oligosaccharide molecules. Branching increases with age, leading to the conversion of i antigen to I antigen.
QCCP2, **Lewis blood group,** p 112

28. A. **fucosyltransferase that adds fucose to type 1 oligosaccharides.**

Similar to the H (whose function is described in choice B), the Le gene product catalyzes the addition of fucosyl groups to the secretory type 1 oligosaccharides to make Le^a antigen. This antigen is then passively absorbed onto the surface of red blood cells (remember that type 1 precursors are secreted).
QCCP2, **Lewis blood group,** p 112

29. C. **Le (a-b+).**

Irrespective of race, the most common phenotype is a-b+. Le^b is made from Le^a precursor by the action of the Secretor gene product. This means that the levels of each are inversely proportional. If an individual has just the Le gene, he or she will be Le (a+b-); if the individual expresses both Le and Se, he or she will be Le (a-b+). Lacking both Le and Se leads to the phenotype Le (a-b-). Note that the phenotype Le (a+b+) cannot exist except transiently.
QCCP2, **Lewis blood group, T2.7,** p 113

30. D. **Fy (a-b-).**

The absence of Duffy a and b confers resistance to *P vivax* malaria. The Fy (a-b-) phenotype is found in more than 2/3 of people of African descent, while it is rare otherwise.
QCCP2, **Duffy,** p 114

31. A. **anti-M.**

Of all the MNS antibodies, only anti-M and anti-N are naturally occurring and clinically insignificant IgM antibodies. Anti-S, anti-s, and anti-U are all acquired IgG antibodies and can pose a threat of hemolytic transfusion reactions.
QCCP2, **MNS,** p 114

32. C. **Kell.**

McLeod phenotype is a chronic hemolytic anemia due to RBC structural abnormalities. The Kx gene on the X chromosome encodes a support protein that stabilizes Kell expression. Without Kx protein, the expression of Kell proteins is greatly diminished. In addition to decreased Kell expression and reduced RBC survival, there is an association with X-linked chronic granulomatous disease.
QCCP2, **Kell blood group,** p 114

33. A. **the cause of acquired B phenotype.**

There are three major things to remember about P antigens. They are agglutinated by pigeon egg and hydatid cyst fluids. They are receptors for the parvovirus B19. Finally, they are the target of antibodies that cause paroxysmal cold hemoglobinuria (which should not be confused with paroxysmal nocturnal hemoglobinuria).
QCCP2, **P blood group,** p 115

2: Blood Banking and Transfusion Answers

34.   C.   **PKHD1.**

    While the gene encoding PKHD1 is located on chromosome 6, it is not located within the major histocompatibility complex like the the genes in the rest of the choices are.
    QCCP2, **HLA,** p 115

35.   B.   MEGAKARYOCYTES.

    While Class I HLA is expressed on virtually all nucleated cells, Class II expression is much more restricted. This is fitting as MHC Class I functions as a "general alarm" and presentation antigen which can be recognized by potential cytotoxic CD8+ T cells. MHC Class II, however, facilitates humoral and cell-mediated immunity by recruiting helper CD4+ T cells to "professional" antigen-presenting cells.
    QCCP2, **HLA,** p 115

36.   D.   **A & B.**

    Either hemolysis or agglutination is needed in order to call a reaction positive. Hemolysis is detected by a pink-colored supernatant, while agglutination is graded on a scale from m+ (microscopic) to 4+.
    QCCP2, **Types of reactions,** p 116

37.   B.   ANTIHUMAN GLOBULIN.

    The easiest way to remember the difference (and function) between a direct antiglobulin test (DAT) and an indirect antiglobulin test (IAT) is that a DAT "directly" tests for the presence of antibodies bound to RBCs by adding antiglobulin. The IAT requires the extra step of adding specific antibodies (serum or purified) prior to the addition of antiglobulin.
    QCCP2, **Phases of testing,** p 118

38.   B.   A WARM-REACTING IgG ANTIBODY.

    For the most part, warm-reacting IgG antibodies are clinically significant, while IgM cold-reacting antibodies are usually insignificant. Some notable exceptions include the IgM anti-ABO and the cold-reacting IgG against the P antigen seen in paroxysmal cold hemoglobinuria.
    QCCP2, **Clinical significance of detected antibodies,** p 118

39.   E.   POSITIVITY WITH 3 CELLS, NEGATIVITY WITH 3 CELLS.

    In most instances, a confirmation of the identity of an antibody requires positivity in at least 3 cells with the antigen and negativity with at least 3 cell lines without the antigen. This of course excludes autoantibodies.
    QCCP2, **Routine panel,** p 118

40.   B.   HIGH IONIC STRENGTH SALINE.

    Nonroutine panels may be due to numerous causes - multiple antibodies, antibodies displaying dosage, high-titer low-avidity (HTLA) antibodies, or antibodies against reagents in the assay. Various techniques have been successfully used to aid with identification - adsorption can be used to selectively remove a confounding antibody, enzymes can be used to enhance or destroy certain antigens, and neutralization can also be used to remove certain antibodies.
    QCCP2, **The nonroutine panel,** p 118

2: Blood Banking and Transfusion Answers

41.   E.   **ALL OF THE ABOVE.**

Certain antibodies very predictably display dosage. The panel can help with the identification of these antibodies. Typically, they will exhibit a stronger reaction to panel cells that are homozygous for the antigen than against cells that are heterozygous. For example, a Fya antibody will react more strongly against an Fy (a+b-) panel cell than against an Fy (a+b+) cell.
QCCP2, **Nonroutine panel,** p 118-119

42.   B.   **THEY EXHIBIT IRREVERSIBLE BINDING TO TEST CELLS.**

HTLA antibodies are usually found as weakly reacting to all the panel cells after AHG is added. This is due to the fact that the antigen is so common that it is present in all panel cells. In addition, they are usually high-titer so that whenever diluted, they are still reactive. For the most part, their only significance is that they can mask a clinically significant antibody.
QCCP2, **Antibodies to high incidence antigens, or HTLA,** p 119

43.   B.   **TN.**

Polyagglutination of adult cells can occur when the T (or Tn or Tk) antigens are present. These antigens are revealed by the action of bacterial neuraminidase on the red cells and are positive for agglutination only in the adult, not in cord serum.
QCCP2, **Polyagglutination,** p 119

44.   B.   **BREAST MILK; I.**

There are a number of odd substances that one can only believe serendipitously found their way into red cell testing. Both hydatid cyst fluid and pigeon egg fluid can neutralize the P antigen. Breast milk neutralizes the I antigen, saliva neutralizes H and Le^a, guinea pig urine neutralizes Sda, and plasma neutralizes Chido and Rodgers.
QCCP2, **T2.9 Neutralizing substances and lectins,** p 120

45.   A.   *DOLICHOS BIFLORUS,* **B.**

I hope that you weren't tricked by this question by not reading it carefully. Read it carefully! The most commonly used lectins (and the ones that you should know) are *Ulex europeaus* which agglutinates O RBCs and are used to detect secretor patients. *Dolichos biflorus,* which binds A1, effectively helps to separate A1 from A2 red blood cells.
QCCP2, **T2.9 Neutralization substances and lectins,** p 120

46.   E.   *FY^A.*

"Lewis is a Rhotten Peeing Kidd" helps me remember the antigens that are enhanced by enzyme treatment.
QCCP2, **Other special techniques,** p 120

47.   B.   **ANTI-ABO.**

Alloantibodies, such as anti-c, anti-Le^a, and anti-Kell, are usually identified on an antibody screen as a cause of a positive crossmatch. The same goes for anti-reagent antibodies. Anti-ABO is not tested on a routine antibody screen, nor can certain low-incidence antigens. As a result, they both are commonly undetected on an antibody screen, despite a positive crossmatch.
QCCP2, **The positive crossmatch,** p 120

2: Blood Banking and Transfusion Answers

48. A. **ACQUIRED B PHENOTYPE.**

The acquired B phenotype occurs when bacterial deacetylases remove the acetyl group from the A1 antigen, making it resemble somewhat the B antigen. As a result, patients will forward type as having both A and B antigens, but retain their anti-B antibodies. Any condition that could lead to bacteremia can cause acquired B phenotype.
QCCP2, **Unusual findings in pre-transfusion testing,** p 121

49. D. **IS THE PATIENT HEMOLYZING RBCs?**

The very first question that should <u>always</u> be asked when a positive DAT shows up (or in a suspected transfusion reaction) is whether or not the patient's red blood cells are hemolyzing. The other questions presented, though important, are clearly not as important as ruling out hemolysis.
QCCP2, **Autoantibodies,** p 122

50. D. **4+.**

Most people's first instinct is to state that there is no correlation between the grade of agglutination and the risk of hemolysis. However, it has been shown that the stronger the agglutination, the greater the risk for hemolysis. In addition, detection of strong C3 reaction is correlated with an increased risk of hemolysis.
QCCP2, **Warm-reacting antibodies,** p 122

51. C. **BENIGN COLD AUTOAGGLUTININS.**

Benign cold agglutinins, most commonly anti-I, are the most frequent source of autoantibodies. There are some cold-reacting antibodies seen with paroxysmal cold hemoglobinuria that are clinically significant, but for the most part, cold-reacting antibodies are not clinically significant.
QCCP2, **Cold-reacting autoantibodies,** p 123

52. E. **37°C.**

The Donath-Landsteiner antibody, first described in syphilis, but now associated with pediatric viral infections, is a unique biphasic antibody that preferentially binds at cold temperatures (such as in the extremities) but then hemolyzes at body temperature (such as when blood from the periphery returns centrally).
QCCP2, **Paroxysmal cold hemoglobinuria,** p 122-123

53. E. **A, B, C.**

A cold autoantibody should be worked up. There is a possibility of a high titer antibody that can react over a wide temperature range and be pathologic. All of the above-named tests are potential means of alleviating a confounding cold autoantibody.
QCCP2, **Blood banking considerations with a cold autoantibody,** p 124

54. D. **COLD AUTOANTIBODY.**

A number of drugs are associated with each mechanism and it's helpful to remember 1 or 2 for each mechanism. The prototypical drug for immune complex-mediated reactions is quinidine. Cephalosporins are known for causing a positive DAT through the immune complex mechanism. Nonimmune protein adsorption is associated with cephalothin. True autoimmune hemolytic anemia is associated with procainamide and aldomet, while hapten-associated positive DAT is associated with penicillin.
QCCP2, **Drug-induced positive DAT,** p 124

2: Blood Banking and Transfusion Answers

55. C. **PLATELET PLA1.**

Both maternal ITP and neonatal alloimmune thrombocytopenic purpura (NATP) are associated with antibodies directed against the platelet antigen, PLA1. Unlike hemolytic disease of the newborn, neonatal alloimmune thrombocytopenic purpura sensitization and hemolysis can occur in the first pregnancy.
QCCP2, **Maternal ITP and NATP,** p 125

56. D. **50%.**

The risk of hemorrhage is extremely high, especially intracranial hemorrhage. The treatment of NATP is washed maternal platelets because the maternal platelets are presumably PLA1 negative.
QCCP2, **NATP,** p 125

57. B. **IgG2.**

In addition to dimeric IgA and pentameric IgM, IgG2 is unable to cause hemolytic disease of the newborn. Like IgA and IgM, IgG2 is unable to cross the placental membrane and is therefore unable to initiate hemolysis.
QCCP2, **Hemolytic disease of the newborn,** p 125

58. B. **ABO.**

Great success has been made with anti-D prophylaxis for Rh-negative women. So much so that ABO incompatibility, especially in A or B children born to O mothers, is the predominant cause of hemolytic disease of the newborn. Luckily, the hemolysis is very mild. Severe HDN is most often due to anti-Kell, followed by anti-c.
QCCP2, **Hemolytic disease of the newborn,** p 126

59. D. **1:16.**

A titer of less than 1:16 is associated with a very low risk of hemolysis. Titers greater than 1:16 become a cause for monitoring fetal hemolysis with either Liley curves and delta OD450 of amniotic fluid or transcranial Doppler ultrasound blood velocity flow.
QCCP2, **Rh hemolytic disease of the newborn,** p 126

60. D. **8% TO 0.1%.**

A single full dose of RhIg - 300 micrograms - delivered at 28 weeks gestation to a Rh-negative mother is capable of decreasing the risk of developing anti-D from 8% to 0.1%.
QCCP2, **Rh hemolytic disease of the newborn,** p 126

61. C. **30 ML.**

1 vial of RhIg can routinely protect against 30 mL of whole blood, 15 mL of red blood cells, or 5 apheresis platelet units. For this reason, when calculating the dose of RhIg, one first calculates the amount of fetal blood in circulation (mother blood volume times percentage fetal blood), then divides that amount by 30 to get the number of vials needed to protect against IgG anti-D development.
QCCP2, **Rh hemolytic disease of the newborn,** p 127

2: Blood Banking and Transfusion Answers

62. **E. STROKE.**

The risk of stroke in sickle cell disease is not due to the chronic transfusions per se, but rather due to the disease itself. Many of the potential risks have been minimized with the use of chelation and cytapheresis, but some risk remains.

QCCP2, **Transfusion in sickle cell disease,** p 127-128

63. **D. RAISED BODY TEMPERATURE.**

The exposure of an individual to massive amounts of blood, whether cross-matched or not, is associated with a number of potential adverse outcomes. If an Rh-negative patient receives Rh (D) + blood without prophylaxis, there is a significant risk of developing anti-D. The use of large amounts of blood is known to cause dilution of many serum proteins and substances, such as coagulation factors, ATP, and 2,3 DPG. Also, there is the risk of transfusing older blood, which can result in increased potassium. Overall, the risk of decreased body temperature is more likely than increased body temperature, which suggests a transfusion reaction in the absence of any other potential source of fever.

QCCP2, **Emergency and massive transfusion,** p 128

64. **C. 75%.**

This figure is used for the calculation of allowable storage time for different storage media and additives.

QCCP2, **RBC components,** p 128

65. **E. GRANULOCYTE CONCENTRATE.**

Frozen products, such as cryoprecipitate and fresh frozen plasma have the longest storage life - around one year. They are followed by refrigerated products, like whole blood or packed red cells, whose lifetime varies with the preservative used, but is in the neighborhood of 1-2 months. Finally, the room temperature-stored products, platelets, and granulocytes have the shortest life-span - 5 days in the case of platelets and 1 day for granulocyte concentrate.

QCCP2, **T2.14,** p 129

66. **D. AS-1.**

Citrate by itself is not used as a preservative, but rather as an anticoagulant. Heparin, too. Heparin, however, has been used in the past to extend the shelf life of blood by a few days. CPD (citrate phosphate dextrose) and CPDA-1 (CPD + adenine) extend to 21 and 35 days, respectively. AS-1 is similar to CPDA-1, but instead of citrate, there is mannitol and sodium chloride, and it extends the most to 42 days.

QCCP2, **T2.15, Additive solutions,** p 129

67. **D. A & B.**

While both Factor V and Factor VII are labile *in vitro*, Factor VII is most labile *in vivo*.

QCCP2, **Red cell components,** p 129

68. **C. 80%.**

The final hematocrit of the red blood cells after centrifugation of whole blood must be no greater than 80%. Above that, the viscosity is too great. The prepared RBCs must be stored at 4°C within 8 hours of being collected. Additive solutions can increase the storage life (see question 66).

QCCP2, **Red cell components,** p 130

2: Blood Banking and Transfusion Answers

69.　A.　**$<5 \times 10^6$.**

At least a 3 log reduction of the white cell count (from 5×10^9) must be achieved in order for a unit to qualify to prevent HLA alloimmunization or CMV transmission. Only a single log reduction is required to prevent febrile non-hemolytic transfusion reactions.
QCCP2, **Red blood cell products,** p 130

70.　B.　**24 HOURS.**

The process of washing cells involves opening the closed system of the unit, washing, and resuspending in normal saline. As a result of opening the system, the shelf life is reduced to 24 hours.
QCCP2, **Red blood cell products,** p 130

71.　A.　**200 MG.**

Each red blood cell unit contains approximately 200 mL red blood cells, with each mL of red blood cells containing 1mg of iron. This means that each RBC unit has 200mg of iron.
QCCP2, **Red blood cell products,** p 131

72.　C.　**0.9% (ISOTONIC) SALINE.**

Only isotonic saline (without medications) may be infused through the same line as red blood cells. Many products, such as lactated Ringer solution, affect the red blood cells (hemolysis, anticoagulation, etc.).
QCCP2, **Red blood cell products,** p 131

73.　A.　**3×10^{11}.**

An apheresis platelet unit is approximately equal to 6 single whole blood-collected units (the "6 pack"). Each individual platelet unit must contain at least 5.5×10^{10} platelets in at least 75% of the units tested. It makes sense that a "6 pack" would contain 6x more platelets than a single unit.
QCCP2, **Platelets,** p 131

74.　B.　**20-24°C.**

Granulocyte concentrates must be collected and used within 24 hours. For that reason, the product is not routinely collected until it is needed. The optimal temperature at which to keep the product is 20-24°C (room temperature).
QCCP2, **Granulocyte concentrates,** p 132

75.　B.　**24 HOURS.**

There are a lot of numbers to remember with FFP preparation, storage, and use. The plasma separated from platelets by a hard spin must be frozen within 8 hours of collection to be considered "fresh frozen plasma." The frozen product can be stored for up to 1 year as such, but then must be used within 24 hours of thawing. The product can be refrigerated and stored for 5 days, but it must be relabeled as thawed plasma with the expectation that it contains lower levels of coagulation factors, especially Factor V and VIII.
QCCP2, **FFP,** p 132

2: Blood Banking and Transfusion Answers

76. E. **HEMOPHILIA A.**

FFP is best used in the situation of coagulopathy that results from the loss of multiple coagulation factors. Loss of single factors, such as Factor VIII in hemophilia A, is better treated with recombinant Factor VIII, or if needed, cryoprecipitate/FFP is also useful in TTP to return ADAMTS-13, in hereditary angioedema, to replace C1q, and in antithrombin deficiency.
QCCP2, **FFP,** p 132

77. D. **FACTOR V.**

More numbers to remember. Each unit of cryo must contain at least 150 mg of fibrinogen and 80IU of Factor VIII. This is the same amount as in FFP (cryo is made from FFP), but instead of a volume of 200 mL, cryo has the factors in 15 mL. Cryo can be used to treat hemophilia, though for a number of reasons, recombinant Factor VIII is the preferred treatment.
QCCP2, **Cryoprecipitated anti-hemophilic factor,** p 133

78. E. **15 GY.**

At least 15 Gy must be delivered to any point of the product while at least 25 Gy must be delivered to the middle of the product. After irradiation, it must be noted that the expiration date cannot exceed 28 days.
QCCP2, **Irradiated products,** p 134

79. A. **CELLULAR PRODUCTS TO IMMUNOCOMPROMISED HOSTS.**

The only clear indication for irradiation is to prevent transfusion-associated graft v. host disease. By irradiating white blood cells, they are rendered incapable of engrafting in an immunocompromised host. Irradiated products do not prevent CMV transmission, alloimmunization, or recurrent febrile non-hemolytic transfusion reactions, like leukoreduction does. Furthermore, irradiating granulocytes would destroy your product. Don't do that.
QCCP2, **Irradiated products,** p 134

80. D. **RED BLOOD CELLS LEUKOREDUCED TO <5×10^8 WHITE BLOOD CELLS.**

Red cell unit can contain up to 5×10^9 white blood cells/unit and should be reduced one order of magnitude in order to prevent febrile nonhemolytic transfusion reactions and three orders of magnitude to prevent CMV transmission or alloimmunization. Washed red blood cells are considered leukoreduced. Most experts believe that leukoreduced and CMV negative by serology units are equivalent in prevention of CMV transmission.
QCCP2, **Leukoreduced products,** p 134

81. B. **STOP THE TRANSFUSION.**

The first step in all transfusion reactions should be always be the same. STOP THE REACTION. Always, every time, always, always. The most important factor in determining the severity of reactions is the amount of product that is delivered to the patient.
QCCP2, **Transfusion complications,** p 135

82. C. **PAPERWORK ERRORS.**

Unfortunately, clerical errors still account for a significant number of hemolytic transfusion reactions - patient ID, sample mislabeling, etc.
QCCP2, **Transfusion complications,** p 135

83.   A.   **FEBRILE NONHEMOLYTIC TRANSFUSION REACTION.**

Luckily, the least severe reaction is the most common, reportedly seen in 0.5% of all transfusions. The most common cause of FNHTRs is cytokines elaborated from white blood cells while the unit is stored. A decreased incidence can be achieved with filtration of red blood cells at the time of collection as well as pretransfusion administration of acetaminophen to patients.
QCCP2, **FNHTRs,** p 136

84.   C.   **ANTI-A/ANTI-B.**

Intravascular acute hemolysis is most commonly due to anti-A or anti-B in cases of ABO incompatibility. The only other antibody of significance associated with acute intravascular hemolysis is anti-Kidd. All the other antibodies presented as choices are more commonly associated with extravascular hemolysis, either acute or delayed.
QCCP2, **Acute hemolytic transfusion reactions,** p 136

85.   D.   *STAPHYLOCOCCUS AUREUS.*

While platelet products are associated with contamination from gram-positive cocci, red blood cells are associated with gram-negative organisms, especially those listed in the choices (except Staph). Remember that red blood cells are refrigerated so organisms that grow in the cold will be favored.
QCCP2, **Bacterial contamination,** p 137

86.   B.   **HLA SIMILARITY, NOT IDENTITY.**

TAGVHD occurs most often when the recipient has an antigen that the donor does not, while all the donor's antigens are present in the recipient. This means that the recipient's white blood cells don't see the donor as foreign, however the donor's white blood cells react to the foreign antigen on the recipient's cells.
QCCP2, **TAGVHD,** p 137

87.   E.   **PATIENTS POST-OP FROM LUNG SURGERY.**

In addition, products containing plasma are more commonly associated with TRALI, perhaps due to anti-HLA antibodies from the donor unit. The diagnosis of TRALI is one of exclusion, after volume overload, sepsis, anaphylaxis, hemolysis, etc. have been ruled out.
QCCP2, **TRALI,** p 138

88.   D.   **THE TRANSFUSION CAN BE RESTARTED AFTER TREATING THE PATIENT.**

Allergic transfusion reactions are unique because once it is determined that the patient is experiencing urticaria due to the transfusion, the patient can be treated with anti-histamines and the transfusion restarted. All of the other choices are either untrue or not unique.
QCCP2, **Allergic transfusion reactions,** p 138

89.   B.   **SPLEEN STATUS (PRESENT OR ABSENT).**

The absence of a spleen is associated with the greatest platelet increments following transfusion. All of the other factors, with the exception of patient age, are associated with platelet refractoriness. To prevent the occurrence of refractoriness, one must try to prevent alloimmunization.
QCCP2, **Platelet refractoriness,** p 139

2: Blood Banking and Transfusion Answers

90. A. **HEPATITIS B VIRUS.**

The viruses are presented in the order of risk of infection. HBV risk is at 1:100000, while HCV risk is 10 times lower and HAV mildly lower than HCV. HIV rates vary wildly but are in the same range as HCV and HAV. West Nile virus-associated infection has been reported in case reports.
QCCP2, **Infections,** p 140

91. E. **SURROGATE MARKER OF HIGH-RISK BEHAVIOR.**

RPR is a confirmatory test for *Treponema* infections, but is a very poor screening test (low PPV). Instead, RPR positivity is used as a marker for other diseases associated with high-risk behavior (HIV, HCV).
QCCP2, **Infections,** p 140

92. C. **JK (A-B-).**

Of the major antigens associated with hemolysis, Kidd (Jk) is one of the more difficult to deal with. The Jk (a-b-) phenotype is rare. Jka is most commonly associated with hemolysis and luckily ~20% of the donor population is Jka-.
QCCP2, **T2.19, Frequency of antigens in USA donor population,** p 142

Chapter 3

Microbiology

1. All of the following refer to cases of uncomplicated urinary tract infections, except:
   A. pyelonephritis in an otherwise healthy young woman
   B. cystitis in a paralyzed young man with a spinal injury
   C. cystitis in a young healthy man
   D. a post-menopausal woman with cystitis
   E. a young healthy woman with cystitis

2. Which of the following situations may require treatment?
   A. pregnant woman with asymptomatic bacteriuria
   B. patients with asymptomatic bacteriuria during cystoscopy
   C. pediatric patient with hypospadias and asymptomatic bacteriuria
   D. A & B
   E. A, B, C

3. Which of the following tests for urinary tract infections has the highest specificity?
   A. microscopic hematuria
   B. urine dipstick positive for hemoglobin
   C. microscopic detection of pyuria
   D. urine dipstick positive for nitrite
   E. urine dipstick positive for leukocyte esterase

4. According to the Infectious Disease Society of America (IDSA) what bacterial concentration should be considered the minimum for the diagnosis of cystitis?
   A. $>10^1$ CFU/mL
   B. $>10^2$ CFU/mL
   C. $>10^3$ CFU/mL
   D. $>10^4$ CFU/mL
   E. $>10^5$ CFU/mL

5. All of the following organisms are causes of culture negative urinary tract infections, except:
   A. *Ureaplasma urealyticum*
   B. *Corynebacterium* D2
   C. *Chlamydia* spp
   D. *Mycoplasma hominis*
   E. all of the above are causes of culture-negative UTIs

6. Which of the following organisms is most commonly associated with hemorrhagic cystitis in bone marrow transplant patients?
   A. BK virus
   B. CMV
   C. HSV
   D. adenovirus
   E. *E. coli*

7. What is the most common cause of infectious diarrhea in an otherwise healthy patient?
    A. Hepatitis A
    B. norovirus
    C. *E. coli*
    D. *Salmonella*
    E. *Clostridium* spp

8. Which of the following organisms should be at the top of the differential diagnosis of bloody diarrhea without fecal neutrophils?
    A. norovirus
    B. enterohemorrhagic *E. coli*
    C. *Entamoeba*
    D. *Vibrio*
    E. *Campylobacter*

9. All of the following symptoms are associated with hemolytic uremic syndrome, except:
    A. mental status changes
    B. microangiopathic hemolytic anemia
    C. renal failure
    D. thrombocytopenia
    E. fever

10. All of the following patients are at an elevated risk of salmonellosis, except:
    A. an otherwise healthy 6-month-old baby
    B. a 24-year-old HIV(+) man
    C. a 93-year-old otherwise healthy woman
    D. an otherwise healthy 33-year-old man
    E. a 62-year-old man with a prosthetic hip

11. Which of the following is the most common cause of Guillain-Barre syndrome?
    A. *Campylobacter jejuni*
    B. *Helicobacter pylori*
    C. *Clostridium difficile*
    D. *Escherichia coli*
    E. *Clostridium perfringens*

12. Which of the following HLA haplotypes is associated with the enteropathic arthritis of *Campylobacter jejuni*?
    A. HLA-A4
    B. HLA-B7
    C. HLA-B27
    D. HLA-DR4
    E. HLA-DP7

13. Which of the following serotypes of *Vibrio cholerae* are responsible for the majority of cases of epidemic cholera?
    A. O1
    B. O139
    C. O233
    D. A & B
    E. A, B, C

3: Microbiology Questions

14. Which of the following *Vibrio* species is the most common cause of food-borne diarrhea in Japan?
    A. *V. cholerae*
    B. *V. parahemolyticus*
    C. *V. vulnificus*
    D. *V. enterocolitica*
    E. *V. perfringens*

15. Which of the following plasmids is associated with pathogenicity in *Yersinia enterocolitica* and can be detected with DNA-based assays?
    A. pYE
    B. pYV
    C. pYP
    D. pmecA
    E. pYR5

16. Which of the following routine tests for *Entamoeba histolytica* has the highest sensitivity and specificity?
    A. colonic ulcer biopsy
    B. stool culture
    C. stool microscopy
    D. stool EIA
    E. stool PCR

17. Which of the following agents is the most common cause of pediatric viral gastroenteritis?
    A. adenovirus, serotypes 40 and 41
    B. Norwalk virus
    C. coronavirus
    D. astrovirus
    E. rotavirus

18. Which of the following tests can act as a substitute for microscopic leukocyte detection?
    A. stool nitrite
    B. stool leukocyte esterase
    C. stool culture
    D. peripheral blood smear
    E. stool lactoferrin

19. Which of the following agents is a very common cause of community-acquired pneumonia but is rare in cases of pneumonia in elderly persons living in nursing homes?
    A. *Streptococcus pneumoniae*
    B. *Mycoplasma pneumoniae*
    C. *Haemophilus influenzae*
    D. *Klebsiella pneumoniae*
    E. *Serratia marascesens*

20. Which of the following people is at the greatest risk of coccidiomycosis?
    A. a Missouri cattle rancher
    B. a homeless alcoholic
    C. a Wyoming rabbit rancher
    D. a Central Valley California migrant worker
    E. a pregnant woman with several housecats

3: Microbiology Questions

21. Which of the following organisms is a more common cause of pneumonia in patients with cystic fibrosis than in patients without cystic fibrosis?
    A. *Legionella pneumophila*
    B. *Pseudomonas aeruginosa*
    C. *Coccidioides immitis*
    D. *Coxiella burnetti*
    E. *Moraxella catarrhalis*

22. All of the following are acceptable diagnostic tools for pneumococcal pneumonia, <u>except</u>:
    A. sputum culture
    B. bronchoscopic biopsy
    C. bronchoalveolar lavage
    D. blood culture
    E. all of the above are acceptable

23. Which of the following risk factors increase the risk of *Haemophilus influenzae* pneumonia?
    A. corticosteroid use
    B. antibiotic use
    C. chronic obstructive pulmonary disease
    D. A & B
    E. A, B, C

24. Which of the following electrolyte abnormalities is associated with *Legionella pneumophila* infection?
    A. hypoglycemia
    B. hyperkalemia
    C. hyponatremia
    D. hyperchloremia
    E. hypomagnesemia

25. Which of the following features is associated with pseudomonal pneumonia?
    A. chronic carriage
    B. severe necrotizing pneumonia
    C. empyema formation
    D. A & B
    E. A, B, C

26. What is the most common way to diagnose *Chlamydia pneumoniae* pneumonia?
    A. urine antigen test
    B. bronchoalveolar lavage and culture
    C. bronchoalveolar lavage and microscopy
    D. serology
    E. transbronchial biopsy

27. Hanta, or Sin Nombre, virus is a bunyavirus found in the four corners area of the U.S. (Arizona, New Mexico, Nevada, Colorado). What is the vector?
    A. deer mouse
    B. Norwegian rat
    C. domestic canine
    D. human
    E. *Ixodes* tick

3: Microbiology Questions

28. Which type of virus causes severe acute respiratory syndrome?
    A. paramyxovirus
    B. enterovirus
    C. rhinovirus
    D. coronavirus
    E. calicivirus

29. Which criterion is most helpful in formulating the differential diagnosis of infective endocarditis?
    A. patient age
    B. status of underlying valve
    C. patient gender
    D. medication list
    E. exposure history

30. What is the most common agent causing normal native valve endocarditis?
    A. *S. milleri*
    B. *S. pneumoniae*
    C. viridans *Streptococcus*
    D. *S. aureus*
    E. *S. epidermis*

31. All of the following are causes of blood culture-negative endocarditis (BCNE), except:
    A. prior antibiotic therapy
    B. Libman-Sacks endocarditis
    C. marantic endocarditis
    D. viridans *Streptococcus*
    E. *Coxiella burnetti*

32. Which of the following is included in the Austrian syndrome?
    A. infective endocarditis
    B. pneumonia
    C. meningitis
    D. A & B
    E. A, B, C

33. Which of the following organisms is/are the most common cause of fungal endocarditis?
    A. *Aspergillus fumigatus*
    B. *Aspergillus niger*
    C. *Candida* spp
    D. *Torulopsis glabrata*
    E. *Leptothrix*

34. Which of the following is the optimal specimen for the diagnosis of infective endocarditis?
    A. a single central venous line 50mL sample
    B. paired peripheral blood samples from the same site
    C. three peripheral blood samples drawn every 24 hours
    D. valve biopsy
    E. three peripheral blood samples every 8 hours for first 24 hours

3: Microbiology Questions

35. How does antibiotic therapy most commonly affect the diagnosis of bacterial endocarditis on valvular material?
    A. the causative organisms are completely eradicated
    B. treatment causes a shift toward other non-virulent organism growth
    C. antibiotics bind to organisms and block staining
    D. gram stain morphology of bacteria is often altered by antibiotics
    E. bacteria cannot be identified on valvular material

36. What clinical feature dominates the presentation of encephalitis?
    A. fever
    B. mental status changes
    C. headache
    D. photophobia
    E. stiff neck

37. All of the following CSF findings are consistent with aseptic meningitis, <u>except</u>:
    A. increased protein
    B. increased glucose
    C. low-level (<250/mL) leukocytosis
    D. increased mononuclear cells
    E. no growth on bacterial culture

38. What is the most common cause of meningitis?
    A. mycobacteria
    B. bacteria
    C. fungus
    D. virus
    E. amoeba

39. All of the following are common causes of neonatal bacterial meningitis, <u>except</u>:
    A. Group B strep
    B. gram negative anaerobes
    C. *Neisseria meningitidis*
    D. *Listeria*
    E. enterovirus

40. What is the most common cause of bacterial meningitis in adults?
    A. *Streptococcus pneumoniae*
    B. *Neisseria meningitidis*
    C. *Listeria monocytogenes*
    D. *E. coli*
    E. *Klebsiella pneumoniae*

41. Which of the following viruses most commonly presents with anterior frontotemporal hemorrhagic encephalitis?
    A. HHV6
    B. HHV8
    C. St. Louis encephalitis virus
    D. HSV-1
    E. Coxsackie A virus

3: Microbiology Questions

42. What is the animal reservoir of West Nile virus?
    A. mice
    B. rats
    C. domestic cats
    D. birds
    E. rabbits

43. Which of the following viruses is the most common cause of winter viral encephalitis?
    A. lymphocytic choriomeningitis virus
    B. Coxsackie A virus
    C. Coxsackie B virus
    D. human herpes virus 6
    E. West Nile virus

44. Which feature separates the typeable from non-typeable strains of *Haemophilus influenzae*?
    A. HA antigen
    B. capsule
    C. mecA gene
    D. penicillin binding protein
    E. growth at 42°C

45. Patients with complement deficiencies are at an increased risk for meningitis caused by this infectious agent:
    A. *Streptococcus pneumoniae*
    B. *Haemophilus influenzae*
    C. *E. coli*
    D. *Listeria monocytogenes*
    E. *Neisseria meningitidis*

46. Which of the following organisms typically causes meningitis in a disproportionate number of both very young and very old patients?
    A. group B *Streptococcus*
    B. *Staphylococcus aureus*
    C. *Listeria monocytogenes*
    D. *Streptococcus pneumoniae*
    E. *Haemophilus influenzae*

47. Which of the following amoebae is most commonly the cause of primary amebic encephalitis?
    A. *Entamoeba histolytica*
    B. *Acanthamoeba*
    C. *Entamoeba coli*
    D. *Endolimax nana*
    E. *Naegleria fowleri*

48. Which of the following etiologies of meningitis is consistent with CSF findings of glucose <45 mg/dL, protein >500 mg/dL, and a white blood cell count >1000 WBC/mL?
    A. viral
    B. amebic
    C. aseptic
    D. bacterial
    E. chemical

49. Latex agglutination tests on CSF are commonly used for the diagnosis of all of the following causes of meningitis, <u>except</u>:
    A. *Haemophilus influenzae*, type B
    B. *Neisseria meningitidis*
    C. group B *Streptococcus*
    D. *Listeria monocytogenes*
    E. *Streptococcus pneumoniae*

50. All of the following criteria are used in the diagnosis of prosthetic joint infection, <u>except</u>:
    A. joint pain with positive bacteremia in two successive blood cultures
    B. growth of the same microorganism in two or more synovial fluid or periprosthetic tissue cultures
    C. purulent synovial fluid or periprosthetic tissue
    D. acute inflammation in periprosthetic tissue
    E. presence of a sinus tract

51. What is/are the most common bacterium found in prosthetic joint infections?
    A. *Staphylococcus aureus*
    B. *Staphylococcus epidermidis*
    C. *Streptococci* spp
    D. gram negative bacilli
    E. *Enterococcus*

52. What is the causative agent of visceral larva migrans?
    A. *Ancylostoma brazilensis*
    B. *Loa loa*
    C. *Toxicara canis*
    D. *Francisella tularensis*
    E. *Chlamydia trachomatis*

53. What is the overall most common cause of bacterial cellulitis?
    A. coagulase-negative *Staphylococcus*
    B. group A *Streptococcus*
    C. *Pasteurella multocida*
    D. *Aeromonas hydrophila*
    E. *Vibrio vulnificus*

54. Which of the following organisms is the most common cause viral myocarditis?
    A. adenovirus
    B. JC virus
    C. Coxsackie A
    D. Coxsackie B
    E. human herpes virus 6

55. All of the following viruses are most commonly detected by culture, <u>except</u>:
    A. HSV-1
    B. HSV-2
    C. adenovirus
    D. HPV
    E. EBV

3: Microbiology Questions

56. MRC-5 cells are an example of which kind of cell culture?
    A. primary cell culture
    B. cell line (secondary cell culture)
    C. established cell line
    D. human diploid fibroblast
    E. malignant transformed cell line

57. All of the following organisms utilize the mosquito as a vector, <u>except</u>:
    A. *Loa loa*
    B. *Wuchereria bancrofti*
    C. *Brugia malayi*
    D. *Dirofilaria immitis*
    E. *Plasmodium falciparum*

58. Which of the following viruses grows best in Hep2 cells?
    A. enterovirus
    B. Coxsackie A
    C. Coxsackie B
    D. adenovirus
    E. cytomegalovirus

59. What's the most common cause of false positive hemadsorption in viral culture?
    A. *Mycoplasma* spp
    B. simian virus
    C. mycobacterium
    D. *Acanthamoeba*
    E. *Candida*

60. Which of the following viruses is assayed by injection into suckling mice <u>and</u> observation for flaccid paralysis?
    A. *Clostridium botulinum*
    B. adenovirus
    C. parvovirus
    D. Coxsackie A virus
    E. respiratory syncytial virus

61. Which of the following viruses causes syncytia formation in culture?
    A. RSV
    B. measles
    C. HSV
    D. A & B
    E. A, B, C

62. Which of the following viruses can have both nuclear <u>and</u> cytoplasmic inclusions?
    A. CMV
    B. measles
    C. rabies
    D. A & B
    E. A, B, C

3: Microbiology Questions

63. What magnitude elevation of virus-specific IgG titer is usually considered the minimum for the diagnosis of an acute viral infection?
    A.   2 fold
    B.   4 fold
    C.   10 fold
    D.   100 fold
    E.   1 million billion fold

64. Which of the following herpes virus family members lie latent in the dorsal root ganglia?
    A.   HSV-1
    B.   HSV-2
    C.   VZV
    D.   A & B
    E.   A, B, C

65. Why is caesarean section delivery of children from mothers with prodromal or active genital herpes recommended?
    A.   increased risk of vaginal trauma to the mother
    B.   indication of immunodeficiency in mother and increased risk of secondary infection
    C.   to decrease the risk of neonatal herpes
    D.   to decrease the risk of spreading infection to health care workers
    E.   to decrease risk of puerperal coinfection

66. How can herpes simplex virus definitively be identified in shell vial assay?
    A.   direct fluorescent antibody stain
    B.   cytopathic effect viewed with light microscopy
    C.   reculture (shell vial assay as a starter culture)
    D.   A & B
    E.   A, B, C

67. All of the following features are used to diagnose congenital varicella, except:
    A.   maternal VZV during pregnancy
    B.   skin lesions in newborn in a dermatomal distribution
    C.   serological evidence of newborn infection with elevated specific IgG persisting beyond 7 months
    D.   serological evidence of newborn infection with elevated specific IgM
    E.   all of the above are potentially utilized in the diagnosis of congenital varicella

68. Ramsay-Hunt syndrome is an infection of the facial nerve as caused by which of the following viruses?
    A.   SV40
    B.   CMV
    C.   HSV
    D.   VZV
    E.   HIV

69. In which of the following patient populations is the risk of CMV retinitis, encephalitis, or nephritis at its highest?
    A.   HIV patients with a CD4 counts <100/mL
    B.   HIV patients with CD4 counts between 500 and 1000/mL
    C.   solid-organ transplant recipients
    D.   older children
    E.   elderly adults

3: Microbiology Questions

70.   Which of the following viruses is responsible for the most common congenital infection in the United States?
   A.   VZV
   B.   CMV
   C.   parvovirus B19
   D.   EBV
   E.   adenovirus

71.   All of the following factors affect the rate of CMV seropositivity?
   A.   pregnancy status
   B.   locale
   C.   age
   D.   socioeconomic status
   E.   all of the above affect the seropositivity rate

72.   All of the following techniques are routinely used to diagnose CMV, except:
   A.   culture
   B.   PCR
   C.   flaccid paralysis in suckling mice injected with patient serum
   D.   direct fluorescent antibody
   E.   serology

73.   What's the most common means of transmission of EBV?
   A.   saliva
   B.   blood
   C.   fecal oral
   D.   respiratory droplet
   E.   solid organ transplantation

74.   Which cell surface antigen is the receptor for the Epstein-Barr virus?
   A.   P antigen
   B.   CD21
   C.   insulin-degrading enzyme
   D.   CD4
   E.   Cd81

75.   All of the following clinical syndromes are caused by EBV, except:
   A.   infectious mononucleosis
   B.   shingles
   C.   primary effusion lymphoma
   D.   post-transplant lymphoproliferative disease
   E.   oral hairy leukoplakia

76.   Which of the following disorders, also known as Duncan disease, is characterized by hepatic necrosis with a profound NK/T cell infiltrate?
   A.   Reye syndrome
   B.   immunoreactive cirrhosis
   C.   hepatitis mononucleosis
   D.   primary hepatic lymphoma
   E.   X-linked lymphoproliferative disorder

3: Microbiology Questions

77. All of the following are considered Hoagland criteria for the diagnosis of infectious mononucleosis, <u>except</u>:
    A. leukocytosis >50% lymphocytes, >10% atypical lymphocytes
    B. fever
    C. pharyngitis
    D. positive culture
    E. positive serological testing

78. Which of the following antibodies can be produced in response to EBV infection?
    A. anti-i
    B. ANA
    C. Paul-Bunnell heterophile antibodies
    D. A & B
    E. A, B, C

79. What's the best definition of heterophile antibodies as produced in EBV infections?
    A. IgM antibodies with an affinity for sheep and horse red blood cells
    B. IgM antibodies with an affinity for the capsule of all DNA viruses
    C. IgA antibodies directed against protein-antigens often consumed in a normal diet
    D. IgG antibodies secreted in tears with an affinity pigeon egg antigens
    E. IgG antibodies with an affinity for plant antigens

80. Which of the following antibodies is most helpful in distinguishing an acute EBV infection from a remote EBV infection?
    A. IgM anti-EA
    B. IgM anti-VCA
    C. IgG anti-EA
    D. IgM anti-VCC
    E. IgG anti-EE

81. All of the following EBV-associated lesions have demonstrable EBER (EBV-encoded RNA) by *in situ* hybridization, <u>except</u>:
    A. Hodgkin lymphoma
    B. oral hairy leukoplakia
    C. primary effusion lymphoma
    D. post-transplant lymphoproliferative disorder
    E. nasopharyngeal carcinoma

82. LMP1 and EBER staining show high concordance in which of the following lesions?
    A. Hodgkin lymphoma
    B. post-transplant lymphoproliferative disorder
    C. infectious mononucleosis
    D. A & B
    E. A, B, C

83. Which of the following subtypes of herpes virus is a possible cause of roseola infantum (exanthem subitum)?
    A. HHV6
    B. HHV7
    C. HHV8
    D. A & B
    E. A, B, C

3: Microbiology Questions

84. Which of the following clinical presentations is associated with HHV8?
    A. Kaposi sarcoma
    B. primary effusion lymphoma
    C. multicentric Castleman disease
    D. A & B
    E. A, B, C

85. Members of which of the following families of viruses are responsible for progressive multifocal leukoencephalopathy and viral hemorrhagic cystitis?
    A. herpes viruses
    B. picornaviruses
    C. reoviruses
    D. papovaviruses
    E. bunyaviruses

86. Benign HPV-associated lesions are associated with this form of the virus:
    A. integrated
    B. episomal
    C. mitochondrial
    D. extracellular
    E. intralysosomal

87. Which disease is associated with an inherited defect in the ability to defend against several HPV subtypes?
    A. Li-Fraumeni
    B. recurrent respiratory papillomatosis
    C. progressive multifocal leukoencephalopathy
    D. post-transplant lymphoproliferative disorder
    E. epidermodysplasia verruciformis

88. Oral squamous papillomas, laryngeal papillomas, condyloma acuminatum, and low-grade cervical squamous intraepithelial lesions are associated with this/these type/s of HPV:
    A. HPV6
    B. HPV11
    C. HPV16
    D. A & B
    E. A, B, C

89. In a person vaccinated against hepatitis B virus several years prior, which serological marker would be expected?
    A. HBsAg
    B. HBeAg
    C. IgG anti-HBc
    D. HBsAb
    E. anti-HBc

90. The persistence of which marker is the best evidence of chronic HBV infection:
    A. HBeAg
    B. HBsAg
    C. anti-HBe
    D. anti-HBs
    E. anti-HBc

3: Microbiology Questions

91. To what does the "window period" of HBV infection refer?
    A. the period between the appearance of HBV DNA and infection
    B. the period between the disappearance of HBsAg and appearance of HBsAb
    C. the period between the disappearance of HBcAg and appearance of HBcAb
    D. the period between HBeAg and HBcAg
    E. the period between infection and IgM anti-HBcAb

92. Which HBV antigen has been used to characterize chronic HBV carriers as either replicative or non-replicative?
    A. HBc
    B. HBs
    C. HBe
    D. HBx
    E. HBp

93. What percentage of people infected with hepatitis C virus will go on to chronic infection?
    A. <5%
    B. 25%
    C. 50%
    D. 85%
    E. >99%

94. Which of the following scenarios might explain a conflicting set of results in a patient with a positive anti-HCV antibody result and negative HCV RNA PCR?
    A. no infection
    B. no infection or recovery from acute HCV
    C. early HCV
    D. chronic HCV
    E. infection

95. How is a sustained virological response or a positive HCV treatment outcome defined?
    A. complete absence of detectable HCV RNA for perpetuity
    B. disappearance of anti-HCV antibody
    C. no evidence of chronic HCV on liver biopsy
    D. undetectable HCV RNA for 24 weeks
    E. greater than 10-fold reduction in HCV RNA

96. Which is the best test for determining the likelihood of progression to cirrhosis in a patient with chronic HCV?
    A. liver biopsy
    B. quantitative HCV RNA
    C. qualitative HCV RNA
    D. serial ALT levels
    E. HCV serotype determination

97. Which of the following hepatitis viruses requires coinfection or chronic infection with HBV in order to infect the liver?
    A. HAV
    B. HCV
    C. HDV
    D. HEV
    E. HGV

3: Microbiology Questions

98. Which of the following viruses is hemagglutinin-positive?
    A. influenza A
    B. influenza B
    C. parainfluenza
    D. A & B
    E. A, B, C

99. Which of the following influenza subtypes is associated with pandemic avian influenza?
    A. H1N1
    B. H5N2
    C. H5N1
    D. H2N1
    E. H2N2

100. Which of the following tests for influenza is considered the gold standard?
    A. culture
    B. direct fluorescent antibody
    C. detection of influenza RNA
    D. serology
    E. rapid Monospot

101. What's the most common secondary complication that can arise with measles infection?
    A. otitis media
    B. pneumonia
    C. myocarditis
    D. appendicitis
    E. subacute sclerosing panencephalitis

102. What name is given to the characteristic measles-infected cell in the lungs or appendix?
    A. Anitschow cell
    B. Touton giant cell
    C. floret cell
    D. Warthin-Finkeldey
    E. Hallmark cell

103. This virus is responsible for nearly all cases of infantile respiratory bronchiolitis:
    A. parainfluenza virus
    B. influenza A virus
    C. metapneumovirus
    D. Coxsackie A virus
    E. respiratory syncytial virus

104. What is the gold standard assay for the diagnosis of enteroviral meningitis in CSF samples?
    A. cell culture
    B. RT-PCR
    C. direct fluorescent antibody
    D. EIA
    E. suckling mouse paralysis assay

3: Microbiology Questions

105. What is notable about the culture of rhinovirus?
    A.   several weeks of incubation
    B.   culture must contain support virus
    C.   high salt media is needed
    D.   requires addition of nasal mucus to culture
    E.   must be incubated at 32°C

106. What does hantavirus and the Crimean-Congo hemorrhagic fever viruses have in common?
    A.   they are members of the bunyavirus family
    B.   they are arthropod-borne
    C.   they are found in geographically overlapping areas
    D.   they have extremely long latency
    E.   they have DNA-based genomes

107. Why are yellow fever and rubella viruses different from the other members of the togavirus family?
    A.   they have DNA genomes
    B.   they have hybrid RNA-DNA genomes
    C.   they require coinfection with another virus
    D.   they do not cause arthropod-borne encephalitis
    E.   they both primarily infect the liver

108. All of the following are potential consequences of *in utero* rubella infection, except:
    A.   glaucoma
    B.   congenital heart disease
    C.   sensorineural deafness
    D.   microcephaly
    E.   midzonal hepatic necrosis

109. Which of the following mosquitoes transmit both yellow fever and Dengue fever viruses?
    A.   *Aedes aegypti*
    B.   *Aedes albopictus*
    C.   *Culex pipiens*
    D.   A & B
    E.   A, B, C

110. Negri bodies in Purkinje cells are associated with which of the following viruses?
    A.   paramyxoviruses
    B.   Eastern equine encephalitis
    C.   rhabdovirus
    D.   lymphocytic choriomeningitis virus
    E.   Ebola virus

111. All of the following are endemic areas for the human T cell lymphotropic virus - I, except:
    A.   Norway
    B.   Caribbean
    C.   S. Japan
    D.   Brazil
    E.   S. Africa

112. Which of the following is/are characteristic of adult T cell lymphoma?
    A. peripheral CD4+/CD25+ flower cells
    B. hypercalcemia
    C. high serum IL-2 receptor
    D. A & B
    E. A, B, C

113. Which test is the primary screening test for HIV?
    A. serum enzyme-linked immunosorbent assay
    B. Western blot
    C. quantitative HIV RNA
    D. CD4 count
    E. p24 antigen detection

114. Which of the following HIV tests is the assay for determining response to anti-retrovirals?
    A. serum ELISA
    B. Western blot
    C. quantitative HIV RNA
    D. CD4 count
    E. p24 antigen detection

115. Which test is the best choice for the detection of HIV infection shortly after an infection?
    A. serum ELISA
    B. Western blot
    C. quantitative HIV RNA
    D. CD4 count
    E. p24 antigen detection

116. Which of the following organisms is detectable with modified acid-fast stains?
    A. *Cryptosporidium*
    B. *Cyclospora*
    C. *Isospora*
    D. A & B
    E. A, B, C

117. Which of the following organisms can be detected with the "adhesive tape" test?
    A. *Giardia lamblia*
    B. *Enterobius vermicularis*
    C. *Strongyloides stercoralis*
    D. *Onchocerca volvulus*
    E. *Brugia malayi*

118. Which parasite can be specifically detected serologically after a recent infection?
    A. *Paragonimus westermanii*
    B. *Strongyloides stercoralis*
    C. *Brugia malayi*
    D. *Taenia solium*
    E. *Toxoplasma gondii*

3: Microbiology Questions

119. What is the principal means of distinguishing *Entamoeba histolytica* from *Entamoeba hartmanii* by light microscopy?
    A.   size of trophozoite
    B.   appearance of karyosome
    C.   appearance of nuclear chromatin
    D.   number of nuclei in cyst form
    E.   appearance of chromatoidal bars in cyst

120. What is the most common site of extraintestinal amebic abscess?
    A.   lungs
    B.   liver
    C.   brain
    D.   spleen
    E.   bladder

121. What's the fastest way to identify *Iodamoeba butschlii*?
    A.   the presence of ingested red blood cells in the trophozoite form
    B.   culture on a lawn of inactivated *E coli*
    C.   its small (5-10 micron) size
    D.   the prominent vacuole in the cyst form
    E.   the presence of up to 8 nuclei in the cyst form

122. Which organism causes granulomatous amebic encephalitis?
    A.   *Naegleria*
    B.   *Acanthamoeba*
    C.   *Entamoeba histolytica*
    D.   *Entamoeba hartmanii*
    E.   *Iodamoeba*

123. What is the non-pathogenic flagellate that must be distinguished from *Giardia lamblia*?
    A.   *Chilomastix mesneli*
    B.   *Dientamoeba fragilis*
    C.   *Trichomonas vaginalis*
    D.   *Trypanosoma cruzi*
    E.   *Leishmania donovani*

124. Which amoeba is most often seen as a coinfection with *Enterobius vermicularis*?
    A.   *Naegleria*
    B.   *Acanthamoeba*
    C.   *Entamoeba histolytica*
    D.   *Dientamoeba*
    E.   *Iodamoeba*

125. What feature of *Leishmania* spp helps to distinguish them from *Histoplasma* or *Toxoplasma*?
    A.   small intracellular amastigotes
    B.   bar-like kinetoplast
    C.   central axostyle
    D.   external flagellum
    E.   extracellular forms

3: Microbiology Questions

126. Which species of *Leishmania* is most commonly associated with mucocutaneous leishmaniasis?
    A. *L. major*
    B. *L. tropica*
    C. *L. brazilensis*
    D. *L. donovani*
    E. *L. mexicana*

127. What characteristic feature of *T. cruzi* trypomastigotes helps distinguish it from *T. brucei* in peripheral blood smears?
    A. undulating flagellum
    B. central kinetoplast
    C. culture on Novy-MacNeal-Nicolle medium
    D. presence in lymph nodes
    E. "C" shape

128. The only medically significant ciliate organism is:
    A. *Entamoeba histolytica*
    B. *Balantidium coli*
    C. *Cryptosporidium parvum*
    D. *Chilomastix mesneli*
    E. *Cyclospora cayetenensis*

129. Where can *Cryptosporidium* be found in an infected host?
    A. adherent to small intestinal brush border
    B. within an intracellular apical vacuole
    C. interdigitated between enterocytes
    D. in foveolar gland crypts of the stomach
    E. intracytoplasmically within enterocytes

130. Which of the following organisms is in the differential diagnosis of the bradyzoite of *Toxoplasma gondii*?
    A. *Leishmania*
    B. *Histoplasma*
    C. *Trypanosoma*
    D. A & B
    E. A, B, C

131. What test best helps to differentiate pregnant women at a lower risk for intrauterine *Toxoplasma* infection?
    A. anti-*Toxoplasma* IgM
    B. PCR of CSF
    C. Giemsa staining
    D. anti-*Toxoplasma* IgG
    E. amniotic fluid serology

132. Which species of *Plasmodium* is responsible for quartan (72-hour) fevers?
    A. *P. falciparum*
    B. *P. vivax*
    C. *P. malariae*
    D. A & B
    E. A, B, C

133. Where do *Plasmodium* sporozoites proliferate?
    A. liver
    B. red blood cells
    C. bone marrow
    D. within nucleated erythrocyte precursors
    E. freely within the blood

134. Individuals who lack the Duffy antigen on the surfaces of their red blood cells are protected against which species of *Plasmodium*?
    A. *P. vivax*
    B. *P. falciparum*
    C. *P. malariae*
    D. A & B
    E. A, B, C

135. Which form of *Plasmodium* is described as intraerythrocytic collections of numerous organisms?
    A. merozoites
    B. schizonts
    C. hypnozoites
    D. trophozoites
    E. bradyzoites

136. All of the following features of *Plasmodium falciparum* are helpful in distinguishing it from *P. vivax* or *P. ovale*, except:
    A. multiple ring forms within an erythrocyte
    B. applique trophozoite forms
    C. enlarged infected red blood cells
    D. banana-shaped gametocytes
    E. double chromatin dots in ring forms

137. Extraerythrocytic ring forms are characteristic of which organisms?
    A. *Babesia microti*
    B. *Plasmodium falciparum*
    C. *Plasmodium vivax*
    D. *Plasmodium ovale*
    E. *Plasmodium malariae*

138. Which of the following organisms is/are commonly seen coinfecting patients with babesiosis?
    A. *Borrelia burgdorfei*
    B. *Ehrlichia chaffeensis*
    C. microfilariae
    D. A & B
    E. A, B, C

139. Which of the following is the most common AIDS-defining illness?
    A. cryptosporidiosis
    B. *Pneumocystis* pneumonia
    C. esophageal candidiasis
    D. Kaposi sarcoma
    E. toxoplasmosis

3: Microbiology Questions

140. Which nematode has a characteristic double-operculated egg?
    A. *Trichuris trichuria*
    B. *Ascaris lumbricoides*
    C. *Necator americanus*
    D. *Ancylostoma duodenale*
    E. *Strongyloides stercoralis*

141. Which nematode has a characteristic mammilated bile-stained egg?
    A. *Trichuris*
    B. *Ascaris*
    C. *Necator*
    D. *Ancylostoma*
    E. *Strongyloides*

142. What's the best way to distinguish *Necator americanus* from *Ancylostoma duodenale*?
    A. appearance of eggs
    B. appearance of long buccal cavity
    C. appearance of mouth parts
    D. absence of genital groove
    E. length of worm

143. Which aspects of *Strongyloides* larva help distinguish it from hookworm larva?
    A. short buccal groove
    B. prominent genital primordium
    C. appearance of eggs
    D. A & B
    E. A, B, C

144. What is the most worrisome outcome of *Strongyloides* infection, especially in immunocompromised patients?
    A. autoinfection
    B. Loeffler syndrome
    C. chronic carrier state
    D. larva currens
    E. hyperinfection

145. What is the most characteristic feature of *Enterobius* worms in histological tissue sections?
    A. prominent genital groove
    B. lateral alae
    C. short buccal opening
    D. flattened uterine branches
    E. sheathed tail

146. Which feature(s) of microfilariae are <u>most</u> helpful in categorizing individual species?
    A. sheath/unsheathed
    B. pattern of nuclei in tail
    C. presence in lymphatics
    D. A & B
    E. A, B, C

3: Microbiology Questions

147. Which organism is predominantly responsible for visceral larva migrans?
      A.   *Onchocerca volvulus*
      B.   *Toxocara canis*
      C.   *Toxocara cati*
      D.   *Ancylostoma brazilensis*
      E.   *Dirofilaria immitis*

148. Which organism has the largest egg?
      A.   *Clonorchis*
      B.   *Diphyllobothrium*
      C.   *Fasciola hepatica*
      D.   *Paragonimus*
      E.   *Trichuris*

149. The eggs of which species of *Schistosoma* can be isolated from urine?
      A.   *S. haematobium*
      B.   *S. japonicum*
      C.   *S. mekongii*
      D.   *S. mansoni*
      E.   *S. intercalatum*

150. What is the primary vector for *Schistosoma*?
      A.   *Aedes* mosquitoes
      B.   freshwater snails
      C.   freshwater fish
      D.   freshwater plants
      E.   pork

151. Which of the following features of *Taenia saginata* helps to distinguish it from *Taenia solium*?
      A.   pork tapeworm
      B.   unarmed rostellum
      C.   egg with a radially striated wall
      D.   proglottid with less than 13 uterine branches
      E.   cystercercosis

152. Infection by this organism can be a cause of B_{12} deficiency:
      A.   *Taenia solium*
      B.   *Taenia saginata*
      C.   *Schistosoma mansoni*
      D.   *Diphyllobothrium latum*
      E.   *Echinococcus granulosus*

153. This organism is responsible for hydatid cysts of the liver:
      A.   *Diphyllobothrium*
      B.   *Taenia*
      C.   *Hymenolepis*
      D.   *Echinococcus*
      E.   *Dypylidium*

3: Microbiology Questions

154. All of the following organisms can show respective dual or triple infection, <u>except</u>:
    A.   *Ascaris* and *Trichuria*
    B.   *Enterobius* and *Dientamoeba*
    C.   *Babesia, B. burgdorfei,* and *Ehrlichia*
    D.   *Hymenolepis nana* and *Echinococcus*
    E.   lepromatous leprosy and *Strongyloides*

155. B cell (humoral) immunodeficiency increases susceptibility to this organism:
    A.   *Giardia*
    B.   *Trichomonas*
    C.   *Toxoplasma*
    D.   *Strongyloides*
    E.   *Cryptosporidium*

156. For what purpose is Niger seed agar used?
    A.   detecting melanin pigment in *Cryptococcus*
    B.   selective agar for *Malassezia furfur*
    C.   *Aspergillus* speciation
    D.   to visualize yeast forms
    E.   to detect pigment in *Trichophyton rubrum*

157. All of the following are dimorphic fungi, <u>except</u>:
    A.   *Histoplasma*
    B.   *Cryptococcus*
    C.   *Coccidioides*
    D.   *Blastomyces*
    E.   *Paracoccidioides*

158. All of the following entities are in the differential diagnosis of a fuzzy colony on a plate, <u>except</u>:
    A.   hyaline septate mold
    B.   dematiaceous mold
    C.   dimorphic fungus
    D.   coccoid yeast
    E.   aseptate mold

159. Which of the following characteristics assist with the speciation of molds?
    A.   rate of growth
    B.   type of hyphae
    C.   pigmentation
    D.   A & B
    E.   A, B, C

160. Which of the following media is most helpful in distinguishing the morphology of yeasts?
    A.   cottonseed agar
    B.   cornmeal agar with Tween 80
    C.   urea agar
    D.   brain-heart infusion medium
    E.   potato dextrose agar

3: Microbiology Questions

161. Which of the following fungi are inhibited by cyclohexamide?
    A. Zygomyces
    B. *Aspergillus*
    C. *Cryptococcus*
    D. A & B
    E. A, B, C

162. Which of the following dimorphic fungi needs to be plated on brain-heart infusion media with blood in order to grow as a yeast?
    A. *Blastomyces dermatidis*
    B. *Histoplasma capsulatum*
    C. *Coccidioides immitis*
    D. *Sporothrix schenkii*
    E. *Paracoccidioides brazilensis*

163. Which of the dimorphic yeasts is often confused histologically with the mold form of another dimorphic fungus?
    A. *Histoplasma*
    B. *Blastomyces*
    C. *Coccidioides*
    D. *Sporothrix*
    E. *Paracoccidioides*

164. Which of the dimorphic fungi are associated with sclerosing mediastinitis?
    A. *Histoplasma*
    B. *Blastomyces*
    C. *Coccidioides*
    D. *Sporothrix*
    E. *Paracoccidioides*

165. Which if the following organisms is in the differential diagnosis of *Coccidioides* spherules?
    A. *Rhinosporidium seeberi*
    B. *Histoplasma capsulatum*
    C. *Prototheca wickerhamii*
    D. A & B
    E. A, B, C

166. Which of the following dimorphic fungi presents the highest risk to laboratory personnel during culture?
    A. *Histoplasma*
    B. *Blastomyces*
    C. *Coccidioides*
    D. *Sporothrix*
    E. *Paracoccidioides*

167. Which of the following organisms grows as a mold with smooth, "lollipop"-shaped conidia?
    A. *Chrysosporium*
    B. *Blastomyces*
    C. *Sporothrix*
    D. A & B
    E. A, B, C

3: Microbiology Questions

168. In what patient population has an unusual inhalational form of *Sporothrix* been identified?
    A. the very young
    B. elderly
    C. immunocompromised
    D. chronic alcoholics
    E. smokers

169. The mold form of *Paracoccidioides* is identical to that of which other fungus?
    A. *Histoplasma*
    B. *Blastomyces*
    C. *Coccidioides*
    D. *Sporothrix*
    E. *Chrysosporium*

170. Which of the following dermatophytes is identified by its macroconidia?
    A. *Trichophyton tonsurans*
    B. *Trichophyton rubrum*
    C. *Epidermophyton floccosum*
    D. A & B
    E. A, B, C

171. Which of the following dermatophytes can be identified with its "birds on a wire" microconidia?
    A. *Microsporidium canis*
    B. *Trichophyton rubrum*
    C. *Epidermophyton floccosum*
    D. *Trichophyton mentagrophytes*
    E. *Trichophyton tonsurans*

172. What organism is the most common cause of onychomycosis?
    A. *Epidermophyton floccosum*
    B. *Trichophyton rubrum*
    C. *Trichophyton mentagrophytes*
    D. *Microsporum canis*
    E. *Microsporum gypseum*

173. Which of the following organisms is characterized by blue-green colonies with a white apron?
    A. *Aspergillus terreus*
    B. *A. niger*
    C. *A. fumigatus*
    D. *A. flavus*
    E. *Penicillium marneffei*

174. Which of the following organisms is characterized by two rows of phialides on the conidia?
    A. *A. terreus*
    B. *A. niger*
    C. *A. fumigatus*
    D. *A. flavus*
    E. *P. marneffei*

3: Microbiology Questions

175. Which species is responsible for the majority of cases of aspergilloma and allergic bronchopulmonary aspergillosis?
    A.   *A. flavus*
    B.   *A. fumigatus*
    C.   *A. niger*
    D.   *A. terreus*
    E.   *P. marneffei*

176. Which species of *Aspergillus* is most commonly seen as otitis externa?
    A.   *A. flavus*
    B.   *A. fumigatus*
    C.   *A. niger*
    D.   *A. terreus*
    E.   *P. marneffei*

177. All of the following hyalinohyphomyces have conidia that occur in clusters, <u>except</u>:
    A.   *Acremonium*
    B.   *Penicillium*
    C.   *Gliocladium*
    D.   *Fusarium*
    E.   all of the above occur in clusters

178. Which organism is the cause of adiaspiromycosis?
    A.   *Fusarium*
    B.   *Chrysosporium*
    C.   *Beuveria*
    D.   *Paecilomyces*
    E.   *Gliocladium*

179. Which of the following fungal organisms is a major concern as an opportunistic infection in burn victims?
    A.   *Gliosporium*
    B.   *Paecilomyces*
    C.   *Scopulariopsis*
    D.   *Scedosporium*
    E.   *Fusarium*

180. What is the most common cause of eumycotic mycetoma in the U.S.?
    A.   *Fusarium*
    B.   *Scopulariopsis*
    C.   *Acremonium*
    D.   *Scedosporium*
    E.   *Paecilomyces*

181. Which of the following dematiaceous molds is responsible for chromoblastomycosis?
    A.   *Fonseca*
    B.   *Phialophora*
    C.   *Cladosporiom*
    D.   *Wangiella*
    E.   *Exophiala*

3: Microbiology Questions

182. All of the following are causes of eumycotic mycetoma, <u>except</u>:
    A.   *Madurella*
    B.   *Actinomyces*
    C.   *Scedosporium*
    D.   *Wangiella*
    E.   *Exophiala*

183. Which of the following zygomycetes has sporangiophores that arise between rhizoids?
    A.   *Rhizopus*
    B.   *Absidia*
    C.   *Mucormycosis*
    D.   *Cunninghamella*
    E.   *Circinella*

184. Under what conditions must the germ tube test be run in order to identify *Candida albicans*?
    A.   suspended in broth, incubated 2 hours at 37°C
    B.   suspended in serum, incubated 24 hours at 37°C
    C.   suspended in broth, incubated 2 hours at 32°C
    D.   suspended in serum, incubated 2 hours at 37°C
    E.   suspended in broth, incubated 24 hours at 37°C

185. Which fungal organism is urease (+) and phenol oxidase (+)?
    A.   *Cryptococcus neoformans*
    B.   *Malassezia furfur*
    C.   *Rhodotorula*
    D.   *Candida krusei*
    E.   *Trichophyton mentagrophytes*

186. Which of the following organisms requires the overlay of olive oil in order to culture?
    A.   *Cryptococcus*
    B.   *Malassezia*
    C.   *Rhodotorula*
    D.   *Candida*
    E.   *Trichophyton*

187. Which of the following stains the capsule of *Cryptococcus*?
    A.   mucicarmine
    B.   Fontana-Masson
    C.   Alcian blue
    D.   India ink
    E.   GMS

188. Which of the following organisms causes infections associated with penetrating trauma and is in a class totally by itself?
    A.   *Sporothrix*
    B.   *Fusarium*
    C.   *Prototheca*
    D.   *Rhodotorula*
    E.   *Malassezia*

3: Microbiology Questions

189. What is the optimal specimen collection for bacterial blood culture?
    A. 2 samples, each with more than 20 mL of blood
    B. 1 sample of 5 mL blood
    C. 3 samples with 5 mL blood each
    D. 5 samples with 5 mL blood each
    E. 3 samples with more than 10 mL blood each

190. Which of the following specimens is routinely quantitatively cultured?
    A. blood
    B. urine
    C. stool
    D. sputum
    E. CSF

191. Which one of the following bacterium/additional stain pairs is incorrect?
    A. *H. influenzae* in CSF/methylene blue
    B. *Legionella*/GMS
    C. spirochetes/dark field microscopy
    D. *C. diphtheriae*/Loeffler methylene blue
    E. *Nocardia*/modified acid fast

192. In a gram stain, which compound stains the bacterial cell wall peptidoglycan?
    A. iodine
    B. safranin
    C. decolorant
    D. crystal violet
    E. no compound; staining is an artifact of heat fixation

193. What is the principal difference between the Ziehl-Neelsen acid-fast stain technique with Kinyoun acid-fast stain technique?
    A. the length that the organisms are stained
    B. the type of dye that is used
    C. Kinyoun uses a weaker acid (sulfuric acid) rather than HCl
    D. Kinyoun uses auramine-rhodamine instead of carbolfuschin as a stain
    E. whether or not heat is used to fix slides

194. Nearly all pathogenic bacteria grow on blood agar plates with the notable exception of which of the following:
    A. *H. influenzae*
    B. *S. aureus*
    C. *E. coli*
    D. *Serratia marascesens*
    E. group A *Strep*

195. Which specialized media is specifically used for the culture of *Legionella*?
    A. Thayer-Martin
    B. buffered charcoal yeast extract (BCYE)
    C. chocolate agar
    D. eosin methylene blue agar
    E. MacConkey agar

3: Microbiology Questions

196. What color do lactose non-fermenters appear as on MacConkey agar?
    A. red
    B. white
    C. green
    D. pink
    E. black

197. What accounts for the high selectivity of *Salmonella-Shigella* agar?
    A. low salt
    B. high bile salt and sodium citrate
    C. high growth temperature
    D. inhibitory aniline dye
    E. charcoal

198. Which of the following media is utilized to grow *Bordetella* spp?
    A. Regan-Lowe media
    B. Bordet-Gengeou
    C. CCF agar
    D. A & B
    E. A, B, C

199. Which of the following organisms grows optimally at 42°C?
    A. *Pseudomonas*
    B. *Listeria*
    C. *Mycobacterium marinum*
    D. *Campylobacter*
    E. *Salmonella*

200. Clumping of bacteria on the surface of a slide with the addition of rabbit serum describes which of the following?
    A. a positive furazolidone test
    B. a positive bound coagulase test
    C. a positive free coagulase test
    D. a negative catalase
    E. a negative free coagulase test

201. Which biochemical test is used to distinguish between *S. saprophyticus* and *S. epidermidis*?
    A. catalase
    B. coagulase
    C. NaCl tolerance
    D. CAMP test
    E. novobiocin

202. What is the purpose of the CAMP test?
    A. to identify antibiotic-resistant *Staphylococcus*
    B. to identify *S. aureus*
    C. to identify Group B beta-hemolytic *Strep*
    D. to identify *Enterococci*

3: Microbiology Questions

203. What is the purpose of the optochin (P)-test?
    A. distinguish among alpha hemolytic *Strep*
    B. distinguish among beta hemolytic *Strep*
    C. to confirm PYR test
    D. as a substitute for coagulase
    E. to test for bile solubility

204. All the following organisms are oxidase positive, <u>except</u>:
    A. *Pseudomonas*
    B. *Shigella*
    C. *Vibrio*
    D. *Campylobacter*
    E. *Pasteurella*

205. What organism best fits indole positive, lactose fermenter on MacConkey agar?
    A. *P. aeruginosa*
    B. *E. coli*
    C. *P. multocida*
    D. *H. influenzae*
    E. *Klebsiella*

206. What test, when paired with the Voges-Proskauer, provides the exact opposite results?
    A. CAMP test
    B. Kirby-Bauer
    C. cytochrome oxidase
    D. nitrate reduction test
    E. methyl red test

207. Which of the following organisms is a rapid urea splitter and therefore grows in both Stuart broth and Christensen broth?
    A. *Proteus*
    B. *Klebsiella*
    C. *Haemophilus*
    D. *Neisseria*
    E. *Branhamella*

208. Which of the following organisms has peritrichous flagella?
    A. *Flavobacterium*
    B. *Bordetella*
    C. *Pseudomonas*
    D. *Acinetobacter*
    E. *Moraxella*

209. Which of the following organisms displays the "string sign"?
    A. *Vibrio vulnificus*
    B. *Vibrio cholerae*
    C. *Vibrio parahaemolyticus*
    D. A & B
    E. A, B, C

210. Which of the following organisms utilizes both glucose and maltose when plated on cysteine-tryptic digest semi-solid agar?
    A. *Neisseria gonorrheae*
    B. *Neisseria lactamica*
    C. *Neisseria meningitidis*
    D. *Moraxella catarrhalis*
    E. *Haemophilus aphrophilus*

211. Which of the following organisms isolated from dog bite infections is coagulase positive?
    A. *Staphylococcus saprophyticus*
    B. *Staphylococcus hyicus*
    C. *Staphylococcus delphini*
    D. *Staphylococcus intermedius*
    E. *Staphylococcus epidermidis*

212. Which of the following are alpha-hemolytic strep?
    A. *Streptococcus pneumoniae*
    B. viridans *Streptococcus*
    C. *Streptococcus agalactaiae*
    D. A & B
    E. A, B, C

213. Which of the following profiles best describes *Streptococcus pneumoniae*?
    A. alpha-hemolytic, bile soluble, optochin sensitive
    B. gamma hemolytic, bile esculin positive, PYR hydrolysis negative
    C. gamma hemolytic, bile esculin positive, PYR hydrolysis positive
    D. beta hemolytic, CAMP test positive, hippurate positive
    E. beta hemolytic, bacitracin (A disk) sensitive, PYR hydrolysis positive

214. Which best describes growth conditions for *Neisseria*?
    A. microaerophilic at 37°C
    B. microaerophilic at 30°C
    C. CO_2-rich at 30°C
    D. CO_2-rich at 35°C
    E. anaerobic at 32°C

215. Which DNase positive organism's colony is not easily broken up and therefore displays the "hockey puck" sign where it can be pushed across the plate?
    A. *N. gonorrheae*
    B. *M. catarrhalis*
    C. *N. lactamica*
    D. *V. cholerae*
    E. *N. meningitidis*

216. Which test can be used to differentiate *Nocardia* from *Actinomyces*?
    A. acid fast stain
    B. aerobic v. anaerobic growth conditions
    C. gram stain
    D. A & B
    E. A, B, C

217. Which of the following is an anaerobic spore-forming gram-positive bacillus?
    A. *Actinomyces*
    B. *Clostridia*
    C. *Lactobacillus*
    D. *Bacillus*
    E. *Listeria*

218. Which of the following features of *Bacillus anthracis* can be used in distinguish it from *Bacillus cereus*?
    A. lack of hemolysis
    B. lack of motility
    C. sensitivity to penicillin
    D. A & B
    E. A, B, C

219. Which organism is responsible for granulomatosis infantisepticum?
    A. *Erysipelothrix*
    B. *Streptomyces*
    C. *Rhodococcus*
    D. *Corynebacterium*
    E. *Listeria*

220. Which enterobacteriaceae family member is non-motile at body temperature, but motile at room temperature?
    A. *Shigella*
    B. *Yersinia*
    C. *Kingella*
    D. *Klebsiella*
    E. *Serratia*

221. Which of the following results of the Kligler iron agar/triple sugar iron (KIA/TSI) slant tests excludes enterobacteriaceae?
    A. alkaline slant/alkaline butt
    B. alkaline slant/acid butt
    C. alkaline slant/acid butt with H_2S production
    D. acid slant/acid butt
    E. acid slant/acid butt with H_2S production

222. Which of the following tests is positive in *Shigella*?
    A. lactose fermentation
    B. Voges-Proskauer
    C. methyl red
    D. indole
    E. motility

223. Which of the following is responsible for most cases of red blood cell-transfusion-associated septic transfusion reactions?
    A. *Yersinia enterocolitica*
    B. *Yersinia pestis*
    C. *Yersinia pseudotuberculosis*
    D. *Citrobacter*
    E. *Edwardsiella*

3: Microbiology Questions

224. This organism can be distinguished from *E. coli* by its H_2S production and from *Salmonella* by a positive indole test:
    A. *Citrobacter*
    B. *Acinetobacter*
    C. *Yersinia*
    D. *Edwardsiella*
    E. *Proteus*

225. Infection with which strain of *E. coli* most closely resembles infection with *V. cholerae*?
    A. ETEC
    B. EIEC
    C. EPEC
    D. EHEC
    E. EAggEC

226. Which of the following results is most consistent and specific for *E. coli* O157:H7?
    A. inability to ferment lactose
    B. inability to ferment sorbitol
    C. indole positivity
    D. growth on MacConkey
    E. positive string test

227. Which of the following organs act as a reservoir for *Salmonella typhi,* leading to intermittent bacteremia?
    A. liver
    B. gall bladder
    C. spleen
    D. A & B
    E. A, B, C

228. Which of the following *V. cholerae* O antigen types are associated with clinical cholera?
    A. O1
    B. O139
    C. O232
    D. A & B
    E. A, B, C

229. What is the optimal growth temperature for *Pseudomonas*?
    A. 22°C
    B. 30°C
    C. 37°C
    D. 42°C
    E. 55°C

230. Which of the following amino acids is required as a supplement in the growth media for *Francisella tularensis*?
    A. phenylalanine
    B. cysteine
    C. tryptophan
    D. proline
    E. alanine

3: Microbiology Questions

231. What is the preferred assay for the presumptive diagnosis of tularemia?
    A. blood culture
    B. ulcer fluid culture
    C. serology
    D. PCR
    E. rapid EIA toxin test

232. Where do the majority of *Brucella* infections in the U.S. occur?
    A. Alaska
    B. Florida and other gulf states
    C. Texas and California
    D. New Hampshire, Vermont, and Maine
    E. Washington and Oregon

233. Which species of *Haemophilus* requires only X factor (hemin)?
    A. *H. influenzae*
    B. *H. parainfluenza*
    C. *H. parahaemolyticus*
    D. *H. haemolyticus*
    E. *H. ducreyi*

234. The growth characteristics of *Legionella* (no growth on SBA or MacConkey, grows on BCYE) are very similar to this organism:
    A. *C. jejuni*
    B. *F. tularensis*
    C. *C. canimorsus*
    D. *B. pertussis*
    E. *P. multocida*

235. Which test helps distinguish *Campylobacter jejuni* from other species of *Campylobacter*?
    A. hippurate hydrolysis
    B. Campy-BAP plate growth
    C. growth at 42°C
    D. oxidase positivity
    E. catalase positivity

236. Which organism causes rat-bite fever?
    A. *Streptobacillus moniliformis*
    B. *Capnocytophaga canimorsus*
    C. *Campylobacter jejuni*
    D. *Haemophilus parahaemolyticus*
    E. *Tropheryma whippelli*

237. Which of the following diagnostic tests for *H. pylori* <u>cannot</u> be used to document post-therapeutic eradication?
    A. serologic IgG anti-*H. pylori*
    B. urea breath test
    C. stool antigen test
    D. stool culture
    E. histologic examination of biopsy tissue

3: Microbiology Questions

238. Which criteria help to distinguish *T. whippelli* from *Mycobacterium avium-intracellulare*?
    A. PAS stain
    B. AFB stain
    C. intestinal infection
    D. A & B
    E. A, B, C

239. Which of the following is/are considered tertiary syphilis complications?
    A. neurological
    B. gummatous
    C. cardiovascular
    D. A & B
    E. A, B, C

240. Which histologic feature(s) do lesions in all stages of syphilis share?
    A. plasma cell infiltrate
    B. obliterative endarteritis
    C. demonstrable presence of spirochetes
    D. A & B
    E. A, B, C

241. At which stage of syphilis are the non-treponemal tests <u>most</u> sensitive for detection?
    A. primary syphilis
    B. secondary syphilis
    C. tertiary syphilis
    D. treated syphilis
    E. at several stages, the sensitivity is 100%

242. Which animal(s) function as a reservoir for *B. burgdorfei*?
    A. white-footed mouse
    B. white-tailed deer
    C. black rat
    D. A & B
    E. A, B, C

243. What's the most common cardiac manifestations of Lyme disease?
    A. obstructive hypertrophic cardiomyopathy
    B. A-V block secondary to myositis
    C. amyloid deposition
    D. mitral valve prolapse
    E. myocardial infarction

244. How is the diagnosis of *Borrelia recurrentis* (relapsing fever) made?
    A. serological confirmation of anti-*Borrelia* antibodies
    B. culture in Barber-Stoenner-Kelly medium
    C. PCR amplification from wound
    D. identification of organisms in thick blood film
    E. elementary body identification

3: Microbiology Questions

245. Conjunctival suffusion and scleral icterus are pathognomonic for infection with this organism:
    A. *Borrelia burgdorfei*
    B. *Borrelia recurrentis*
    C. *Leptospira interrogans*
    D. *B. aalborgi*
    E. *T. carateum*

246. Which of the following is the intracellular form of *Chlamydia*?
    A. the elementary body
    B. large-cell variant
    C. the reticulate body
    D. the MOMP body
    E. small-cell variant

247. Which serotype of *C. trachomatis* causes lymphogranuloma venereum?
    A. A
    B. B
    C. D
    D. F
    E. L

248. What is the most common cause of infection with *Chlamydia psittaci*?
    A. human contact
    B. bird contact
    C. domestic cat contact
    D. rat contact
    E. cattle contact

249. Members of the *Rickettsiae* have a predilection for infecting which of the following types of cells?
    A. hepatocytes
    B. erythrocytes precursor cells
    C. histiocytes
    D. endothelial cells
    E. myoepithelial cells

250. Which of the following conditions predisposes patients to a more severe form of Rocky Mountain Spotted Fever?
    A. sickle cell trait
    B. absence of Duffy antigen
    C. hemoglobin C disease
    D. beta-thalassemia
    E. glucose-6-phosphate deficiency

251. What organism is predominantly found in North America and is seen as a morula form in peripheral blood smears?
    A. *Rickettsia prowazekii*
    B. *Rickettsia typhi*
    C. *Anaplasma phagocytophila*
    D. *Bartonella bacilliformis*
    E. *Coxiella burnetti*

3: Microbiology Questions

252. Which best describes the characteristic granulomas found in Q fever?
   A.   garlanded granulomas
   B.   caseating granulomas
   C.   ring granulomas
   D.   neutrophilic granulomas
   E.   necrotizing granulomas

253. Which of the following variant forms of *Coxiella burnetti* can survive extracellularly?
   A.   reticular body
   B.   small cell variant
   C.   elementary body
   D.   large cell variant
   E.   phase II variant

254. Which of the following organisms is associated with trench fever?
   A.   *Bartonella quintana*
   B.   *Bartonella henselae*
   C.   *Bartonella bacilliformis*
   D.   *Mycoplasma hominis*
   E.   *Ureaplasma urealyticum*

255. Which of the following organisms can cause the formation of stellate microabscesses with parasitized palisading histiocytes?
   A.   *Bartonella henselae*
   B.   *Francisella tularensis*
   C.   *Chlamydia trachomatis*
   D.   A & B
   E.   A, B, C

256. What feature of *Mycoplasma* defines the organism?
   A.   lack of nuclear DNA
   B.   lack of cell wall
   C.   RNA-only genome
   D.   motility
   E.   hyphal growth

257. What non-specific antibody is *M. pneumoniae* associated with?
   A.   cold agglutinin IgM anti-I
   B.   warm anti-i
   C.   antinuclear antibody
   D.   anti-mitochondrial antibody
   E.   anti-liver/kidney microsomal antibody

258. All of the following organisms produce H_2S, <u>except</u>:
   A.   *Salmonella*
   B.   *Proteus*
   C.   *Citrobacter*
   D.   *Shigella*
   E.   *Edwardsiella*

3: Microbiology Questions

259. All of the following species of *Staphylococcus* are coagulase positive, <u>except</u>:
    A. *S. aureus*
    B. *S. hyicus*
    C. *S. delphini*
    D. *S. intermedius*
    E. *S. saprophyticus*

260. Which of the following is considered a major criterion for the diagnosis of acute rheumatic fever as defined by the Jones criteria?
    A. fever
    B. elevated ESR
    C. Sydenham chorea
    D. arthralgia
    E. prolonged PR interval

261. Which mycobacterial species resembles a shepherd's crook?
    A. *Mycobacterium tuberculosis*
    B. *Mycobacterium marinum*
    C. *Mycobacterium gordonae*
    D. *Mycobacterium kansasii*
    E. *Mycobacterium avium-intracellulare*

262. Which of the following features identifies a mycobacterial stain as presumptive *M. tuberculosis*?
    A. positive acid-fast staining with cording in broth culture
    B. NAP-sensitivity of broth-grown mycobacteria
    C. arylsulfatase positivity
    D. A & B
    E. A, B, C

263. Which of the following slow-growing *Mycobacterium* accumulates niacin?
    A. *M. tuberculosis*
    B. *M. bovis*
    C. *M. africanum*
    D. *M. avium-intracellulare*
    E. *M. kansasii*

264. To which of the Runyon classification groups does *M. tuberculosis* belong?
    A. Group I
    B. Group II
    C. Group III
    D. Group IV
    E. none of the above

265. Which of the following *Mycobacterium* species, although technically a Runyon Group II, could also be considered a Class I organism under certain conditions?
    A. *M. kansasii*
    B. *M. szulgai*
    C. *M. scrofulaceum*
    D. *M. gordonii*
    E. *M. thermoresistible*

3: Microbiology Questions

266. What percentage of immunocompetent people infected with primary TB infection develop active TB?
    A.   0%
    B.   10%
    C.   50%
    D.   90%
    E.   100%

267. Which of the following coinfections often lead to smear-negative TB and PPD anergic false-negative results?
    A.   HCV
    B.   *Borrelia burgdorfei*
    C.   *Ascaris lumbricoides*
    D.   HIV
    E.   methicillin-resistant *Staphylococcus aureus*

268. What condition particularly predisposes toward *M. kansasii* pulmonary disease?
    A.   pneumoconiosis
    B.   pre-existing *M. tuberculosis*
    C.   squamous cell carcinoma of the lung
    D.   diabetes mellitus
    E.   congenital pulmonary adenomatoid malformation

269. Which of the following mycobacterial species is the cause of the Buruli ulcer?
    A.   *M. leprae*
    B.   *M. ulcerans*
    C.   *M. fortuitum*
    D.   *M. marinum*
    E.   *M. chelonei*

270. Which of the following features are associated with lepromatous leprosy?
    A.   widespread skin infections
    B.   superinfection with *Strongyloides*
    C.   non-caseating granulomas with few AFB
    D.   A & B
    E.   A, B, C

3: Microbiology Answers

1.   B.   **CYSTITIS IN A PARALYZED YOUNG MAN WITH A SPINAL INJURY.**

The difference between complicated and uncomplicated UTIs is that once an uncomplicated UTI is treated, there is an expectation that the disease will resolve whereas a complicated UTI may have recurrences or long-term consequences - frequently due to an underlying predisposing condition.
QCCP2, **Urinary tract infection,** p 148

2.   E.   **A, B, C.**

For the most part asymptomatic bacteriuria does not require treatment. It is defined as $>10^3$CFU/mL in a voided urine specimen (actually, two consecutive samples in a woman due to the high contamination rate) without the symptoms of cystitis (frequency, urgency, dysuria, etc).
QCCP2, **UTI,** p 148

3.   D.   **URINE DIPSTICK POSITIVE FOR NITRITE.**

All of the tests presented have fairly high sensitivity, but only the presence of nitrite is somewhat specific. Since the nitrite test requires the presence of bacteria capable of reducing nitrate to nitrite any bug unable to do so will not be detected, eg, enterococci. The most sensitive and specific surrogate to detect UTI is a combination of leukocyte esterase and nitrite.
QCCP2, **Lab approach,** p 148

4.   C.   **$>10^3$ CFU/ML.**

It may appear nitpicky, but the traditional teaching has always been $>10^5$ CFU/mL based on studies that showed bacterial levels that high were strongly correlated with pyelonephritis. More recent studies have shown lower levels of bacteriuria may be associated with disease and require treatment.
QCCP2, **Laboratory approach,** p 149

5.   B.   *CORYNEBACTERIUM* **D2.**

Corynebacterium is a common cause of hospital-acquired UTI and is capable of being cultured, unlike the other organisms, which are common causes of culture-negative UTI.
QCCP2, **Specific agents,** p 149

6.   D.   **ADENOVIRUS.**

Adenovirus, especially serotype 11 is associated with the hemorrhagic cystitis that can be seen in immunosuppressed patients, especially those post-bone marrow transplant.
QCCP2, **Specific agents,** p 149

7.   B.   **NOROVIRUS.**

Viruses account for the vast majority of cases of infectious diarrhea, especially the members of the norovirus family. Bacterial causes are responsible for 10% of the cases with *E. coli* accounting for the majority of those cases.
QCCP2, **Infectious diarrhea,** p 149

3: Microbiology Answers

8. B. **ENTEROHEMORRHAGIC *E COLI*.**

   E. coli O157:H7, or enterohemorrhagic *E. coli* (EHEC), should be considered in the presentation of bloody diarrhea without neutrophils. The presence of neutrophils with bloody diarrhea suggests other causes, such as *Clostridium difficile, Salmonella, Campylobacter,* and *Shigella.*
   QCCP2, **Infectious diarrhea, Differential diagnosis,** p 149

9. A. **MENTAL STATUS CHANGES.**

   The hemolytic uremic syndrome associated with *E. coli* O157:H7 bears many similarities to the thrombotic thrombocytopenic purpura due to decreased amounts of ADAMTS-13 protein. The major difference in the clinical presentation between HUS and TTP is that patients with TTP will exhibit neurological symptoms, which usually manifest as mental status changes.
   QCCP2, **Infectious diarrhea - specific agents,** p 150

10. D. **AN OTHERWISE HEALTHY 33-YEAR-OLD MAN.**

    A number of groups are at an increased risk of *Salmonella* bacteremia, the primary cause of morbidity in patients infected with *Salmonella*. These include the immunocompromised (choice B), the very young (choice A), the very old (choice C), and those with permanent prosthetic devices (choice E).
    QCCP2, **Infectious diarrhea - specific agents,** p 150

11. A. **CAMPYLOBACTER JEJUNI.**

    Overall, the majority of cases of GBS (~70%) have either no identifiable cause or are due to a multitude of different organisms. *C. jejuni* accounts for the largest percentage of cases due to a single identifiable organism.
    QCCP2, **Infectious diarrhea - specific agents,** p 150

12. C. **HLA-B27.**

    The reactive arthropathy, or Reiter syndrome ("Can't see [uveitis], can't pee [urethritis], can't climb a tree [arthritis]"), is seen predominantly in patients expressing the HLA-B27 allele.
    QCCP2, **Infectious diarrhea - specific agents,** p 150

13. D. **A & B.**

    While O1 and O139 cause epidemic cholera (voluminous rice water stools), other non-O1, non-O139 strains can cause self-limited colitis or, less commonly, wound infections. Most cases of cholera are due to the consumption of contaminated shellfish or rice.
    QCCP2, **Specific agents - *Vibrio*,** p 150

14. B. **VIBRIO PARAHAEMOLYTICUS.**

    Both *V. parahaemolyticus* and *V. vulnificus* are associated with exposure to contaminated seafood or seawater. A common history of eating seafood or getting cut while either swimming in the sea or cleaning a fish tank is often seen. *V. parahaemolyticus* is much more common than *V. vulnificus*.
    QCCP2, **Specific agents,** p 150

3: Microbiology Answers

15.   B.   ᴘYV.

This may be more detail than many people want about *Yersinia enterocolitica*, but it is an easy subject for a test question. Another important fact about *Yersinia* is that, like *Campylobacter*, infections can be seen in a higher percentage of patients expressing the HLA-B27 allele and the associated reactive arthropathy.
QCCP2, **Infectious diarrhea - specific agents,** p 150-1

16.   D.   ꜱᴛᴏᴏʟ EIA.

Neither culture nor PCR are routinely performed in cases of suspected *Entamoeba histolytica*. Biopsy and stool microscopy are limited by both the paucity of organisms and the possible presence of related non-pathogenic *Entamoeba* species, such as *E. dispar*. Enzyme-linked immunoassay has the highest sensitivity and specificity.
QCCP2, **Infectious diarrhea, specific agents,** p 151

17.   E.   ʀᴏᴛᴀᴠɪʀᴜꜱ.

While Norwalk virus is a common cause of viral gastroenteritis in all age groups, pediatric patients are most often infected with rotavirus. Norwalk virus is the most common cause of adult viral gastroenteritis and is often responsible for the diarrheal outbreaks on cruise ships, resorts, or nursing homes. Norwalk viruses are spread by food and person-to-person contact.
QCCP2, **Infectious diarrhea, specific agents,** p 150

18.   E.   ꜱᴛᴏᴏʟ ʟᴀᴄᴛᴏꜰᴇʀʀɪɴ.

Stool microscopy is a laborious process utilized to detect the presence of leukocytes as well as ova and parasites. Instead of searching for leukocytes, one can perform assays that detect the production of a protein produced by neutrophilic lactoferrin.
QCCP2, **Infectious diarrhea, specific agents,** p 150

19.   B.   *Mᴙᴄᴏᴘʟᴀꜱᴍᴀ ᴘɴᴇᴜᴍᴏɴɪᴀᴇ.*

Atypical causes of community-acquired pneumonia, such as *Mycoplasma pneumoniae* and *Chlamydia pneumoniae*, are much less often a cause of pneumonia in the nursing home. *S. pneumoniae* tops the list, followed by *Haemophilus influenzae*, but also other causes, such as aspirated oral flora (aerobic gram-negative bacilli and anaerobes), are common causes of pneumonia in the communally-living elderly.
QCCP2, **Pneumonia, differential diagnosis,** p 152

20.   D.   ᴀ Cᴇɴᴛʀᴀʟ Vᴀʟʟᴇʏ Cᴀʟɪꜰᴏʀɴɪᴀ ᴍɪɢʀᴀɴᴛ ᴡᴏʀᴋᴇʀ.

Valley fever, or San Joaquin fever, are caused by *Coccidioides immitis*, which is seen in high, dusty deserts, such as those found in S.E. California, Arizona, and New Mexico. Sandstorms are responsible for spreading the spores.
QCCP2, **T3.1, Risk factors for agents of pneumonia,** p 152

21.   B.   *Pꜱᴇᴜᴅᴏᴍᴏɴᴀꜱ ᴀᴇʀᴜɢɪɴᴏꜱᴀ.*

Pseudomonas (both *P. aeruginosa* and *P. cepaciae*), *Burkholderia*, and *Stenotrophomonas*, all gram-negative, lactose non-fermenting organisms - as well as *Staphylococcus aureus* - are often seen as causes of pneumonia in patients with cystic fibrosis.
QCCP2, **T3.1,** p 152

3: Microbiology Answers

22. A. **SPUTUM CULTURE.**

A very high percentage (up to 10%) of normal healthy adults are colonized with *Streptococcus pneumoniae,* leading to a very high false positive rate. Bacteremia occurs at a very high rate with *Pneumococcus,* making blood culture a viable tool to diagnose pneumonia. In addition, a urine antigen that tests similar to the one utilized for the diagnosis of *Legionella* has a potential use in the future.
QCCP2, **Pneumonia, specific agents,** p 152

23. E. **A, B, C.**

Haemophilus influenzae causes a severe pneumonia seen most often in patients with COPD, especially those with more chronic bronchitis than emphysema and those who are treated with antibiotics or steroids
QCCP2, **Pneumonia, specific agents,** p 152

24. C. **HYPONATREMIA.**

Patients with Legionnaire disease develop very severe illness with very high fever, mental status changes and hyponatremia. Diagnosis can be made with culture, but a rapid urinary antigen test is also available.
QCCP2, **Pneumonia, specific agents,** p 153

25. D. **A & B.**

It is important to note that *Pseudomonas* often leads to a chronic state with frequent re-infections, even with treatment. Also, the pneumonia associated with *Pseudomonas* is severe, with necrosis and an acute respiratory distress syndrome presentation.
QCCP2, **Pneumonia, specific agents,** p 153

26. D. **SEROLOGY.**

While culture is the gold standard, it is difficult to obtain appropriate specimens, so culture is not often performed. Serology is the most often used means to diagnose *C. pneumoniae,* with either a 4-fold increase in IgG or an IgM titer >1:16.
QCCP2, **Pneumonia, specific agents,** p 153

27. A. **DEER MOUSE.**

Peromyscus maniculatus, or the deer mouse, spreads the virus in its infected feces. People living in close contact with animals are at a particularly high risk. Infected individuals experience a flu-like prodrome with thrombocytopenia, followed by additional peripheral blood findings, such as increased immunoblastic lymphocytes (>10%). Finally, patients develop ARDS where more than 1/3 of patients don't survive.
QCCP2, **Viral pneumonia,** p 153

28. D. **CORONAVIRUS.**

SARS is a severe respiratory disease spread from human to human and caused by a coronavirus (SARS-CoV). After a 1-2 week incubation, patients develop acute respiratory distress syndrome.
QCCP2, **Viral pneumonia,** p 154

3: Microbiology Answers

29. B. **STATUS OF UNDERLYING VALVE.**

The differential diagnosis of organisms that cause infective endocarditis can be divided according to valve status: the organisms that infect normal valves are different from those that infect abnormal native valves and those that infect prosthetic valves.
QCCP2, **Infective endocarditis, differential diagnosis**, p 154

30. D. *STAPHYLOCOCCUS AUREUS.*

The most common cause of normal native valve endocarditis is *S. aureus*, which leads to a severe and destructive infection. Other potential causes of normal native valve endocarditis can include *S. milleri* and enterococci. Abnormal native valves are usually victim to less severe, subacute endocarditis, caused by viridans *Strep* or the HACEK organisms. Prosthetic valves are most commonly infected by *Staphylococcus epidermidis*.
QCCP2, **Infectious endocarditis, differential diagnosis**, p 154

31. D. **VIRIDANS** *STREPTOCOCCI.*

In addition to carcinoid heart syndrome and other difficult-to-culture infectious causes, such as *Bartonella*, *Chlamydia*, and *Legionella*, are common causes of blood culture-negative endocarditis. Viridans *Streptococci* infections typically occur on damaged native valves and can be cultured.
QCCP2, **Infectious endocarditis, differential diagnosis**, p 155

32. E. **A, B, C.**

Austrian syndrome refers to the triad of endocarditis, typically caused by *S. pneumoniae*, with pneumonia and meningitis. The syndrome was first described by Robert Austrian in 1957 and has been shown to be most closely associated with alcoholism.
QCCP2, **Infectious endocarditis, specific agents**, p 155

33. C. *CANDIDA* **SPP.**

While *Torulopsis glabrata* and *Aspergillus* spp account for a significant number of cases of fungal endocarditis, *Candida* spp are responsible for the majority. Certain factors predispose toward fungal endocarditis - immunodeficiency, long term antibiotic use, and IV drug use.
QCCP2, **Infective endocarditis, specific agents**, p 155

34. E. **THREE PERIPHERAL BLOOD SAMPLES EVERY 8 HOURS FOR THE FIRST 24 HOURS.**

In addition, the samples should be from 3 different sites and taken approximately 1 hour before a fever spike. Also, paired samples are encouraged (one aerobic, one anaerobic). The documentation of continuous bacteremia is an important diagnostic tool.
QCCP2, **Laboratory approach to diagnosis**, p 156

35. D. **GRAM STAIN MORPHOLOGY OF BACTERIA IS OFTEN ALTERED BY ANTIBIOTICS.**

Often, antibiotic therapy leads to a change in the morphology of bacteria, including their gram stain characteristics (positive, negative), which makes identification difficult.
QCCP2, **Laboratory approach to diagnosis**, p 156

3: Microbiology Answers

36. B. **MENTAL STATUS CHANGES.**

The CNS infections can present along the spectrum from meningitis, both bacterial and viral, to encephalitis, often with overlapping features. The principal presentation of encephalitis is usually mental status changes, whereas the other choices presented tend to dominate the presentation of meningitis.
QCCP2, **Meningitis, differential diagnosis,** p 156

37. B. **INCREASED GLUCOSE.**

Meningitis can be classified by CSF laboratory as well as microscopic results. Aseptic meningitis, which is most often viral in nature, typically presents with all the features listed above, with the exception that glucose levels are usually normal or even slightly decreased.
QCCP2, **Meningitis,** p 156

38. D. **VIRUS.**

Overall, aseptic meningitis is more common than bacterial meningitis and the most common causes of aseptic meningitis are viral. Of the viral causes, the most common are in the family of *Enteroviridae*, such as poliovirus, Coxsackie A and B, and echovirus. The viruses cause encephalitis with a summer- and fall-predominant distribution.
QCCP2, **Meningitis,** p 157

39. C. *N. MENINGITIDIS.*

Neisseria meningitidis is a common cause of meningitis in infants through adults. *H. influenzae* used to be the predominant bacterial cause, but the advent of universal vaccination led to a decrease in prevalence of *H. influenzae* meningitis.
QCCP2, **Meningitis,** p 157

40. A. *S. PNEUMONIAE.*

The pneumococcus reigns supreme in adults, both in cases of meningitis and pneumonia. The remaining choices are listed in rough order of decreasing prevalence as causes of bacterial meningitis.
QCCP2, **Meningitis,** p 157

41. D. **HSV-1.**

Temporal encephalitis is associated with HSV-1. There is an interesting set of cerebral topographic-related syndromes associated with HSV encephalitis, such as aphasia and phantom perception of odors and tastes. Another tip-off to HSV is RBCs in the CSF. The prognosis for HSV encephalitis is poor.
QCCP2, **Meningitis, specific agents,** p 157

42. D. **BIRDS.**

Remember to stay away from dead birds! The host organism is the bird, which passes on the virus through a mosquito vector to humans. Arboviruses in general (to include Eastern equine, St. Louis, California, etc.) are best diagnosed through serological means.
QCCP2, **Meningitis, specific agents,** p 157

3: Microbiology Answers

43. A. **LYMPHOCYTIC CHORIOMENINGITIS VIRUS.**

     LCMV is the most common cause of winter/spring viral encephalitis, while enteroviruses such as Coxsackie, are the main causes of summer/fall epidemics. LCMV is spread to humans through contact with infected mouse feces.
     QCCP2, **Meningitis, specific agents,** p 158

44. B. **CAPSULE.**

     The presence of a capsule separates the typeable (capsulated) from the non-typeable (unencapsulated). Furthermore, the typeable strains are categorized into serotypes according to the type of capsule protein present - the most prevalent serotype being type B.
     QCCP2, **Meningitis, specific agents,** p 158

45. E. *NEISSERIA MENINGITIDIS.*

     N. meningitidis is associated with outbreaks of meningitis in children and adults in close living conditions, such as schools, dorms, barracks, or nursing homes (though less prevalent in the elderly). Systemic meningococcemia is associated with a petechial rash and hemorrhagic adrenal infarction (Waterhouse-Friedrichsen syndrome), both of which have a poor prognosis.
     QCCP2, **Meningitis, specific agents,** p 158

46. C. *LISTERIA MONOCYTOGENES.*

     Besides age (<1 month and older than 70 years), predisposing factors toward the development of *Listeria* meningitis include diabetes and immunosuppression (steroids, HIV, and transplantation).
     QCCP2, **Meningitis, specific agents,** p 158

47. E. *NAEGLERIA FOWLERI.*

     Naegleria infection is associated with fresh water exposure. The organism migrates through the nasopharynx and invades the brain through the cribriform sinus. Often there is a history of trauma in fresh water (water skiing accident, diving accident). The infection is especially virulent, often causing death within days. *Acanthamoeba* can also cause encephalitis, but with a granulomatous appearance. *Acanthamoeba* is also responsible for the majority of cases of amebic keratitis.
     QCCP2, **Meningitis, specific agents,** p 158

48. D. **BACTERIAL.**

     The cause of meningitis can be narrowed down with the CSF chemistry. Low glucose and high protein/WBC count is consistent with a bacterial meningitis. The WBC differential is typically left-shifted with a predominance of neutrophils.
     QCCP2, **Laboratory evaluation,** p 158

49. D. *LISTERIA MONOCYTOGENES.*

     Listeria is a very difficult organism to identify in CSF. Gram stain sensitivity is less than 50% and there is no commercially available latex agglutination test at this time. Culture is the main source of positive identification.
     QCCP2, **Laboratory evaluation,** p 159

3: Microbiology Answers

50.   A.   **JOINT PAIN WITH POSITIVE BACTEREMIA IN 2 SUCCESSIVE BLOOD CULTURES.**

Each of the applicable criteria is fairly specific for prosthetic joint infection. There are several etiologies of joint infection. The most common is the direct introduction of bacteria, though in a small percentage of late infection, hematogenous spread is the cause.
QCCP2, **Prosthetic joint infection and other clinical syndromes,** p 159

51.   B.   *STAPHYLOCOCCUS EPIDERMIDIS.*

Coagulase-negative staph account for almost 1/2 of the cases of prosthetic joint infections, most often presenting months after surgery. This makes sense since coag-negative staph is a normal skin flora microbe and the majority of joint infections are due to the introduction of bacteria during surgery. On the other hand, since it is normal skin flora, coag-negative staph is a common cause of contamination of cultures.
QCCP2, **Prosthetic joint infections and other clinical syndromes,** p 159

52.   C.   *TOXOCARA CANIS.*

Ancylostoma is the causative agent of cutaneous larval migrans, while *Loa loa* inhabits the subcutis and conjunctiva. *Francisella tularensis* causes ulceroglandular fever. *Chlamydia trachomatis* causes lymphogranuloma venereum and trachoma.
QCCP2, **T3.2,** p 160

53.   B.   **GROUP A *STREP***

Coag-negative strep causes many cases of post-traumatic cellulitis; *Pasteurella* is associated with animal bites, *Aeromonas* with fresh water and *V. vulnificus* with salt water exposure.
QCCP2, **T3.2,** p 160

54.   D.   **COXSACKIE B.**

Coxsackie A and B are frequently confused for each other when it comes to the diseases that they each cause. Coxsackie A causes hand-foot-mouth disease, so named for the most common locations of the lesions. Coxsackie B, on the other hand, is responsible for the majority of cases of viral myocarditis.
QCCP2, **T3.2,** p 160

55.   E.   **EBV.**

EBV, along with rubella and the arboviridae, are not routinely cultured, but rather diagnosed based on the positive serology. Similarly, rota- and rhabdoviruses are not cultured; their diagnosis depends on virus-specific antigen detection.
QCCP2, **Virology Laboratory Methods,** p 162

56.   B.   **CELL LINE (SECONDARY CELL CULTURE).**

MRC-5, named for the Medical Research Council where they were first propagated, are a secondary cell line with limited viability. Cells don't survive after a number of transfers, unlike a primary cell culture, which can't be transferred at all, or an established cell line, which can be transferred nearly illimitably. Human diploid fibroblasts are another type of secondary cell culture.
QCCP2, **Viral lab methods,** p 162

3: Microbiology Answers

57.   **A.** *LOA LOA.*

Loa loa is spread by the mango fly (*Chrysops*). There are a few memorable and significant vector-organism pairs to remember. Lyme disease, ehrlichiosis, and babesiosis are spread by the *Ixodes* tick. *Borrelia recurrentis* is the only borrelial species spread by a louse (the human body louse) rather than a tick. *Trypanosoma cruzi* and the reduviid bug, *Leishmania* (cutaneous) and the sandfly (*Phlebotomus*), and *Onchocerca* and the black fly (*Simulium*) are all high-yield.
QCCP2, **T3.3, Vectors,** p 163

58.   **D.** **ADENOVIRUS.**

Hep2 cells are derived from the upper respiratory tract, a region for which adenovirus has a high tropism (same with RSV).
QCCP2, **T3.4,** p 154

59.   **B.** **SIMIAN VIRUS.**

SV is a very common cause of false positive hemabsorption results. An uninoculated control should be run concurrent with the patient sample as a negative control. Another common contaminant is *Mycoplasma,* which can cause poor growth in cell lines and decreased infective potential of the viruses.
QCCP2, **Virology, lab methods,** p 164

60.   **D.** **COXSACKIE A VIRUS.**

Clostridium botulinum can cause flaccid paralysis in infants, but it's not a virus, and it's not assayed in suckling mice. Adenovirus causes cytopathic effect in Hep2 cells, parvovirus needs erythroid precursors and RSV causes syncytia formation in Hep2 cells.
QCCP2, **T3.5,** p 164

61.   **E.** **A, B, C.**

If you think about the histopathology of these viruses, it helps. RSV of course causes syncytia formation - it's in the name! Measles infection can cause the formation of Warthin-Finkeldey giant cells, and then there's the 3 Ms describing the nuclei of cells infected with HSV - multinucleation, margination, and molding.
QCCP2, **T3.6, viral histology,** p 165

62.   **D.** **A & B.**

Both CMV and measles are known for having nuclear and cytoplasmic inclusions. HSV and adenovirus have nuclear inclusions only, while rabies is the only major human viral pathogen with cytoplasmic inclusions only (Negri bodies).
QCCP2, **T3.6, Viral histology,** p 165

63.   **B.** **4 FOLD.**

Paired sera collected 7-10 days apart is used to measure the elevation of IgG titers between convalescence and acute illness. Elevation of 4-fold is considered strong evidence for an acute infection, while a single elevated IgM titer has similar connotations.
QCCP2, **Virology, laboratory evaluation,** p 165

3: Microbiology Answers

64.   E.   **A, B, C.**

The HSV family of viruses is made up of the prototypical enveloped DNA viruses. Three of the members lie dormant within dorsal root ganglia until they are reactivated.
QCCP2, **Human herpes viruses, T3.8,** p 166

65.   C.   TO DECREASE THE RISK OF NEONATAL HERPES.

Vertical transmission of HSV from genital lesions to an infant can cause neonatal HSV infection, which can manifest as skin lesions to encephalitis, retinitis, even sepsis. There is a very high transmission rate with vaginal birth.
QCCP2, **Human herpes viruses,** p 167

66.   A.   DIRECT FLUORESCENT ANTIBODY STAIN.

The shell vial technique is very popular in virus labs due to its small size, low volume, ease of use, and ability to run multiple samples in parallel. The assay involves centrifugation of the patient sample onto a cover slip coated with a culture monolayer. In a shell vial assay for HSV, cytopathic effect is NOT used as indication of a positive assay, but rather the detection of viral antigens by direct fluorescent antibody staining.
QCCP2, **Human herpes virus,** p 167

67.   E.   ALL OF THE ABOVE ARE POTENTIALLY UTILIZED IN THE DIAGNOSIS OF CONGENITAL VARICELLA.

The incidence of perinatal varicella is highest when the mother contracts VZV within a few days of delivery, with the incidence declining inversely with gestational age. Because of the extremely high infectivity of VZV contracted perinatally (50-60%), VZ immunoglobulin is recommended for prophylaxis, perhaps along with acyclovir.
QCCP2, **VZV,** p 167

68.   D.   **VZV.**

VZV reactivation in a dermatomal pattern is the cause of the painful shingles rash. When reactivation occurs in the facial nerve the Ramsay-Hunt syndrome can result in facial paralysis, vertigo, tinnitus, and otalgia.
QCCP2, **VZV,** p 167-8

69.   A.   HIV PATIENTS WITH CD4 COUNTS <100/ML.

In addition to HIV patients with very low CD4 counts, immunocompromised transplant recipients are at an increased risk, though not as great as that of HIV patients. Typically, primary CMV presents with a mononucleosis-like syndrome, which can progress to a pneumonia - especially in neonates and the immunocompromised.
QCCP2, **CMV,** p 168

70.   B.   **CMV.**

Passed transplacentally, the risk of *in utero* infection is greatest when the mother acquires a primary CMV infection while pregnant. The effects from *in utero* infection can range from severe to mild, with the most common manifestation of sensorineural hearing loss.
QCCP2, **CMV,** p 168

3: Microbiology Answers

71.   A.   **PREGNANCY STATUS.**

While the effects of primary and reactivated CMV infection in pregnant women are potentially dire, there is no statistically significant effect on the rate of seropositivity. The rate of seropositivity in Africa is much greater than most of the rest of the world. The risk of CMV infection increases with age (presumably due to increased risk of exposure). Also, lower socioeconomic status is associated with increased CMV seropositivity.
QCCP2, **CMV,** p 168

72.   C.   **FLACCID PARALYSIS IN SUCKLING MICE AFTER INJECTION.**

In addition to tissue histology looking for the characteristic nuclear owl eye, inclusions can be performed if diagnostic tissue is available. Observation of flaccid paralysis in suckling mice is used to diagnose Coxsackie A virus.
QCCP2, **CMV,** p 169

73.   A.   **SALIVA.**

They don't call it the kissing disease for nothing! A less common means of transmission is through blood transfusion or solid organ transplantation. Nearly 90% of people in the world have been infected with EBV.
QCCP2, **EBV,** p 169

74.   B.   **CD21.**

The C3d receptor, or CD21, functions as the target for EBV cell entry. P antigen (associated with Donath-Landsteiner ab), paroxysmal nocturnal hemoglobinuria, neutralized by pigeon egg and hydatid cyst fluid) is the parvovirus receptor. Insulin-degrading enzyme is the putative receptor for varicella-zoster virus, while CD4 is the receptor for HIV. Recent studies suggest that CD81 may have a role as a receptor for HCV.
QCCP2, **EBV,** p 169

75.   B.   **SHINGLES.**

Shingles is associated with VZV infection. There are myriad clinical syndromes associated with EBV infection, especially long-term latent effects. In addition to the conditions presented above, primary CNS lymphoma, Burkitt lymphoma, Hodgkin lymphoma, lymphomatoid granulomatosis, and nasopharyngeal carcinoma are all associated with latent EBV infection.
QCCP2, **T3.9,** p 168

76.   E.   **X-LINKED LYMPHOPROLIFERATIVE DISORDER.**

As an X-linked disorder, primarily men are affected. The range that disease can manifest extends from the previously mentioned hepatic necrosis and death to less severe agammaglobulinemia or B-cell lymphoma. The disorder is due to a defect in the SAP gene, which leads to uncontrolled NK/T cell activation.
QCCP2, **EBV,** p 169

77.   D.   **POSITIVE CULTURE.**

Adenopathy is the missing criterion. While positive culture can occur with EBV, it is neither routinely performed, nor required for the diagnosis. These criteria are very restrictive and may miss many cases. Partial fulfillment of criteria can be seen in many other diseases, such as strep pharyngitis, which can have both fever and adenopathy, while the leukocytosis can be seen with CMV or *Toxoplasma* infections.
QCCP2, **EBV,** p 169

3: Microbiology Answers

78.   E.   **A, B, C.**

In addition, rheumatoid factor levels may be increased. For this reason and because the culture of EBV is difficult, routine diagnosis is usually made serologically.
QCCP2, **EBV,** p 169

79.   A.   **IgM antibodies with an affinity for sheep and horse red blood cells.**

Heterophile antibodies are a fairly specific, though not very sensitive indicator of EBV infection. They are also the basis of the Monospot EBV detection agglutination assay.
QCCP2, **EBV,** p 170

80.   B.   **IgM anti-VCA.**

Anti-viral capsid antibodies (VCA) are the only EBV antibodies with a high specificity for the acute phase of infection. This IgM antibody is the first antibody to appear with acute infection but quickly decreases in titer with time. IgM anti-VCA recedes to undetectable titers with convalescence but quickly reappears with virus reactivation.
QCCP2, **EBV,** p 170

81.   B.   **oral hairy leukoplakia.**

In addition to tumors and pre-tumoral lesions, EBER can be shown in the reactive hyperplastic lymphoid tissue of infectious mononucleosis. In some tumors, it is not strongly expressed (~1/2 of Hodgkin disease cases are positive) versus other tumors where it is very strongly expressed (nasopharyngeal carcinoma, NK-T cell lymphoma - nasal type, and endemic-type Burkitt lymphoma).
QCCP2, **EBV,** p 170

82.   E.   **A, B, C.**

The positive correlation between the two stains is highest when observed in the cells that are of interest. LMP1 has a modest false positive rate which can be overcome by narrowing the observation to the cells of interest.
QCCP2, **EBV,** p 171

83.   D.   **A & B.**

Both HHV6 and HHV7 cause overlapping and similar clinical syndromes. A small percentage of those infected develop the characteristic roseola infantum rash. In addition, they are both responsible for a significant number of cases of juvenile febrile seizures, presumably due to their tropism for the CNS.
QCCP2, **HHV6,** p 171

84.   E.   **A, B, C.**

Especially in the immunocompromised patient, HHV8, or KSHV, is responsible for a number of disease processes. The etiologic agent in these cases is identified by FISH, PCR, IHC, or serological means.
QCCP2, **HHV8,** p 171

3: Microbiology Answers

85. D. PAPOVAVIRUS.

The papovaviridae are a family of DNA viruses including the <u>papilloma</u> viruses, <u>poly</u>oma viruses, and <u>va</u>cuolating viruses (SV40) JC, a member of the polyoma virus family, is responsible for progressive multifocal leukoencephalopathy, while another polyoma virus, BK, can cause hemorrhagic cystitis. The BK-induced cystitis is notable for the presence of virus-infected "decoy" cells, so named because they can be easily confused for exfoliated high-grade urothelial carcinoma.
QCCP2, **Papovaviruses,** p 171

86. B. EPISOMAL.

In most benign HPV lesions, the virus DNA is maintained in circular extrachromosomal episomes. The process of integration into the host genome by HPV is more often associated with malignant disease.
QCCP2, **HPV,** p 171

87. E. EPIDERMODYSPLASIA VERRUCIFORMIS.

An autosomal recessive condition mapped to a gene on chromosome 17, EV manifests with upper extremity lesions within the first 10 years, which can progress to invasive squamous cell carcinoma.
QCCP2, **HPV,** p 171

88. D. A & B.

Subtypes 6 and 11 are often associated with low-grade lesions, while the more oncogenic subtypes, such as 16 and 18, are associated with the higher-grade lesions. HPV18 is most commonly associated with cervical adenocarcinoma.
QCCP2, **HPV, T3.11,** p 172

89. D. HBsAb.

All of the other choices, with perhaps the early appearance post-vaccination of HBsAg, should not be seen in a vaccinated individual. HBeAg is present during active viral replication, while anti-HBc is present only in someone who has resolved an acute infection. It is the same with anti-HBe, though this is less associated with resolution than with someone who has just had the HBeAg turn negative in testing.
QCCP2, **HBV,** p 174

90. B. HBsAg.

The persistence of surface antigen is an excellent indicator of chronicity. With acute infection and resolution, surface antigen peaks 2-3 months post-infection and before symptoms, but is completely gone before 6 months, to be replaced by anti-surface antibody (HBsAb) and the clinical symptoms of acute hepatitis. In chronic infection, the surface antibody does not appear, while the surface antigen persists.
QCCP2, **F3.2-3.3,** p 173-4

91. B. THE PERIOD BETWEEN THE DISAPPEARANCE OF HBsAg AND APPEARANCE OF HBcAb.

Less sensitive assays of the past may have missed the diagnosis of HBV if performed in the brief period around 5-6 months post-infection. Serologically, this corresponds to the period between the disappearance of the surface antigen and the appearance of the surface antibody. Nowadays, we can measure IgM anti-HBc during this time period and expect it to be positive.
QCCP2, **HBV,** p 175

3: Microbiology Answers

92. C. HBE.

In the past, HBe antigen was used to classify patients. However, there are issues with the consistency of HBe serology, so now the measurement of HBV DNA copy number has replaced HBe. A copy number of $>10^5$/mL is needed to classify a chronic HBV carrier as "replicative."

QCCP2, **HBV molecular assays,** p 176

93. D. 85%.

The vast majority of people infected with HCV develop chronic infections. Of these, 10-15% become cirrhotic, and of the cirrhotics, 5% (if non-drinkers) will develop hepatocellular carcinoma. Alcohol consumption greatly increases the risk of HCC, especially in the cirrhotic with chronic infection.

QCCP2, **HCV,** p 176

94. B. NO INFECTION OR RECOVERY FROM ACUTE HCV.

A positive anti-HCV could be either a false positive, in the case of non-infection, or it could indicate the patient was one of the 15% of cases where HCV did not develop chronic infection.

QCCP2, **HCV,** p 176

95. D. UNDETECTABLE HCV RNA FOR 24 WEEKS.

A sustained virologic response (SVR) is used to define patients who have responded positively to treatment (IFN/ribavirin). The single most important prognostic predictor of response to IFNs is the genotype of HCV. Types 2 and 3 respond well while type 1, the more common type seen in the U.S., tends to respond poorly.

QCCP2, **HCV,** p 177

96. A. LIVER BIOPSY.

All of the tests mentioned have a role in the diagnosis and management of HCV. However, only liver biopsy can provide the data required to grade inflammation and stage fibrosis of liver infection.

QCCP2, **HCV,** p 177

97. C. HDV.

HDV can only infect hepatocytes that are infected with HBV. Coinfection of patients with HBV and HDV results in a more severe disease and significantly increases the risk of cirrhosis and hepatic failure.

QCCP2, **HBV,** p 175

98. E. A, B, C.

A viral surface protein, hemagglutinin, binds to sialic acid receptors on the surface of respiratory epithelial cells and in turn are expressed on the surface of infected cells. The hemagglutinin has the ability to agglutinate red blood cells, which is the basis of the diagnostic hemadsorption test.

QCCP2, **Orthomyxoviruses,** p 177-8

3: Microbiology Answers

99.   C. H5N1.

There are currently over 15 H and 9 N subtypes, with the numbers growing steadily due to antigenic shifts. Birds are the more common reservoir for influenza, for example, the chickens in S.E. Asian H5N1 avian influenza. The virus can cause an ARDS clinical appearance with a 50% mortality, predominantly affecting teenagers.
QCCP2, **Orthomyxoviruses,** p 178

100.   A.   CULTURE.

Nasopharyngeal, sputum, or throat samples can be used to culture virus, either in cell culture or in the more rapid shell vial assay. All the other tests mentioned, with the exception of the Monospot test, have shown utility in the diagnosis of influenza.
QCCP2, **Orthomyxovirus, diagnosis,** p 178

101.   A.   OTITIS MEDIA.

Superinfection can cause otitis media or pneumonia, especially in immunocompromised patients. All of the other choices can happen with measles infection but for the most part are rare, especially SSPE.
QCCP2, **Measles,** p 179

102.   D.   WARTHIN-FINKELDEY CELL.

The Anitschow cell is seen in rheumatic fever. The Touton giant cell with its wreath-like arrangement of nuclei can be seen with several lesions, including juvenile xanthogranuloma and atypical fibroxanthoma. The floret cell is seen with pleomorphic liposarcoma and the hallmark cell is usually associated with anaplastic large cell lymphoma.
QCCP2, **Measles,** p 179

103.   E.   RESPIRATORY SYNCYTIAL VIRUS.

Respiratory syncytial virus also causes 1/2 of all cases of lower respiratory tract infections in children. Persistence of immunity does not often occur, so reinfection is common. Among other techniques, the characteristic formation of syncytia in Hep-2 cells is used in the diagnosis of RSV.
QCCP2, **RSV,** p 179

104.   B.   RT-PCR.

As of now, RT-PCR is the most rapid and sensitive assay available for the detection of enterovirus in the CSF. However, backup culture should be done in tandem as well. DFA and EIA are not commonly used, and I just wanted an excuse to use the suckling mouse assay again, which you may recall can be used in the diagnosis of Coxsackie A, an enterovirus.
QCCP2, **Picornaviruses,** p 179

105.   E.   MUST BE INCUBATED AT 32°C.

The only unique property of rhinovirus is that it should be cultured in a temperature slightly lower than body temperature. The thought of adding nasal mucus to a culture is a little more than I can bear.
QCCP2, **Rhinovirus,** p 179

3: Microbiology Answers

---

106. A. **THEY ARE MEMBER OF THE BUNYAVIRUS FAMILY.**

Hantavirus and the Congo-Crimean hemorrhagic fever virus are both members of the bunyavirus family, along with other hemorrhagic fever viruses, such as Rift Valley fever and La Crosse viruses. Most other hemorrhagic fever viruses belong to other virus families, such as the filoviruses Marburg and Ebola.
QCCP2, **Family *Bunyaviridae*,** p 180

107. D. **THEY DO NOT CAUSE ARTHROPOD-BORNE ENCEPHALITIS.**

Yellow fever and rubella virus are both RNA virus members of the *Togaviridae.* Unlike all other togaviruses, such as alphaviruses and other flaviviruses, they are not predominantly arthropod-borne causes of encephalitis. Yellow fever favors the heart, GI tract, liver, and kidneys, while rubella causes lymphadenopathy and rash.
QCCP2, **Family *Togaviridae*,** p 180

108. E. **MIDZONAL HEPATIC NECROSIS.**

Congenital rubella is a potentially devastating infection, especially if acquired in the first trimester. While hepatosplenomegaly can occur, midzonal necrosis is not seen. It is, however, a prominent feature of yellow fever infection.
QCCP2, **Rubella virus,** p 180

109. D. **A & B.**

The *Aedes* mosquitoes are responsible for transmission of the viruses that cause yellow fever and Dengue fever, as well as some of the causative agents of filariasis and viral encephalitis. *Culex pipiens* is also a vector for many of the *Arboviridae,* such as Eastern and Western equine encephalitis, but it is not been shown transmit yellow or Dengue fever viruses.
QCCP2, **Dengue and yellow fever,** p 180

110. C. **RHABDOVIRUS.**

Rabies virus is transmitted through bites by contaminated animals. In most of the world, that means dogs and cats. In areas where the domestic causes are controlled, non-domestic animals, such as bats, skunks, and foxes are responsible for the transmission of the majority of cases.
QCCP2, **Family *Rhabdoviridae*,** p 180

111. A. **NORWAY.**

HTLV-I is spread primarily through IV drug use and sexual contact. It is the causative agent of the demyelinating disease, tropical spastic paraparesis and adult T cell lymphoma through the infection of CD4+ T cells.
QCCP2, **HTLV-I,** p 181

112. E. **A, B, C.**

Patients can also have skin rash and extreme thirst. Interestingly, the neoplastic cells express CD25, which is the IL-2 receptor, as well as high levels of free IL-2 receptor in the serum. The usual incubation time for ATCL is 20-30 years.
QCCP2, **HTLV-I,** p 180

3: Microbiology Answers

113.   A.   **SERUM ENZYME-LINKED IMMUNOSORBENT ASSAY.**

The extremely high sensitivity of the serum ELISA test makes it the screening test of choice. There can be a window period between the infection and seroconversion, usually 6-8 weeks, leading to possible false negative results. The confirmation of a positive result is usually done with Western blot, which is read positive if at least two bands (p24, gp41, and gp120/160) are positive.
QCCP2, **HTLV-3 [HIV-1 and -2],** p 180

114.   C.   **QUANTITATIVE HIV RNA.**

Quantitative HIV RNA is an assessment of viral load. Quantitation of RNA levels is an excellent prognostic tool to predict progression, especially long-term.
QCCP2, **HIV,** p 182-3

115.   C.   **QUANTITATIVE HIV RNA.**

The sensitivity of quantitative HIV RNA approaches 100%; however, the specificity is less. In a confirmatory test, you would like optimal specificity, unlike screening tests where you would like the sensitivity to be high.
QCCP2, **HIV,** p 183

116.   E.   **A, B, C.**

All of the above parasites are potentially positive for acid-fast staining, improving the chances of detection notably. The related organism microsporidium is not acid-fast and may require more invasive means for diagnosis.
QCCP2, **Parasites, specimens,** p 184

117.   B.   *ENTEROBIUS VERMICULARIS.*

The adult female worm migrates to the anal verge at night to lay eggs. This accounts for the nocturnal anal pruritus that is a symptom of enterobial infection. Some of the eggs that are laid by the female worm can be collected with adhesive tape applied to the anus at night.
QCCP2, **Cellophane tape,** p 184

118.   E.   *TOXOPLASMA GONDII.*

For the most part, specific serology beyond elevated IgE following parasitic infection is not available. The exception is *Toxoplasma*, which is a potentially catastrophic cause of transplacental (the "T" in TORCH) infection if it is primarily acquired by a woman during pregnancy.
QCCP2, **Laboratory methods,** p 185

119.   A.   **SIZE OF TROPHOZOITE.**

The only selection that is different between the related organisms is the size of the trophozoite. *Entamoeba histolytica* is roughly twice the size at 20-30 microns diameter than *E. hartmanii*, which is only 5-10 microns in diameter. Also, though non-specific, *E. histolytica* tends to be the most common trophozoite to contain ingested RBCs.
QCCP2, **T3.16, Amoeba that resemble *E. histolytica*,** p 184

3: Microbiology Answers

120. B.   LIVER.

The gray-white purulence or anchovy paste amebic abscess is most often in the liver, though the brain and spleen are not uncommon sites for abscess formation.
QCCP2, **E. histolytica,** p 185

121. D.   THE PROMINENT VACUOLE IN THE CYST FORM.

Iodamoeba beutschlii, at risk of sounding indelicate, has a "butt" or a large clear vacuole in the cyst form. *Naegleria* is grown on inactivated *E. coli, Entamoeba hartmanii* is small, and *Entamoeba coli* has up to 8 nuclei in the cyst form.
QCCP2, **Protozoa,** p 185

122. B.   *ACANTHAMOEBA.*

Acanthamoeba is known for causing GAE as well as a severe keratitis in contact lens users who make their own contact lens cleaning solution or use tap water.
QCCP2, **Acanthamoeba,** p 186

123. A.   *CHILOMASTIX MESNELI.*

Unlike the "falling leaf" motility of *Giardia, C. mesneli* has a rotary motion and a cyst form with only one nucleus (*Giardia* cysts have 4. The other choices are all pathogenic organisms.
QCCP2, **Chilomastix mesneli,** p 186

124. D.   *DIENTAMOEBA.*

With two nuclei and a fractured central karyosome, *Dientamoeba* is often seen coinfecting with *Enterobius.* Like *Enterobius, D. fragilis* causes diarrhea and pruritus ani.
QCCP2, **Dientamoeba,** p 186

125. B.   BAR-LIKE KINETOPLAST.

Especially in the intracellular amastigote forms of the three organisms, the one feature of *Leishmania* that helps to distinguish it from the others is the bar-like kinetoplast adjacent to the nucleus. Specific culture media, such as Novy-MacNeal-Nicolle medium, can be used to isolate *Leishmania* where the flagellated promastigote form can be identified.
QCCP2, **Leishmania,** p 186-7

126. C.   *L. BRAZILENSIS.*

A number of species of *Leishmania* are pathogenic, often causing distinct disease entities. *L. tropica* and *L. major* are associated with solitary cutaneous lesions, while *L. donovani* is associated with systemic disease (Kala-azar). *L. mexicana* is the causative agent of the self-limiting Chiclero ulcer of the ear lobe, while *L. brazilensis* causes mucosal and cutaneous lesions.
QCCP2, **Leishmania,** p 187

3: Microbiology Answers

127.   E.   "C" SHAPE.

The other features mentioned are shared to some extent by both species of trypanosomes. The characteristic "C" shape (remember - Cruzi, Chagas, "C"-shape) helps to identify *Trypanosoma cruzi* compared to the more randomly curved trypomastigotes of *T. brucei*.
QCCP2, **Trypanosoma spp,** p 187

128.   B.   *BALANTIDIUM COLI.*

A 50-70 micron organism with circumferential ciliation and a lenticulate nucleus, *B. coli* is the most medically significant ciliate (and the only one you probably have to be aware of).
QCCP2, **Ciliates,** p 187

129.   B.   WITHIN AN INTRACELLULAR APICAL VACUOLE.

On light microscopy, the *Cryptosporidia* appear to be small (8-15 micron), round organisms attached to the extracellular brush border. However, ultrastructural studies have determined that the organism is located in a unique position within an intracellular, yet extracytoplasmic apical vacuole. Very strange. *Isospora* interdigitates, *Microsporidium* is intracellular, and *Strongyloides* is found within the crypt epithelium.
QCCP2, *Cryptosporidiosis*, p 188

130.   E.   A, B, C.

The bradyzoite forms of *Toxoplasma* are small intracellular organisms seen within the cytoplasm of histiocytes, while the tachyzoites are curved extracellular organisms. A histiocyte filled with *Toxoplasma* bradyzoites resembles *Leishmania, Histoplasma, Trypanosoma,* and *Coccidioides,* and must be distinguished.
QCCP2, *Toxoplasma*, p 188

131.   D.   ANTI-TOXOPLASMA IgG.

Less than 1/5 of pregnant women have been previously infected by *Toxoplasma*, a fact which is confirmed with positive IgG anti-toxo serology. These previously infected women are at an extremely low risk of transplacental transmission of *Toxoplasma* compared to those who have not been previously exposed.
QCCP2, *Toxoplasma*, p 189

132.   C.   *P. MALARIAE.*

P. malariae differs from the other species of *Plasmodium* by having 72 hour or quartan fever spikes rather than the 48 hour tertian fevers. *P. malariae* can also have nephrotic syndrome and prefers to infect older red blood cells.
QCCP2, *Plasmodium* **spp** , p 189

133.   A.   LIVER.

After sporozoites are introduced into the blood stream by an anopheline mosquito, they travel to the liver to proliferate. The infected hepatocytes rupture and release the merozoites, which infect RBCs. Hypnozoites are the forms that maintain a latent infection in the liver.
QCCP2, *Plasmodium*, p 189

3: Microbiology Answers

134.   A.   *P. VIVAX.*

The Duffy antigen is the receptor for *P. vivax;* therefore, loss of the receptor affords some protection against infection. G6PD deficiency provides some protection against all species of *Plasmodium,* while sickle cell trait protects individuals predominantly against *P. falciparum.*
QCCP2, **Plasmodium,** p 189-190

135.   B.   SCHIZONTS.

The schizont is the form that contains numerous merozoites within the erythrocyte. With the rupture of the schizont, merozoites are released to infect other RBCs. The hemolysis corresponds to the clinical fever spikes.
QCCP2, **Plasmodium,** p 190

136.   C.   ENLARGED INFECTED RBCs.

Unlike *P. ovale* and *P. vivax, P. falciparum*-infected RBCs tend not to be enlarged. Schuffner dots are also a characteristic of *P. vivax* and *P. ovale.*
QCCP2, **Plasmodium,** p 190

137.   A.   *BABESIA MICROTI.*

Only *Babesia* has extraerythrocytic forms. In addition, there aren't gametocytes or schizonts present in the peripheral blood with babesiosis.
QCCP2, **Babesia microti,** p 191

138.   D.   A & B.

Lyme disease, babesiosis, ehrlichiosis, and even some flaviviruses are transmitted by the deer tick, *Ixodes scapularis,* on the east coast and the western black-legged tick, *Ixodes pacificus,* on the west coast.
QCCP2, **Babesia microti,** p 191

139.   B.   *PNEUMOCYSTIS* PNEUMONIA.

PCP, or *Pneumocystis carinii* pneumonia, is the most common AIDS-defining illness. Now renamed *Pneumocystis jiroveckii,* the organism presents with a characteristic bilateral "bat-wing" distribution of lung opacity with frothy alveolar exudate. Within the exudate, the organisms can be seen either in relief (Wright-Giemsa) or as positively-staining "crushed ping-pong balls" (GMS).
QCCP2, **Pneumocystis,** p 191

140.   A.   *TRICHURIS TRICHURIA.*

Trichuris, the whipworm, has an extremely tapered anterior end and double-operculated egg. It may coinfect with *Ascaris.*
QCCP2, **Trichuris,** p 191-2

3: Microbiology Answers

141.   B.   *ASCARIS.*

Without the unique outer shell, *Ascaris* eggs resemble those of hookworms or *Strongyloides*. *Ascaris* is also significant for its lifecycle - eggs are ingested, hatch in the intestine, migrate to the lungs, and, after being expectorated, are in turn swallowed and take up residence in the duodenum. During the lung stage, they can cause the hypereosinophilic Loeffler syndrome.
QCCP2, *Ascaris*, p 192

142.   C.   APPEARANCE OF MOUTH PARTS.

Necator has cutting plates (the "*Necator* grater") while *Ancylostoma* has teeth. Otherwise, the other features presented in the question are remarkably similar in both organisms. Other difference not mentioned include the geographic distribution - *A duodenale* is not present in the U.S.
QCCP2, **Hookworms**, p 192

143.   D.   A & B.

The short buccal groove and prominent genital primordium help distinguish *Strongyloides* larva. Again recall that the eggs of the hookworms, a decorticate *Ascaris* egg, and the eggs of *Strongyloides* are, for all intents and purposes, identical.
QCCP2, **Strongyloides**, p 192

144.   E.   HYPERINFECTION.

Hyperinfection is a potentially lethal complication where infective worms break through the intestinal barrier (autoinfection) and then disseminate intravascularly. Needless to say, that's bad.
QCCP2, **Strongyloides**, p 193

145.   B.   LATERAL ALAE.

The lateral alae should be searched for especially in cases of appendicitis, which is a common location to find the adult worm. Eggs can be identified via the cellophane tape test.
QCCP2, **Enterobius**, p 193

146.   E.   A, B, C.

All are potential means of categorizing the microfilariae - the sheathed worms are *Wuchereria*, *Brugia*, and *Loa loa*. The unsheathed are *Mansonella* and *Onchocerca*. Both *Onchocerca* and *Wuchereria* lack terminal nuclei, while *Loa loa* & *Mansonella* have nuclei to the tip and *Brugia* has two isolated nuclei at the tip Finally, *Wuchereria* and *Brugia* can be found in the lymphatics, while the rest are not. In addition, the worms can be categorized according to their periodicity in the blood.
QCCP2, **T3.19, Filariae**, p 193

147.   B.   *TOXOCARA CANIS.*

Most cases of visceral larva migrans (and ocular larva migrans) are due to *Toxocara canis*. A small percentage is due to *T. cati*. *Onchocerca* causes corneal opacities, *A. brazilensis* causes cutaneous larva migrans, and *Dirofilaria* causes lung infection in humans and heart infections in dogs and cats.
QCCP2, **Toxocara canis & cati**, p 194

3: Microbiology Answers

148. C. *FASCIOLA HEPATICA.*

Fasciola hepatica (and *buskii*) have the largest human parasite eggs known (~150 microns in diameter). The eggs have a non-shouldered operculum and lack an abopercular knob.
QCCP2, **T3.20,** p 194

149. A. *S. HAEMATOBIUM.*

S. intercalatum and *S. haematobium* are very similar, but while *S. intercalatum* infects the intestine, *S. haematobium* prefers the veins of the bladder. *S. mansoni* and *S. japonicum* primarily infect the liver and can lead to cirrhosis. *S. mekongii* is very similar to *S. japonicum* but in a more limited distribution in Laos and Cambodia.
QCCP2, **Schistosoma (bilharziasis),** p 195

150. B. FRESH WATER SNAILS.

The cercariae of *Schistosoma* infest fresh water snails in water where they can freely swim. The cercariae penetrate the skin and migrate to the blood vessels of the bladder (*S. haematobium*), liver (*S. mansoni, japonicum, mekongii*) or intestine (*S. intercalatum*).
QCCP2, **Schistosoma,** p 195

151. B. UNARMED ROSTELLUM.

The *Taenia* species have several features to distinguish them from each other. *T. saginata* is the beef tapeworm; *T. solium* is the pork tapeworm. *T. saginata* has an unarmed rostellum, unlike the armed rostellum of the pork tapeworm. The proglottid of the beef tapeworm has more than 13 uterine branches (as visualized by India ink injection), where the pork tapeworm has less than 13 branches. In addition, the pork tapeworm can cause cystercercosis, which the beef tapeworm doesn't. The eggs of both tapeworms are identical, with thick radially-striated walls.
QCCP2, **Cestodes,** p 196

152. D. *D. LATUM.*

Diphyllobothrium latum is noted for its ability to cause vitamin B_{12} deficiency by competing for binding the vitamin. It occurs primarily in Scandinavia and E. Europe.
QCCP2, **Diphyllobothrium,** p 197

153. D. *ECHINOCOCCUS.*

The definitive host is the dog. Ingestion of infected dog stool (oh, boy!) through intermediate hosts, such as sheep or cattle, causes the disease. The primary manifestation is multilocular hepatic cysts, and there are several species.
QCCP2, **Echinococcus spp,** p 197

154. D. *HYMENOLEPIS NANA* AND *ECHINOCOCCUS.*

There is no known association between *Hymenolepis* and *Echinococcus*. All the other groups have been shown to coinfect, some due to common vectors (*Babesia*, Lyme, *Ehrlichia*), some due to host immune status (leprosy and *Strongyloides* hyperinfection).
QCCP2, **Take-home points,** p 197

3: Microbiology Answers

155. A. *GIARDIA.*

Cryptosporidium, Toxoplasma, and *Strongyloides* infections are affected by T-cell immunodeficiency, while *Trichomonas* is not significantly affected by immunodeficiency.
QCCP2, **Parasitic infections in immunodeficient patients,** p 197

156. A. DETECTING MELANIN PIGMENT IN *CRYPTOCOCCUS.*

Bird seed (Niger) is used to selectively demonstrate *Cryptococcus neoformans,* where it will form brown/black colonies due to enzymatic (phenol oxidase) conversion of caffeic acid to melanin, within a week.
QCCP2, **T3.21,** p 198

157. B. *CRYPTOCOCCUS.*

Cryptococcus does not have a mold form, only yeast. Therefore, unlike *Histoplasma, Coccidioides, Blastomyces, Paracoccidioides,* and *Sporothrix,* it is not one of the dimorphic yeasts. Other medically relevant fungi of the coccoid yeast-type, like *Cryptococcus,* include *Torulopsis* and *Malassezia.*
QCCP2, **T3.22, Classification of fungi,** p 198

158. D. COCCOID YEAST.

The presence of a fuzzy colony implies the presence of a mold. Based on that, one would not expect a coccoid yeast to be in the differential diagnosis. It is important to also note that most dimorphic fungi will grossly appear as a mold by yeast conversion.
QCCP2, **Identification of a fungal isolate,** p 198-9

159. E. A, B, C.

Each of these features - and also type of sporulation - will help to categorize molds into discrete families.
QCCP2, **Identification of a fungal isolate,** p 199

160. B. CORNMEAL AGAR WITH TWEEN 80.

Cottonseed agar is used specifically to convert the mold phase of *Blastomyces* to the yeast form. Cornmeal with Tween 80 stimulates conidiation and chlamydospore production, aiding in speciation. Urea agar is helpful in detecting urease which is produced by *Cryptococcus neoformans.* Brain-heart infusion is a non-selective medium which will support the growth of saprophytic and pathogenic fungi. Potato dextrose agar is useful in demonstrating the production of pigment by *Trichophyton rubrum.*
QCCP2, **T3.21, Special fungal culture techniques,** p 198

161. E. A, B, C.

Most fungal pathogens, especially dimorphic fungi or dermatophytes will grow, albeit slowly, in cyclohexamide. Zygomyces, *Aspergillus,* and *Cryptococcus* won't grow.
QCCP2, **Identification of a fungal isolate,** p 199

162. B. *HISTOPLASMA CAPSULATUM.*

Blastomyces grows as a yeast on cottonseed agar while *Coccidioides* requires specialized media to grow as a yeast. The rest of the dimorphic fungi readily grow as yeast.
QCCP2, **Laboratory methods,** p 199

163.   E.   *PARACOCCIDIOIDES.*

The yeast form of *Paracoccidioides* contains the characteristic "Mariner's wheel" configuration of irregular circumferential cytoplasmic blebbing. Similarly, the mold form of *Histoplasma* has circumferential cytoplasmic buds which are more frequent and regular than those of the *Paracoccidioides* yeast.
QCCP2, **F3.14, Dimorphic fungi,** p 200

164.   A.   *HISTOPLASMA.*

Most dimorphic fungi with the notable exception of *Sporothrix* are infective through pulmonary aspiration - *Histoplasma* can cause the formation of pulmonary nodules, or sclerosing mediastinitis. It can also be disseminated through the reticuloendothelial system, where it can migrate to the spleen or bone marrow.
QCCP2, **Dimorphic fungi and molds,** p 201

165.   E.   A, B, C.

All resemble the 50-200 micron spherules that contain the small 2-5 micron endospores. *Rhinosporidia* is larger and found in the nasal sinus, *Prototheca* in the olecranon bursa. The wall of the spherule of *Coccidioides* is thick, but when the spherules are released. they can resemble those of *Histoplasma*.
QCCP2, **Dimorphic fungi and molds,** p 201

166.   C.   *COCCIDIOIDES.*

The mold form of *Coccidioides* forms barrel-shaped arthroconidia of live cells alternating with empty shells. The shell portions break easily, releasing the infective arthroconidia into the air where they can be freely inhaled unless proper precautions are taken.
QCCP2, **Dimorphic fungi and molds,** p 202

167.   D.   A & B.

A number of other molds, such as *Paracoccidioides* and *Scedosporium* can produce "lollipop" conidia. *Sporothrix*, however, produces a very characteristic "daisy-head" conidia that is not easily confused with *Blastomyces*.
QCCP2, **Blastomyces,** p 202

168.   D.   CHRONIC ALCOHOLICS.

Although *Sporothrix* is unique among the dimorphic because its primary means of infection is percutaneous, a less common means of inhalation (like the rest of the dimorphic fungi) has been documented in chronic alcoholics.
QCCP2, **Sporothrix,** p 203

169.   B.   *BLASTOMYCES.*

Paracoccidioides has been called the "South American *Blastomyces*" because it looks and behaves very similarly to *Blastomyces*.
QCCP2, **Paracoccidioides,** p 203

3: Microbiology Answers

170.   C.   *EPIDERMOPHYTON FLOCCOSUM.*

Trichophyton species (*T. rubrum, T. tonsurans, T. mentagrophytes*) are identified by their <u>micro</u>conidia, while
E. floccosum and the *Microsporum* spp are identified by their <u>macro</u>conidia. *E. floccosum* has "beaver tail"
macroconidia with transverse septae; *Microsporum canis* has transverse septa also, but with serrated edges ("dog
teeth") and pointed ends. *Microsporum gypseum* is very similar to *M. canis* but without the serrations.
QCCP2, **Dermatophytes,** p 203

171.   B.   *T. RUBRUM.*

The *Trichophyton* spp have microconidia and, of them, each has unique morphological features. *T. rubrum*
has "birds on a wire" microconidia spaced along hyphae; *T. tonsurans* has widely variable microconidia, while
T. mentagrophytes has grape-like clusters and occasional spiral hyphae.
QCCP2, **Dermatophytes,** p 203

172.   B.   *TRICHOPHYTON RUBRUM.*

The *Trichophyton* spp, especially *T. rubrum,* cause the majority of cases of onychomycosis. Individuals with HIV
and diabetes are at an increased risk for onychomycosis. In addition, it is important to note that other fungi, such
as *Candida,* can cause onychomycosis.
QCCP2, **Dermatophytes,** p 204

173.   C.   *ASPERGILLUS FUMIGATUS.*

Each of the *Aspergillus* spp has a distinct appearance on plates. *A. fumigatus* is blue-green, *A. terreus* has a
cinnamon-buff colony, *A. niger* has a black colony, and *A. flavus* has a brown colony with lateral striations.
QCCP2, **Aspergillus,** p 204

174.   A.   *ASPERGILLUS TERREUS.*

Just like the discrete gross appearance on plates, each of the *Aspergillus* spp can be speciated by the appearance
of the conidia. *A. terreus* has 2 rows of phialides. *A. niger* has black circumferential phialides. *A. fumigatus* has a
single row of phialides. *A. flavus* has a circumferential row of phialides (a "flavorful lollipop"). *P. marneffei* looks
like *A. fumigatus* but lacks the swollen vesicle at the base of the phialides that all the members of *Aspergillus* have.
QCCP2, **Aspergillus,** p 204-5

175.   B.   *ASPERGILLUS FUMIGATUS.*

There are 3 principle pulmonary diseases caused by *Aspergillus* spp, primarily *A. fumigatus*: Aspergilloma, a
fungal ball that grows in the site of a pre-existing cavitary lesion; Allergic bronchopulmonary aspergillosis, an
exaggerated allergic response to noninvasive *Aspergillus* colonization that's seen mostly in patients with cystic
fibrosis; and finally, invasive aspergillosis, a vascular-invasive disease seen mostly in the immunocompromised.
QCCP2, **Aspergillus,** p 205

176.   C.   *ASPERGILLUS NIGER.*
QCCP2, **Aspergillus,** p 205

3: Microbiology Answers

177. B. *PENICILLIUM.*

If anything called for a mnemonic, it would be all these genera of hyaline molds - a "GAF" is a tool to grab things and hold them together in a cluster. The organisms with clustered conidia are <u>G</u>liocladium, <u>A</u>cremonium, and <u>F</u>usarium. The branching chain conidia are a further reach - imagine looking through a pay telescope to see a pen hanging from a chain on a tree branch. Interpretation - the <u>branching</u> <u>chain</u> conidia are <u>P</u>enicillium, <u>P</u>aecilomyces, and <u>Sc</u>opulariopsis. All the rest occur singly - Scedosporium, Beuveria, Sepedonium, and Chrysosporium.
QCCP2, **Hyalinohyphomyces,** p 206

178. B. *CHRYSOSPORIUM.*

Adiaspiromycosis is a benign granulomatous infection with characteristic large thick-walled spherules.
QCCP2, **Conidia occurring singly,** p 206

179. E. *FUSARIUM.*

In addition to the myriad of infections including a disseminated infection in immunocompromised hosts, *Fusarium* can cause infections in burn victims, pulmonary infections, skin infections, and fungemia.
QCCP2, *Fusarium,* p 207

180. D. *SCEDOSPORIUM.*

It is also a common cause of disseminated infection in near-drowning victims and infections related to penetrating trauma.
QCCP2, **Hyalinohyphomyces,** p 207

181. E. A, B, C.

Chromoblastomycosis is a cutaneous fungal infection with the "copper penny" sclerotic or Medlar bodies that represent pigmented subcutaneous septated yeast forms.
QCCP2, **Pigmented (demaitiaceous) molds,** p 208

182. B. *ACTINOMYCES.*

Mycetomas, or deep subcutaneous infections, can be categorized as either true (eumycotic - caused by fungus) or actinomycotic (caused by non-fungal organisms). All of the choices presented, with the exception of *Actinomyces,* are fungal, or eumycotic, causes of mycetoma. The bacterial causes also can include *Streptomyces* and *Nocardia.*
QCCP2, **Mycetoma,** p 208

183. B. *ABSIDIA.*

Absidia and *Rhizopus* are the only zygomycetes that produce rhizoids or little rootlets from their hyphae. While the rhizoids in *Rhizopus* lie directly below the sporangiophores, those of *Absidia* are offset.
QCCP2, **Zygomyces,** p 208-9

3: Microbiology Answers

184.   D.   SUSPENDED IN SERUM, INCUBATED 2 HOURS AT 37°C.

It's actually important to understand the conditions under which the germ tube test is performed. The reason is that overincubation will greatly decrease the nearly 100% specificity that the assay has for *Candida albicans*. Unlike the pseudohyphae that *Candida* can form in tissue, the germ tube is a true hypha (there is no "pinch" between the germ tube and the mold).
QCCP2, **The germ tube test**, p 209

185.   A.   *CRYPTOCOCCUS NEOFORMANS*.

All of the organisms mentioned, with the exception of *Malassezia*, are urease positive, but *Cryptococcus* is the only one that is also phenol oxidase positive. The presence of phenol oxidase can be demonstrated on bird (Niger) seed agar where the phenol oxidase will convert the caffeic acid in the agar into melanin pigment, yielding the characteristic brown/black pigment.
QCCP2, **Yeast identification**, p 210

186.   B.   *MALASSEZIA*.

Malassezia furfur is the cause of tinea versicolor, a skin infection usually found on greasy back skin, and is also associated with total parenteral nutrition (lipid-rich) line infections. *Malassezia* requires a source of long-chain fatty acids to grow in culture. An olive oil overlay provides the required fatty acids.
QCCP2, **Yeast identification**, p 210

187.   B.   FONTANA-MASSON.

Remember, the phenol oxidase converts caffeic acid to melanin, which is what Fontana-Masson stains. The polysaccharides in the thick capsule of *Cryptococcus* can be stained with mucicarmine or Alcian blue. India ink works by forming a white negative space of the organism against a black-stained background.
QCCP2, **Cryptococcus**, p 210

188.   C.   *PROTOTHECA*.

Prototheca wickerhamii is the only known algal cause of human infections. Most commonly, the infection takes the form of olecranon bursitis or a cutaneous skin infection. The organism is said to resemble soccer balls or hub caps, referring to the morulated appearance. The organism is associated with exposure to water and dolphins.
QCCP2, **Prothecosis**, p 212

189.   E.   3 SAMPLES WITH MORE THAN 10mL EACH.

Preferably, the samples should be collected within 24 hours and, if possible, preceding or coincident with a febrile episode. Having less than three samples decreases sensitivity and having more doesn't improve sensitivity.
QCCP2, **Bacteriology laboratory methods**, p 213

190.   B.   URINE.
QCCP2, **Laboratory methods, specimens**, p 213

191.   B.   *LEGIONELLA*/GMS.

Several bacterial species are notable for the special requirements they have for growth or identification. All of the mentioned choices are correct except *Legionella*, which is best visualized with a Dieterle stain rather than GMS.
QCCP2, **T3.27, Additional bacterial stains**, p 213

3: Microbiology Answers

192.   D.   **CRYSTAL VIOLET.**

The crystal violet in a gram stain is applied after heat fixation (which gets the bugs to stick to the slide). Crystal violet stains the peptidoglycans of the bacterial cell wall. After that, iodine is applied as a mordant to enhance the crystal violet staining. This is followed by decolorization where gram-positive organisms retain the violet due to their thick cell wall and gram negatives lose the violet stain. Finally, safranin is added to stain the decolorized gram-negative organisms.
QCCP2, **Direct examination,** p 213

193.   E.   **WHETHER OR NOT HEAT IS USED TO FIX SLIDES.**

Acid-fast organisms are defined as those that retain carbolfuschin stain despite acid decolorization. That makes choices B and D wrong. The Fite technique differs from Kinyoun and Ziehl-Neelsen by using a weaker acid to decolorize, and thereby stains "weakly" acid-fast organisms, such as *Nocardia.* The only difference between Ziehl-Neelsen and Kinyoun stains is the type of fixation - ZN uses heat, Kinyoun does not.
QCCP2, **Acid-fast stains,** p 214

194.   A.   *HAEMOPHILUS INFLUENZAE.*

Blood agar is a non-selective media used often as the initial growth media from which colonies can be subcultured onto selective media for identification. An exception is *Haemophilus influenzae,* which requires factors X (hemin) and V (NAD) that is present only when the RBCs are lysed. Therefore, to grow *H. influenzae* chocolate (lysed RBC) agar or with a streak of *Staphylococcus* to provide the required factors.
QCCP2, **Culture media,** p 214

195.   B.   **BUFFERED CHARCOAL YEAST EXTRACT (BCYE).**

There are a number of specialized media utilized for the isolation of specific organisms. BCYE is for *Legionella* (I remember a "legion of bicycles"), Thayer-Martin for the growth of *Neisseria,* MacConkey for gram negatives, chocolate agar for *Haemophilus.* Eosin methylene blue is similar to MacConkey.
QCCP2, **Culture media,** p 214

196.   D.   **PINK.**

MacConkey agar is both selective for gram-negative organisms and differential for lactose fermenters v. non-lactose fermenters. The lactose non-fermenters appear as light pink colonies, and include organisms such as *Pseudomonas, Serratia,* and *Burkholderia.*
QCCP2, **Culture media,** p 213

197.   B.   **HIGH BILE SALT AND SODIUM CITRATE.**

The selective nature of SS agar is due to the high bile salt and sodium citrate, but also to the lack of any carbohydrate except lactose, so that only lactose-fermenting gram-negative organisms can grow. *Shigella* and *Salmonella* are distinguished as colorless colonies, whereas other gram-negative fermenters are usually red. Finally, *Salmonella* is distinguished from *Shigella* by the presence of a black center in the otherwise clear colony.

198.   D.   **A & B.**

CCF, or cycloserine-cefoxitin fructose-egg yolk agar, is a fairly selective medium for growing *Clostridium difficile,* which is a dying practice due to the high specificity and sensitivity of immunologic testing for toxins A and B.
QCCP2, **T3.29,** p 215

3: Microbiology Answers

199.   D.   *CAMPYLOBACTER.*

Pseudomonas and *Mycobacterium marinum* prefer cooler temperatures (25°-30°C) while *Campylobacter* likes it warm (42°C). Most others grow best at body temperature, including *Listeria.* The characteristic tumbling motility of *Listeria,* however, is best observed at 25°C.
QCCP2, **Culture temperature,** p 216

200.   B.   A POSITIVE BOUND COAGULASE TEST.

The description of the test sounds like coagulation, things sticking together. Rabbit serum provides the fibrinogen that bound coagulase converts to fibrin. A more sensitive and time-consuming test is the tube test for free coagulase, which should be performed whenever the slide or bound test is negative. It is important to examine the test tube at both 4 hours and 20 hours (but only if negative at 4 hours). Some strains break down clots with time (false negative at 20 hours), or some other strains take longer to make clots (false negative at 4 hours).
QCCP2, **Coagulase,** p 216

201.   E.   NOVOBIOCIN.

Once the catalase test is positive, indicating *Staphylococcus,* and coagulase is negative (coagulase-negative *Staph*), the next test to do is the novobiocin test. The common skin floral *Staphylococcus epidermidis* is susceptible to the antibiotic novobiocin, while *S. saprophyticus* is resistant. "Saprophyticus" means that it grows on dead material. I remember that *S. saprophyticus* is "resistant" to "new (novo) life (bio)."
QCCP2, **Novobiocin susceptibility,** p 216

202.   C.   TO IDENTIFY GROUP B BETA-HEMOLYTIC *STREPTOCOCCUS.*

In the CAMP test, a single streak of *Staphylococcus aureus* is plated perpendicular to a streak of presumptive Group B beta-hemolytic *Strep* on a sheep blood agar plate. A positive test is indicated by an "arrowhead" zone of beta hemolysis pointing toward the *Staph* streak. The reason is that the Group B *Strep* produce "CAMP Factor," which synergizes with the beta hemolysin of *S. aureus. S. aureus* is identified with the coagulase test; *Enterococci* can be identified with a number of tests including bile esculin and 6.5% NaCl tolerance.
QCCP2, **Biochemical tests,** p 216

203.   A.   DISTINGUISH AMONG ALPHA HEMOLYTIC *STREP*

The optochin, or P-disk test, is used to distinguish between alpha hemolytic *Strep* such as *S. pneumoniae,* which is optochin-sensitive, and the viridans *Strep,* which are optochin-resistant. As a matter of fact, the optochin disk has a "P" on it for its relative specificity for pneumococcus.
QCCP2, **Optochin,** p 217

204.   B.   *SHIGELLA.*

Organisms of the Enterobacteriaceae family (*E. coli, Shigella, Salmonella, Klebsiella, Proteus,* etc.) are uniformly oxidase negative. It's actually part of the definition of the family - oxidase negative glucose fermenters. The set of gram-negative oxidase-positive organisms include *Pseudomonas, Campylobacter, Pasteurella, Vibrio, Aeromonas, Neisseria,* and *Brucella.* One can hallucinate on PCP, a VAN driven by an OX named "Bruce." *Moraxella* is also oxidase-positive, but it doesn't fit into my mnemonic. Sorry, *Moraxella.*
QCCP2, **Cytochrome oxidase,** p 217

3: Microbiology Answers

205.   B.   *E. COLI.*

The indole test indicates the presence of bacterial tryptophanase, which metabolizes tryptophan into indole. While *E. coli*, *Pasteurella*, and *H. influenzae* are all positive for indole, only *E. coli* is a lactose fermenter on MacConkey. *Pseudomonas* is indole (-) and a lactose non-fermenter, *Klebsiella* is a strong lactose fermenter, but is also indole (-).
QCCP2, **Indole,** p 217

206.   E.   METHYL RED TEST.

Bacteria use one of two pathways to utilize pyruvate - one pathway results in mixed acid production, yielding a positive methyl red test, while if butylene glycol is produced, they yield a positive Voges-Proskauer test. The two are mutually exclusive and therefore have opposite results.
QCCP2, **Test,** p 217

207.   A.   *PROTEUS.*

Due to the high amount of buffer in Stuart broth, only strong urea-splitters, such as the *Proteus* spp, turn positive. There is less buffer in Christensen, and therefore it is less selective, allowing weaker urea-splitting organisms, such as *Klebsiella,* to turn positive (red).
QCCP2, **Laboratory methods,** p 217

208.   B.   *BORDETELLA.*

All of the choices are flagellated, but *Bordetella* is the only one of them with peritrichous, or circumferential, flagella. *Acinetobacter, Moraxella,* and *Flavobacterium* have non-motile flagella, while *Pseudomonas aeruginosa* has a polar monotrichous flagellum.
QCCP2, **Laboratory Methods,** p 217

209.   B.   *VIBRIO CHOLERAE.*

V. cholerae can be distinguished from other species of *Vibrio* with the string test. When added to 0.5% deoxycholate (bile salt), *V. cholerae* will string out from the mixture and stay that way. Other species of *Vibrio* will cease to string out after a minute.
QCCP2, **Laboratory Methods,** p 218

210.   C.   *NEISSERIA MENINGITIDIS.*

The carbohydrate tests for *Neisseria* are easily remembered - *N. gonorrheae* utilizes only glucose, *N. meningitidis* uses maltose and glucose, while *N. lactamica* utilizes lactose, maltose, and glucose. *Moraxella* can't use any of those sugars as carbohydrate sources. *Moraxella* does however produce DNase, unlike the *Neisseria* spp.
QCCP2, **Laboratory Methods,** p 218

211.   D.   *S. INTERMEDIUS.*

S. saprophyticus and *S. epidermidis* are both coagulase-negative *Staph* species. *S. hyicus, S. delphini,* and *S. intermedius* are all coagulase-positive *Staph* species (along with the more common *S. aureus*). *S. intermedius* is the most commonly isolated of the coagulase-positive *Staph* species isolated from infected dog bite sites.
QCCP2, **Specific bacteria key characteristics,** p 219

3: Microbiology Answers

212. D. **A & B.**

Alpha hemolysis is defined as a partial hemolysis or green discoloration on sheep blood agar. The most important of the alpha-hemolytic *Strep* spp are the viridans *Strep* and *S. pneumoniae*. *S. agalactiae* and *S. pyogenes* are true, or beta-hemolytic, organisms, while gamma, or non-hemolytic, *Strep* include the enterococci and *S. bovis*.
QCCP2, **Specific bacteria key characteristics,** p 219

213. A. ALPHA-HEMOLYTIC, BILE SOLUBLE, OPTOCHIN-SENSITIVE.

S. pneumoniae is among the green, or alpha-hemolytic, *Strep*, which also includes many of the viridans (which means "green") *Strep*. Remember that *S. pneumoniae* is optochin-sensitive, unlike viridans *Strep*.
QCCP2, **Group D,** p 219

214. D. CO$_2$-RICH AT 35°C.

Neisseria is not hardy and requires careful handling and growth conditions. It prefers chocolate agar (Thayer-Martin) with antibiotics. Cotton swabs inhibit the growth of *Neisseria*, so Dacron swabs should be used to collect samples.
QCCP2, **Gram-negative cocci,** p 219

215. B. *M. CATARRHALIS.*

M. catarrhalis looks very similar to *Neisseria* spp (gram-negative kidney bean-shaped diplococci) and is also non-motile, oxidase positive and catalase positive. Unlike *Neisseria,* it's DNase positive and displays the "hockey puck" sign (colonies stay intact and, when pushed, move along the media intact, like a hockey puck).
QCCP2, **Gram-negative cocci,** p 219-220

216. D. **A & B.**

Both are gram-positive, but *Nocardia* is weakly acid-fast and prefers aerobic conditions, while *Actinomyces* is not acid-fast and prefers anaerobic culture.
QCCP2, **Gram-positive bacilli,** p 220

217. B. *CLOSTRIDIA.*

All are gram positive bacilli, but only *Actinomyces, Clostridia,* and *Lactobacillus* are anaerobes. Of those three, only *Clostridia* makes spores, too. *Listeria* and *Bacillus* are aerobic, with *Bacillus* producing spores and *Listeria* not.
QCCP2, **Gram-positive bacilli,** p 220

218. D. **A & B.**

Bacillus cereus is beta hemolytic and motile, unlike *B. anthracis*. Both are sensitive to penicillin and form spores. Also unlike *B. cereus, B. anthracis* forms medusa-head colonies on sheep blood agar and produces a toxin containing edema factor, protective antigen, and lethal factor.
QCCP2, **Aerobic gram-positive bacilli,** p 220

3: Microbiology Answers

219.　E.　*LISTERIA.*

The tumbling motility, the cold enrichment and the preference for infecting pregnant women are all characteristics of *Listeria*. Because of the predilection for pregnant women, there is the risk to infants born to infected mothers of granulomatosis infantisepticum, a condition described as multiple, disseminated suppurative abscesses affecting numerous organs.
QCCP2, **Listeria**, p 220-1

220.　B.　*YERSINIA.*

Most enterobacteriaceae are motile with the exception of *Shigella* and *Klebsiella. Yersinia* is unique in only being motile at 22°C.
QCCP2, **Gram-negative bacilli**, p 221

221.　A.　ALKALINE SLANT/ALKALINE BUTT.

The KIA/TSI test is a weird and wonderfully complex assay. Multiple characteristics are assayed simultaneously - aerobic (slant) v. anaerobic (butt) growth, fermentation of sugar (pH change), and whether the organism produces H_2S or gas. Glucose fermenters result in an alkaline slant and acid butt at 24 hours; lactose-fermenters have an acid slant and acid butt. Given that enterobacteriaceae ferment glucose with or without lactose fermentation, an alkaline slant and alkaline butt excludes them.
QCCP2, **Anaerobic gram-negative bacilli**, p 221-2

222.　C.　METHYL RED.

Testmanship and knowledge of some test characteristics would narrow down your choices to Voges-Proskauer and methyl red. Because the results of each test are always opposites, one of them must be the positive, while the other is negative.
QCCP2, **Shigella**, p 222

223.　A.　*YERSINIA ENTEROCOLITICA.*

Because of its preference to grow in the cold, *Yersinia* contamination is a problem with blood products that are stored in the refrigerator, such as RBCs, and not so much with platelets, which are stored at room temperature. Of the *Yersinia* spp, Y *enterocolitica* is most often isolated.
QCCP2, **Yersinia**, p 222

224.　D.　*EDWARDSIELLA.*

Citrobacter also resembles *Salmonella,* but unlike *Salmonella,* it is positive in ONPG (beta-galactosidase) assay. *Edwardsiella* is also notable for coinfection with *Entamoeba* and for its affinity to infect people with iron overload.
QCCP2, **Edwardsiella**, p 222

225.　A.　ETEC.

Enterotoxigenic *E. coli* makes a toxin that functions similarly to *Cholera* toxin by stimulating the G proteins in the small intestine, leading to a profuse, watery secretory diarrhea.
QCCP2, **Escherichia**, p 222-3

3: Microbiology Answers

226. B. **INABILITY TO FERMENT SORBITOL.**

E. coli O157:H7 is similar to other *E. coli* in that it can ferment lactose, grow on MacConkey agar, and is indole positive. Unlike other strains of *E. coli,* when O157:H7 is plated on modified sorbitol: MacConkey agar substituted for lactose, the colonies grow clear instead of yellow.
QCCP2, **EHEC,** p 223

227. E. **A, B, C.**

S. typhi is picked up by the reticuloendothelial system once it transverses the bowel wall. It can then remain hidden in macrophages in the liver, gall bladder, and spleen.
QCCP2, **Salmonella,** p 223

228. D. **A & B.**

V. cholerae can be divided into strains that cause cholera (O1) and those that do not (non-O1). On the Indian subcontinent, subtype O139 is now recognized as a cause of cholera.
QCCP2, **V. cholerae,** p 223

229. D. **42°C.**

Pseudomonas grows at a temperature that would induce the expression of heat-shock proteins in most other bacteria.
QCCP2, **Pseudomonas,** p 224

230. B. **CYSTEINE.**

Francisella tularensis is a gram negative coccobacillus that doesn't grow on MacConkey and requires cysteine and cystine to grow.
QCCP2, **Francisella,** p 224

231. D. **PCR.**

Serology is most common, but it is slow and non-specific. PCR is faster and can be performed on samples and fixed tissue. Culture is not performed because it is difficult to grow and potentially dangerous.
QCCP2, **F. tularensis,** p 224

232. C. **TEXAS AND CALIFORNIA.**

More than 1/2 of cases occur in Texas and California, states with a high cattle population. *Brucella* is transmitted from infected livestock, primarily. A pathognomonic feature of systemic brucellosis is foul-smelling sweat.
QCCP2, **Brucella,** p 224

233. E. *HAEMOPHILUS DUCREYI.*

H. ducreyi, the causative agent of chancroid, requires only X factor ("X-rated"), while *H. parainfluenzae* and *H. parahemolyticus* require only V factor (NAD) (the "P's" need "V's"), and *H. influenzae* and *H. haemolyticus* require both X and V.
QCCP2, **T3.32 and T3.24**

3: Microbiology Answers

234. B. *FRANCISELLA TULARENSIS.*

Recall that *Francisella* requires cysteine and cystine, which helps to distinguish it from most other organisms.
*QCCP2, **Legionella**,* p 225

235. A. HIPPURATE HYDROLYSIS.

All of the choices are shared by *Campylobacter* spp except hippurate hydrolysis, which is specific for *C. jejuni.*
*QCCP2, **Campylobacter**,* p 225

236. A. *STREPTOBACILLUS MONILIFORMIS.*

S. moniliformis grows as cotton ball aggregates in liquid culture and is the cause of rat-bite fever.
*QCCP2, **S. moniliformis**,* p 225

237. A. SEROLOGIC IgG ANTI-*HELICOBACTER PYLORI.*

Antibody levels remain elevated long after the infection is eradicated, making serological testing, which can be performed on urine or serum, a very poor choice for documenting post-therapeutic success.
*QCCP2, **H. pylori**,* p 226

238. A. A & B.

Tropheryma whippelli is typically PAS (+)/non acid-fast; the opposite is true for MAI. Both are very commonly found in the intestine.
*QCCP2, **T. whippelli**,* p 226-7

239. E. A, B, C.

All are considered manifestations of tertiary syphilis. Some of the classic neurological symptoms are tabes dorsalis and optic neuritis, classic gummas affecting the gingiva, skin, and bones. The most common cardiovascular manifestation is aortic insufficiency.
*QCCP2, **T3.35, Clinical stages of syphilis**,* p 226

240. D. A & B.

From primary to tertiary syphilis, including congenital syphilis, all lesions share the presence of a dense plasmacytic infiltrate and an obliterative endarteritis. The identification of spirochetes is not always a required feature and their presence is not usually easily demonstrated. Serology is usually more dependable.
*QCCP2, **T3.35, Clinical stages of syphilis**,* p 226

241. B. SECONDARY SYPHILIS.

Diagnostic sensitivity for both non-treponemal and treponemal tests is highest during secondary syphilis, while the lowest sensitivity is during primary syphilis and treated syphilis.
*QCCP2, **T3.36, Sensitivity of serological tests for syphilis**,* p 227

242. **D. A & B.**

Most often, the white-footed mouse acts as a natural reservoir for *Borrelia burgdorfei*. The *Ixodes* tick acts as a vector for Lyme disease, babesiosis, and certain *Ehrlichia* spp. In addition to the mouse, deer act as an important reservoir in areas endemic to the disease.
*QCCP2, **Borrelia**,* p 227

243. **B. A-V BLOCK SECONDARY TO MYOSITIS.**

Stage 2 (following hematogenous spread and the erythema chronicum migrans of Stage 1) has many systemic manifestations, which accounts for the frequent confusion with autoimmune or neoplastic disease. Among the Stage 2 manifestations are a lymphocytic CSF pleocytosis and A-V block secondary to myocarditis.
*QCCP2, **Borrelia**,* p 227

244. **D. IDENTIFICATION OF ORGANISMS IN THICK BLOOD FILMS.**

Unlike *Borrelia burgdorfei,* which is almost never seen in peripheral blood, *B. recurrentis* can be seen in peripheral blood smear and detected by darkfield exam or by Wright-Giemsa staining.
*QCCP2, **Borrelia**,* p 228

245. **C. *LEPTOSPIRA INTERROGANS.***

Weil disease is defined by meningitis, nephritis, and hepatitis. The presence of icterus portends a poor prognosis. Leptospirosis is histopathologically defined by non-specific features of vasculitis, endothelial damage, and inflammatory infiltrates.
*QCCP2, **Leptospira interrogans**,* p 228

246. **C. THE RETICULATE BODY.**

Chlamydia is an intracellular bacteria present in 2 forms, on of which is a smaller elementary body that is able to live extracellularly, which explains why it is the infectious form. The larger form is the reticulate body, which is found exclusively within infected cells. MOMP refers to the diagnostic major outer membrane protein. Small cell and large cell variants are seen with *Coxiella burnetti*.
*QCCP2, **Chlamydiae**,* p 229

247. **E. L.**

While trachoma, or conjunctival, *Chlamydia* infection is caused by serotype A, LGV is caused by serotype L. Pneumonia and the myriad other manifestations of *Chlamydia* infection are caused by the other serotypes.
*QCCP2, **Chlamydiae**,* p 229

248. **B. BIRD CONTACT.**

Chlamydia psittaci is the causative agent behind psittacosis. The most common contact is from household domestic birds, such as parrots. While person-to-person spread can occur, it is very rare.
*QCCP2, **Chlamydia**,* p 230

3: Microbiology Answers

249. D. **ENDOTHELIAL CELLS.**

Because of the affinity for endothelial cells, all rickettsial organisms share common histological findings of endothelial swelling and a disseminated vasculitis with thrombi formation.
*QCCP2, **Rickettsiae***, p 230

250. E. **GLUCOSE-6-PHOSPHATASE DEFICIENCY.**

A rapidly fatal fulminant infection with *Rickettsia rickettsiae* can be seen in patients with G6PD.
*QCCP2, **Rocky Mountain Spotted Fever***, p 230

251. C. *ANAPLASMA PHAGOCYTOPHILA.*

Ehrlichiosis is caused by *Ehrlichia chaffeensis,* which causes the monocytic disease, and *A. phagocytophila,* which causes granulocytic ehrlichiosis. Because it is more likely that granulocytes will be found in peripheral blood, *Anaplasma* is easier to diagnose with that modality.
*QCCP2, **Ehrlichia***, p 230

252. C. **RING GRANULOMAS.**

The granulomas associated with Q fever appear like napkin rings with peripheral macrophages and central clearing. They are most often seen in the liver, associated with hepatitis, but also can be seen in the bone marrow.
*QCCP2, **Q fever***, p 230

253. B. **SMALL CELL VARIANT.**

The large cell and small cell variants describe the ultrastructural appearance of the extracellular/intercellular small form and the exclusively intercellular large form. Both forms can exist within the monocyte, but only the small cell variant can survive extracellularly.
*QCCP2, **Q fever***, p 230

254. A. *BARTONELLA QUINTANA.*

B. quintana is spread by the body louse, of which there were many cases among troops during World War I. *B. henselae* causes cat-scratch disease, bacillary angiomatosis in the immunocompromised, and Parinaud oculoglandular syndrome. *B. bacilliformis* causes Oroya fever and verruga peruana, spread by the sandfly. *M hominis* and *U urealyticum* are causes of nongonococcal urethritis.
*QCCP2, **Bartonella***, p 231

255. E. **A, B, C.**

All of the organisms mentioned can produce tissue lesions that are very similar. With *Bartonella*, especially in bacillary angiomatosis, lesions with large pockets of organisms can be demonstrated with Warthin-Starry staining.
*QCCP2, **Bartonella***, p 231

256. B. **LACK OF CELL WALL.**

All mycoplasma lack cell walls and are therefore unlike other bacteria and are resistant to beta-lactam antibiotics. In addition, they are different from bacteria and similar to fungi in that they have sterol-containing cell membranes.
*QCCP2, **Mycoplasma***, p 232

257. A. COLD AGGLUTININ IGM ANTI-I.

The presence of anti-I is associated with the majority of cases of atypical pneumonia caused by *Mycoplasma pneumonia* and can be used as a nonspecific indicator of infection.
QCCP2, **Mycoplasma,** p 232

258. D. *SHIGELLA.*

Shigella and *Salmonella* are separable on SS media due to the presence of H$_2$S in *Salmonella,* represented by a black dot center of the *Salmonella* colony.
QCCP2, **Other bacterial facts,** p 232

259. E. *STAPHYLLOCOCCUS SAPROPHYTICUS.*

The coagulase test is a major tool in the *Staphylococcus* workup, separating *S. aureus* from the coagulase-negative *Staph.* However, it is important to appreciate that *S. aureus* is not the only coagulase-positive species of *Staphylococcus* and that a positive coagulase reaction is not equivalent to a presumptive diagnosis of *S. aureus.*
QCCP2, **Other bacterial facts,** p 233

260. C. SYNDENHAM CHOREA.

Sydenham chorea, the condition of choreathetoid movements of the upper extremities, tongue, and eyes, fulfills one of the criteria for the diagnosis of acute rheumatic fever. The other major criteria are carditis, polyarthritis, erythema marginatum, and subcutaneous nodules. The minor criteria in addition to those listed include history of antecedent *Strep* infection. In order to diagnose acute rheumatic fever, there should be 2 major criteria or 1 major and 2 minor criteria.
QCCP2, **T3.39, Jones criteria,** p 233

261. D. *MYCOBACTERIUM KANSASII.*

M. kansasii is a photochromagen-producing species, Group I by the Runyon classification system for non-tuberculous *Mycobacteria.*
QCCP2, **Mycobacteria,** p 233

262. D. A & B.

Cording refers to the ability of *Mycobacterium tuberculosis* to clump when cultured, resulting in strings or cords of organisms, a feature due to cord factor - a virulence factor. Also, NAP-sensitivity is a suspicious finding that is consistent with *M. tuberculosis.* Arylsulfatase is used to separate fast-growing *Mycobacterium* between the positive *M. fortuitum* and *M. chelonei,* and the nonpathogenic and arylsulfatase-negative *M. phlei* and *M. smegmatis.*
QCCP2, **Mycobacteria,** p 233-4

263. A. *MYCOBACTERIUM TUBERCULOSIS.*

Of all the known major species of *Mycobacteria,* only *M. tuberculosis, M. simiae,* and to a lesser extent, and *M marinum,* are able to accumulate niacin as demonstrated with a yellow colony on media with a detection compound (cyanogen chloride) that reacts with the free niacin.
QCCP2, **Mycobacteria,** p 234

3: Microbiology Answers

264.   E.   **NONE OF THE ABOVE.**

The Runyon classification system is expressly used for the classification of non-tuberculous mycobacteria. Group I is the photochromagens (yellow pigment when grown in the light), including *Mycobacterium kansasii, M. simiae, M. marinum,* and *M. asiaticum,* lending itself to the mnemonic, "SMAK the photographer." Group II is scotochromagens, that is, they make pigment in the dark and include *M. gordonae, M. scrofulaceum, M. thermoresistable,* and *M. flavescens.* (They get in "FiGhTS" in the dark). Group III is the non-pigmented, and includes *M. avium-intracellulare, M. hemophilium, M. terratriviale, M. malmoense, M. gastri, M. bovis, M. xenopii.* Finally, Group IV is the fast growers and the only significant organisms to human infections in this group are *M. chelonei* and *M. fortuitum.*
*QCCP2, **Mycobacteria**,* p 234

265.   B.   *MYCOBACTERIUM SZULGAI.*

M. szulgai is a scotochromagen at 35°-37°C and a photochromagen at 25°C.
*QCCP2, **Mycobacteria**,* p 234

266.   B.   **10%.**

Actually, 10% is on the high side of estimates as the vast majority of people (90%) infected with respiratory TB resolve the infection. The remaining 5-10% (higher in the immunocompromised) go on to develop active disease, which most often is pulmonary, but can also be extrapulmonary.
*QCCP2, **M. tuberculosis**,* p 235

267.   D.   **HIV.**

TB is a difficult disease to diagnose - screening tests like PPC and sputum smears have high false-negative rates and culture often takes weeks. Nucleic acid amplification tests may be more sensitive and rapid, but long-term validation is lacking. HIV makes diagnosis even more difficult.
*QCCP2, **M. tuberculosis**,* p 235

268.   A.   **PNEUMOCONIOSIS.**

Behind *Mybacterium tuberculosis* and *M. avium-intracellulare, M. kansasii* is one of the most common causes of mycobacterial pulmonary disease.
*QCCP2, **Mycobacteria**,* p 236

269.   B.   *MYCOBACTERIUM ULCERANS.*

The necrotizing ulcerative cutaneous Buruli ulcer is caused by infection with *M. ulcerans.* All the choices are notable for causing skin disease without pulmonary disease. Most are associated with penetrating trauma - *M. marinum* with fresh water fish tanks.
*QCCP2, **Mycobacteria** causing skin and soft tissue infections,* p 236

270.   D.   **A & B.**

Lepromatous leprosy is associated with anergy and therefore a more widespread involvement with the presence of large numbers of acid-fast bacilli and foamy macrophages. The tuberculoid form is associated with a robust granulomatous reaction to infection. In tuberculoid form, there is a small number of organisms present. Two leprosy factoids: *Mycobacterium leprae* grows on armadillo footpads and the most consistent signs are anesthetic skin lesions with palpable prominent peripheral nerves.
*QCCP2, **M. leprae**,* p 236

Chapter 4

Hematopathology

1. The hemiglobin cyanide technique of measuring hemoglobin can detect all forms of hemoglobin, <u>except</u>:
    A. methemoglobin
    B. carboxyhemoglobin
    C. deoxyhemoglobin
    D. sulfhemoglobin
    E. oxyhemoglobin

2. Which of the following values is calculated from red blood cell indices in an automated red blood cell count?
    A. red blood cell count (RBC)
    B. hematocrit
    C. mean corpuscular volume (MCV)
    D. red cell distribution width (RDW)
    E. total hemoglobin

3. For the automated counting of leukocytes by the Coulter principle, what is usually done to the blood sample?
    A. filtering out red blood cells
    B. lysis of red blood cells
    C. clumping agent added to remove platelets
    D. sample is clotted
    E. leukocytes selectively filtered before counting

4. Which leukocyte has the highest side scatter?
    A. monocytes
    B. neutrophils
    C. basophils
    D. eosinophils
    E. lymphocytes

5. Where is the platelet window as counted by electrical impedance?
    A. 1-2 fL
    B. 2-20 fL
    C. 20-50 fL
    D. 30-36 fL
    E. 36-360 fL

6. What feature of reticulocytes is the most helpful in distinguishing them from mature red blood cells?
    A. size
    B. shape
    C. color
    D. RNA
    E. DNA

4: Hematopathology Questions

7. Which feature of a reticulocyte is most helpful at determining its age?
    A. presence/absence of a nucleus
    B. RNA content
    C. enumeration of ribosomes
    D. presence/absence of mitochondria
    E. presence/absence of Golgi bodies

8. For which of the following hematocrits is the correction factor = 3.0 for calculating the reticulocyte proliferation index?
    A. 40%
    B. 30%
    C. 15%
    D. 5%
    E. 2%

9. In the hemoglobin solubility (dithionate) test, which form(s) of hemoglobin cause(s) turbidity (positive reaction)?
    A. HbSS
    B. HbSC
    C. HbSA
    D. A & B
    E. A, B, C

10. Which of the following patterns of eosinophilia in the acid elution test for detection of fetal hemoglobin is most consistent with hereditary persistence of fetal hemoglobin?
    A. heterocellular
    B. pancellular
    C. centrocellular
    D. paucicellular
    E. acellular

11. Which pair of hemoglobin variants cannot be resolved with hemoglobin electrophoresis on cellulose acetate at pH 8.6?
    A. HbS, HbD
    B. HbS, HbA
    C. HbA, HbF
    D. HbC, HbS
    E. HbG. HbF

12. Which of the following are consistent with the diagnosis of beta-thalassemia?
    A. increased red blood cell
    B. low MCV
    C. decreased HbA_2
    D. A & B
    E. A, B, C

13. Which of the following hemoglobins is routinely quantified by HPLC? (Choose all possible answers)
    A. HbS
    B. HbA
    C. HbA_2
    D. HbC
    E. HbF

4: Hematopathology Questions

14. Which of the following chemicals are present in Wright stain?
    A. eosin
    B. methylene blue
    C. alcohol
    D. A & B
    E. A, B, C

15. What type of leukocytes are stained by Sudan black B?
    A. granulocytes
    B. monocytes
    C. lymphocytes
    D. A & B
    E. A, B, C

16. Which of the following cell types is predominantly stained by non-specific esterases (alpha naphthyl acetate esterase and alpha naphthyl butyrate esterase) and is inhibited by sodium fluoride?
    A. monocytes
    B. megakaryocytes
    C. lymphocytes
    D. granulocytes
    E. erythrocytes

17. Which of the following description best fits the method of determining leukocyte alkaline phosphatase (LAP) score?
    A. the sum of scoring of 100 monocytes, lymphocytes, and granulocytes 0 to 4+ based on intensity of LAP staining
    B. the sum of scoring of 100 monocytes and lymphocytes 0 to 4+ based on intensity of LAP staining
    C. the sum of scoring of 100 eosinophils 0 to 4+ based on intensity of LAP staining
    D. the sum of scoring of 100 bands and polymorphonuclear cells 0 to 4+ based on intensity of LAP staining
    E. the sum of scoring of 100 lymphocytes 0 to 4+ based on intensity of LAP staining

18. Why is it important to use fluorochromes that absorb light at one wavelength and emit at another wavelength in flow cytometry?
    A. the intensity of light at the original wavelength in flow cytometry
    B. for simultaneous analysis of cell size and complexity
    C. the change in wavelength and consequently color indicates the velocity of the particle
    D. the original wavelength used is not at a detectable wavelength
    E. the shift in wavelength allows for greater particle resolution

19. Which of the following stains expressed by pre-B cells are typically lost in B cells?
    A. TdT
    B. CD34
    C. HLA-DR
    D. A & B
    E. A, B, C

20. Which of the following B cell markers is expressed along with IgM expression?
    A. CD19
    B. CD34
    C. TdT
    D. CD38
    E. CD10

4: Hematopathology Questions

21. What is the normal peripheral blood and tissue ratio of T to B cells?
    A. 1:5
    B. 1:10
    C. 3-4:1
    D. 10:1
    E. 100:1

22. The surface expression pattern of CD3 follows the surface expression of this other T cell marker:
    A. CD2
    B. TdT
    C. CD34
    D. T cell receptor
    E. CD4

23. In which of the following locations are gamma-delta T cells most commonly found?
    A. spleen
    B. dermis
    C. intestine
    D. A & B
    E. A, B, C

24. All of the following neoplasms express high levels of bcl-6, except:
    A. nodular sclerosis Hodgkin lymphoma
    B. Burkitt lymphoma
    C. follicular lymphoma
    D. nodular lymphocyte-predominant Hodgkin lymphoma
    E. t(3;14) diffuse large B-cell lymphoma

25. All of the following cells express CD1a, except:
    A. Langerhans cells
    B. Touton giant cells
    C. dendritic reticular cells
    D. interdigitating reticulum cells
    E. cortical thymocytes

26. Which of the following T-cell phenotypes is most likely to be associated with a neoplasm?
    A. CD4+/CD8-
    B. CD4-/CD8+
    C. CD4+/CD8+
    D. CD4-/CD8-
    E. all of the above are normal phenotypes

27. In which of the following types of cells is CD5 usually expressed?
    A. mature T cells
    B. small lymphocytic lymphoma/chronic lymphocytic leukemia
    C. rheumatoid arthritis
    D. A & B
    E. A, B, C

28. Leu-M1 expression is commonly seen in all of the following, <u>except</u>:
    A. Reed-Sternberg cells
    B. mature monocytes
    C. anaplastic large cell lymphoma hallmark cells
    D. most adenocarcinomas
    E. granulocytes

29. What is the typical CD20 staining pattern in chronic lymphocytic leukemia?
    A. strong and diffuse
    B. dim
    C. absent
    D. cytoplasmic restriction
    E. nuclear

30. Which of the following surface markers is the IL-2 receptor?
    A. CD20
    B. CD21
    C. CD23
    D. CD25
    E. CD30

31. Which of the following cell surface markers is associated with a more aggressive subtype of CLL/SLL?
    A. CD13
    B. CD20
    C. FMC-7
    D. CD38
    E. CD125

32. Which of the following surface markers is expressed on nearly all cells but is decreased in paroxysmal nocturnal hemoglobinuria?
    A. CD19
    B. CD57
    C. CD59
    D. CD99
    E. CD123

33. CD99 expression is present in all the following, <u>except</u>:
    A. Ewing sarcoma
    B. lymphoblastic lymphoma
    C. granulosa cell tumor
    D. synovial sarcoma
    E. CD99 is expressed in all of the above

34. Which of the following malignancies can be positive for CD117?
    A. GI stromal tumor
    B. seminoma
    C. mastocytoma
    D. A & B
    E. A, B, C

4: Hematopathology Questions

35. In which of the following is HLA-DR most consistently expressed?
    A. acute promyelocytic leukemia
    B. B cell acute lymphocytic leukemia
    C. T cell acute lymphocytic leukemia
    D. immature T cells
    E. granulocytes

36. Which of the following immunoglobulin domains are expressed on the heavy chain and not the light chains?
    A. V
    B. D
    C. J
    D. C
    E. all of the above are expressed in both

37. Which of the following patterns best represents the order in which immunoglobulin chains rearrange in B cells?
    A. heavy chains, kappa light chain, lambda light chain
    B. kappa light, heavy, lambda
    C. kappa, lambda, heavy
    D. lambda, kappa, heavy
    E. heavy, lambda, kappa

38. What general rule of thumb is used for lower limit of detection of a clonal rearrangement implying malignancy?
    A. clone composing 0.1-0.5% of total cells
    B. clone composing >1-5% of total cells
    C. clone composing >5-10% of total cells
    D. clone composing >10-50% of total cells
    E. clone composing >50%

39. Which of the following procedures represents the second step of Southern blotting?
    A. apply DNA to agarose gel and subject to electrophoresis
    B. digest DNA with restriction endonucleases
    C. transfer DNA to membrane
    D. apply labeled probe
    E. extract DNA from cells with interest

40. All of the following translocations are suited for diagnosis by PCR, except:
    A. t(14;18)
    B. t(2;5)
    C. t(15;17)
    D. t(11;14)
    E. t(9;22)

41. Which of the following modalities is best suited for detecting translocations involving bcl-1 (cyclin D) gene?
    A. cytogenetics
    B. PCR
    C. fluorescence *in situ* hybridization (FISH)
    D. Southern blot
    E. immunohistochemistry

4: Hematopathology Questions

42. What is the most common mode of inheritance of hereditary spherocytosis?
    A.   autosomal recessive
    B.   autosomal dominant
    C.   X-linked recessive
    D.   X-linked dominant
    E.   it is not inherited; it is sporadic

43. Which RBC index is most consistently abnormal in cases of hereditary spherocytosis?
    A.   RBC count
    B.   MCV
    C.   Hct
    D.   Hgb
    E.   MCHC

44. Which of the following tests is most often performed to diagnose hereditary spherocytosis?
    A.   osmotic fragility test
    B.   DAT
    C.   Ham's test
    D.   flow cytometry
    E.   oxidative stress test

45. What protein is most commonly mutated in hereditary elliptocytosis?
    A.   ankyrin
    B.   spectrin
    C.   band 3
    D.   protein 4.2
    E.   elliptocin

46. What is the most common etiology in hereditary stomatocytosis?
    A.   abnormal Na/K permeability
    B.   deficient cytoskeletal structural proteins
    C.   inability to repair oxidative stress damage
    D.   hemoglobin mutation resulting in qualitative defects in hemoglobin
    E.   ATP depletion due to glycolytic enzyme deficiency

47. All of the following features of G6PD deficiency are typically seen on a Wright-Giemsa-stained peripheral smear, except:
    A.   poikilocytosis
    B.   spherocytosis
    C.   bite cells
    D.   blister cells
    E.   Heinz bodies

48. What is the best time to perform diagnostic testing for G6PD deficiency?
    A.   during a hemolytic crisis
    B.   3 days after a hemolytic crisis
    C.   3 weeks after a hemolytic crisis
    D.   1 month after a hemolytic crisis
    E.   3 months after a hemolytic crisis

4: Hematopathology Questions

49. Which of the following abnormal RBC morphologies is associated with pyruvate kinase deficiency?
    A. acanthocytes
    B. dacrocytes
    C. echinocytes
    D. drepanocytes
    E. stomatocytes

50. This condition is also known by a more descriptive acronym:
    A. CDA, type I
    B. CDA, type II
    C. CDA, type III
    D. pyruvate kinase deficiency
    E. paroxysmal nocturnal hemoglobinuria

51. What is the method of inheritance of paroxysmal nocturnal hemoglobinuria?
    A. X-linked recessive
    B. X-linked dominant
    C. autosomal recessive
    D. autosomal dominant
    E. it's not inherited; it's sporadic

52. All of the following test results are consistent with a diagnosis of paroxysmal nocturnal hemoglobinuria, except:
    A. decreased conversion of NADH to NAD
    B. increased hemolysis in isotonic sucrose
    C. increased hemolysis in acidified heterologous and homologous serum
    D. diminished CD55/59 on leukocytes, platelets, and red blood cells
    E. decreased LAP score

53. Which of the following RBC inclusions are seen in sideroblastic anemia and contain high amounts of iron?
    A. Cabot rings
    B. Howell-Jolly bodies
    C. Heinz bodies
    D. Pappenheimer bodies
    E. Hunt bodies

54. What accounts for the majority of cases of sideroblastic anemia?
    A. clonal stem cell defect
    B. medications
    C. alcohol
    D. irradiation
    E. copper deficiency

55. At which stage of erythroid development does parvovirus arrest?
    A. erythroblast
    B. normoblast
    C. pronormoblast
    D. reticulocyte
    E. erythrocyte

4: Hematopathology Questions

56. All of the following are true about Blackfan-Diamond syndrome, <u>except</u>:
     A. it is an inherited constitutional red cell aplasia
     B. erythroid precursors in the bone are decreased
     C. it usually responds to corticosteroids
     D. leukocytes are also decreased, platelets are unaffected
     E. i antigen is often present in high levels on red blood cells

57. To what class of disorders does Fanconi anemia belong?
     A. autosomal dominant proto-oncogenic activation
     B. X-linked recessive
     C. autosomal recessive chromosome breakage
     D. X-linked dominant
     E. mitochondrial

58. What do Blackfan-Diamond, Kostman, and thrombocytopenia with absent radii syndromes have in common?
     A. all are inherited in an autosomal dominant fashion
     B. all are associated with horseshoe kidney
     C. all have associated thrombocytopenia
     D. all are aplastic disorders of a single cell line
     E. the cells are all hypersensitive to clastogenic agents

59. What is the approximate prevalence of sickle cell trait among African-Americans?
     A. 0.01%
     B. 0.1%
     C. 2%
     D. 10%
     E. 33%

60. What is the average lifespan of red blood cells with HbSS?
     A. 5 days
     B. 17 days
     C. 38 days
     D. 56 days
     E. 120 days

61. The increased HbF often present in patients with sickle cell disease is protective. How?
     A. since there is no beta globin cells don't sickle as readily
     B. HbF binds O_2 with greater affinity than most other hemoglobins increasing RBC O_2 delivery
     C. HbF inhibits HbSS polymerization
     D. A & B
     E. A, B, C

62. What single etiology accounts for the majority of aplastic crises in children with sickle cell disease?
     A. *Salmonella*
     B. parvovirus B19
     C. repeated microthrombotic episodes
     D. low oxygen stress
     E. high oxygen stress

4: Hematopathology Questions

63. All of the following neurological conditions are associated with HbS disease, <u>except</u>:
    A. meningitis
    B. cerebral infarction
    C. Lhermitte-Duclos
    D. sensorineural hearing loss
    E. moyamoya disease

64. All of the following nephropathies are associated with sickle cell disease, <u>except</u>:
    A. papillary necrosis
    B. renal infarction
    C. thin basement membrane disease
    D. pyelonephritis
    E. renal medullary carcinoma

65. Which of the following complications of sickle cell disease occurs more frequently in patients with HbSC and HbS-beta thalassemia than in those with HbSS?
    A. pre-eclampsia
    B. chronic nonspecific hepatomegaly
    C. hyperhemolytic crisis
    D. priapism
    E. proliferative retinopathy

66. What is the effect of coinheritance of beta thalassemia on the HbS proportion in patients with HbS mutation?
    A. decreased
    B. no change
    C. elevated
    D. it depends
    E. there is no HbS in HbS-beta thalassemia

67. Which of the following hemoglobinopathies is associated with rod-shaped crystals?
    A. HbS
    B. HbC
    C. HbSC
    D. HbD
    E. HbE

68. This hemoglobinopathy is due to a fusion product of the delta and beta as well as a characteristic HbS proportion of less that 30%:
    A. HbD
    B. HbG
    C. Hb_{Lepore}
    D. $Hb_{Constant\ Spring}$
    E. HbE

69. All of the following hemoglobins are unstable, <u>except</u>:
    A. $Hb_{Chesapeake}$
    B. $Hb_{Hasharon}$
    C. Hb_{Koln}
    D. Hb_{Zurich}
    E. $Hb_{Hammersmith}$

4: Hematopathology Questions

70. Which of the following ions is bound to hemoglobin in methemoglobin?
    A. Ca^{++}
    B. Fe^{+++}
    C. Fe^{++}
    D. Mg^{++}
    E. Mn^{++}

71. What is the treatment of methemoglobinemia?
    A. methylene blue
    B. cyanide
    C. desferroxamine
    D. phenacetin
    E. EDTA

72. All of the following are part of the beta-globin cluster, <u>except</u>:
    A. delta globin gene
    B. beta globin gene
    C. alpha globin gene
    D. gamma globin gene
    E. beta pseudogene

73. What's the most frequent genetic cause of beta° allele production?
    A. nonsense mutations
    B. promoter mutations
    C. locus control region mutations
    D. point mutations
    E. 5' untranslated region mutations

74. Which of the following genotypes is associated with alpha thalassemia trait?
    A. --/-alpha
    B. -alpha/-alpha
    C. --/alpha^{cs}alpha
    D. A & B
    E. A, B, C

75. All of the following are considered "thalassemic indices," <u>except</u>:
    A. decreased RBC count
    B. low MCV
    C. lot Hct
    D. normal to slightly increased RDW
    E. MCV/RBC ratio <13

76. What's the most common confounding factor that causes beta-thalassemia to be diagnosed as alpha-thalassemia based on hemoglobin electrophoresis?
    A. concomitant sickle cell disease
    B. concomitant sickle cell trait
    C. concomitant congenital dyserythropoietic anemia
    D. iron deficiency
    E. hereditary elliptocytosis

ASCP Quick Compendium Companion for Clinical Pathology

4: Hematopathology Questions

77. How is beta-thalassemia major defined?
    A. beta/beta$^+$
    B. beta/beta$^\circ$
    C. beta$^\circ$/beta$^\circ$
    D. beta$^\circ$/beta$^+$
    E. none of the above

78. What's the most common cause of warm autoimmune hemolytic anemia?
    A. IgM anti-I
    B. IgG anti-I
    C. IgM anti-Rh
    D. IgG anti-Rh
    E. IgM anti-H

79. All of the following antibodies are capable of fixing complement, except:
    A. IgA
    B. IgM
    C. IgG1
    D. IgD
    E. IgG3

80. What's the specificity of the most common cause of cold autoagglutinins?
    A. anti-i
    B. anti-H
    C. anti-Pr
    D. anti-I
    E. anti-IH

81. What's the only reliable CBC index in the presence of cold agglutinins?
    A. Hct
    B. hemoglobin
    C. RDW
    D. platelets
    E. reticulocyte index

82. Which of the following reagents can be used to detect antibodies directed against the i antigen?
    A. type O cord blood
    B. type O adult blood
    C. type A1 adult blood
    D. A & B
    E. A, B, C

83. What is the most common modern presentation of paroxysmal cold hemoglobinuria?
    A. older people with Reynaud syndrome
    B. in children following a viral illness
    C. older person several years following a syphilis infection
    D. neonates with congenital syphilis
    E. alcoholics with advanced cirrhosis

4: Hematopathology Questions

84. What description best fits the Donath-Landsteiner antibody?
    A. IgM cold agglutinin/hemolysin
    B. biphasic IgM hemolysin
    C. IgG biphasic hemolysin
    D. IgG warm agglutinin/ hemolysin
    E. cold IgM agglutinin

85. Which describes the best way to detect cryoglobulins?
    A. run serum electrophoresis at 4°C
    B. clot blood at 4°C then immediately subject serum to electrophoresis
    C. incubate serum at 4°C with non-specific IgM, subject immunoprecipitate to electrophoresis
    D. clot blood at 37°C, store serum for 3 days at 4°C, collect precipitate and subject to electrophoresis
    E. spin down unclotted blood at 37°C, store supernatant at 4°C, subject precipitate to electrophoresis

86. Which of the following types of cryoglobulins are most commonly associated with Waldenstrom macroglobulinemia?
    A. type I
    B. type II
    C. type III
    D. types II and III
    E. type IV

87. All of the following are associated with the clinical presentation of cryoglobulinemia, except:
    A. palpable purpura
    B. petechiae
    C. arthralgias
    D. glomerulonephritis
    E. anemia

88. What is the most common renal manifestation of cryoglobulinemia?
    A. minimal change
    B. membranous glomerulopathy
    C. post-infectious glomerulonephritis
    D. membranoproliferative glomerulonephritis, type I
    E. membranoproliferative glomerulonephritis, type II

89. What is typically the earliest laboratory evidence of an iron-deficiency anemia?
    A. decreased transferrin
    B. decreased ferritin
    C. decreased serum iron
    D. increased zinc protoporphyrin
    E. decrease in hemoglobin

4: Hematopathology Questions

90. Which of the following patterns is most consistent with iron-deficiency anemia?
   A.   increased soluble serum transferrin receptor, zinc protoporphyrin, free erythrocyte protoporphyrin, and decreased ferritin
   B.   decreased soluble serum transferrin receptor, zinc protoporphyrin, free erythrocyte protoporphyrin, and increased ferritin
   C.   increased soluble serum transferrin receptor, decreased zinc protoporphyrin, free erythrocyte protoporphyrin, and ferritin
   D.   decreased soluble serum transferrin receptor, zinc protoporphyrin, free erythrocyte protoporphyrin, and ferritin
   E.   increased soluble serum transferrin receptor, zinc protoporphyrin, free erythrocyte protoporphyrin, and ferritin

91. What's the best estimate of iron concentration of packed red blood cells?
   A.   0.1 mg iron/unit pRBCs
   B.   0.2 mg iron/unit pRBCs
   C.   0.5 mg iron/unit pRBCs
   D.   1.0 mg iron/unit pRBCs
   E.   10 mg iron/unit pRBCs

92. What is the relationship between iron and lead levels in children?
   A.   no correlation
   B.   increased iron, and increased lead independent of socioeconomic status
   C.   decreased iron and increased lead independent of socioeconomic status
   D.   increased iron and increased lead dependent on socioeconomic status
   E.   decreased iron and increased lead dependent on socioeconomic status

93. Where does intrinsic factor bind vitamin B_{12}?
   A.   oral cavity
   B.   stomach
   C.   duodenum
   D.   ileum
   E.   jejunum

94. Where in the body is folate absorbed?
   A.   oral cavity
   B.   stomach
   C.   duodenum
   D.   ileum
   E.   jejunum

95. All of the following are features of megaloblastic anemia, except:
   A.   marked oval macrocytosis
   B.   left-shifted leukocytosis
   C.   decreased RBC count
   D.   hypersegmented neutrophils
   E.   large platelets

4: Hematopathology Questions

96. Which of the following represent residual nuclear fragments?
    A. Pappenheimer bodies
    B. Cabot rings
    C. Heinz bodies
    D. target cells
    E. basophilic stippling

97. Which of the following is the most common cause of anemia in hospitalized patients?
    A. inadequate iron intake
    B. inadequate folate intake
    C. hemolytic anemia
    D. inherited membrane or enzyme defects
    E. anemia of chronic disease

98. All of the following can cause intravascular hemolysis, except:
    A. ABO incompatibility
    B. penicillin-mediated immune hemolysis
    C. mechanical heart valve
    D. snake evenomation
    E. paroxysmal nocturnal hemoglobinuria

99. All of the following are in the differential diagnosis of hyporegenerative microcytic anemia, except:
    A. iron deficiency
    B. hereditary spherocytosis
    C. thalassemia
    D. sideroblastic anemia
    E. anemia of chronic disease

100. All of the following tumors are associated with erythrocytosis due to erythropoietin production, except:
    A. renal cell carcinoma
    B. cerebellar hemangioblastoma
    C. uterine leiomyoma
    D. hepatocellular carcinoma
    E. squamous cell carcinoma of the lung

101. All of the following are characteristics of a peripheral smear with reactive neutrophilia, except:
    A. toxic granulation
    B. up to 1% blasts
    C. Dohle bodies
    D. cytoplasmic vacuoles
    E. band forms and metamyelocytes

102. All of the following are suggestive of a myeloproliferative disorder, except:
    A. basophilia
    B. persistent neutrophilia
    C. normal LAP score
    D. lack of granulation/Dohle bodies
    E. myelocyte bulge

4: Hematopathology Questions

103. Which of the following infections is notable for a neutrophilia with a lack of toxic granulation, thrombocytopenia, hemoconcentration, and >10% immunoblastic lymphocytes?
    A.   hantavirus
    B.   *Cryptococcus*
    C.   *Yersinia pestis*
    D.   parvovirus B19
    E.   *Prototheca wickerhamii*

104. Which type of lymphocyte is most commonly the major component of a reactive lymphocytosis?
    A.   immature uncategorized lymphocytes
    B.   B cells
    C.   T cells
    D.   NK cells
    E.   follicular dendritic cells

105. Which demographic is most likely to experience the syndrome of persistent polyclonal B lymphocytes?
    A.   older men with chronic illness
    B.   young women with inborn errors of metabolism
    C.   neonates with congenital defects
    D.   young female smokers
    E.   pregnant woman with pre-eclampsia

106. Which of the following infections is classically associated with Reider cells with small mature clefted nuclei?
    A.   parvovirus B19
    B.   EBV
    C.   HIV
    D.   CMV
    E.   pertussis

107. Which of the following is/are suggestive of a monocytic neoplasm rather than a reactive monocytosis?
    A.   persistent monocytosis
    B.   promonocytes in the peripheral blood
    C.   splenomegaly
    D.   A & B
    E.   A, B, C

108. Which of the following cytokines is most responsible for eosinophil differentiation and release from the bone marrow?
    A.   IL-1
    B.   IL-2
    C.   IL-4
    D.   IL-5
    E.   IL-6

109. Which of the following features is most helpful in the lineage of blasts?
    A.   size of nuclei
    B.   Auer rods
    C.   prominent cytoplasmic vacuolization
    D.   presence of nucleoli
    E.   color of cytoplasm

4: Hematopathology Questions

110. What is the most common cause of neutropenia?
    A. medications
    B. lymphoid neoplasms
    C. infection
    D. non-lymphoid neoplasms
    E. congenital defects

111. Which of the following are required for the diagnosis of Felty syndrome?
    A. rheumatoid arthritis
    B. neutropenia
    C. splenomegaly
    D. A & B
    E. A, B, C

112. All of the following are associated with lymphopenia, except:
    A. systemic lupus erythematosus
    B. severe acute respiratory syndrome
    C. steroid therapy
    D. Kostmann syndrome
    E. Bruton agammaglobulinemia

113. In normal reactive lymph nodes where is the staining for bcl-2 strongest?
    A. follicle germinal center
    B. mantle zone
    C. marginal zone
    D. subcapsular region
    E. internodal zone

114. Which of the following infections is associated with florid follicular hyperplasia?
    A. syphilis
    B. HIV
    C. CMV
    D. HHV8
    E. HTLV-I

115. All of the following are associated with hyaline vascular Castleman disease, except:
    A. "lollipop" germinal center - germinal centers with perforating hyalinized vessels
    B. hyperplastic mantle "onion-skinning"
    C. multiple germinal center within a follicle
    D. HHV8 infection
    E. lack of systemic manifestations

116. Which of the following best characterizes Kimura disease?
    A. young Asian man with soft tissue head/neck mass, cervical lymphadenopathy, peripheral eosinophilia, and increased IgE
    B. woman with increased serum Ig and serum IgE
    C. young Asian man with mucocutaneous ulcers, "strawberry" tongue, edema, rash, coronary artery disease, and cervical lymphadenopathy
    D. sinus histiocytosis with massive lymphadenopathy in an older patient
    E. middle aged man with foamy macrophage infiltration into multiple organs

4: Hematopathology Questions

117. All the following are characteristic of Rosai-Dorfman disease, <u>except</u>:
    A. hemophagocytosis
    B. massive lymphadenopathy
    C. plasma cell-rich lymph node infiltrate
    D. S100, CD31, and CD11b positive histiocytes
    E. sinus histiocytosis

118. Which of the following infections is characterized by suppurative granulomas?
    A. cat-scratch disease
    B. lymphogranuloma venereum
    C. tularemia
    D. A & B
    E. A, B, C

119. Which of the following neoplastic lymphocytic expansions is most often confused with the diffuse pattern of nodal expansion associated with EBV and several other viruses?
    A. nodular lymphocyte-predominant Hodgkin lymphoma
    B. Hodgkin lymphoma
    C. small lymphocyte lymphoma
    D. follicular lymphoma
    E. mantle cell lymphoma

120. Which of the following immunohistochemical patterns is most consistent with CLL/SLL?
    A. CD5-/CD23-
    B. CD5-/CD23+
    C. CD5+/CD23-
    D. CD5+/CD23+
    E. SLL and CLL stain differently

121. What accounts for the frequent smudge cells in CLL?
    A. increased *in vivo* cell lysis
    B. apoptosis-related changes
    C. artifact due to EDTA
    D. artifact due to heparin
    E. bystander lysis

122. Which pattern of bone marrow infiltration by CLL is associated with the worst prognosis?
    A. diffuse
    B. nodular
    C. interstitial
    D. sparse
    E. homogeneous

123. Which CLL/SLL markers are associated with poor prognosis?
    A. CD38
    B. ZAP-70
    C. FMC7
    D. A & B
    E. A, B, C

124. All of the following changes are associated with CLL transformation to prolymphocytic lymphoma, <u>except</u>:
    A.   weakened CD23 expression
    B.   increased CD5
    C.   increased CD20
    D.   increased sIg
    E.   increased CD22

125. Which of the following clinical features is associated with the worst prognosis in SLL/CLL?
    A.   anemia
    B.   lymphadenopathy
    C.   splenomegaly
    D.   lymphocytosis
    E.   thrombocytosis

126. Which of the following markers is associated with unmutated immunoglobulin heavy chain variable region?
    A.   ZAP-70
    B.   CD38
    C.   CD23
    D.   A & B
    E.   A, B, C

127. Which of the following markers expressed in blastic mantle cell lymphoma helps to distinguish it from lymphoblastic lymphoma/leukemia?
    A.   cyclin D1
    B.   CD5
    C.   TdT
    D.   A & B
    E.   A, B, C

128. What is the fusion partner of bcl-1 that leads to its overexpression of t(11;14) mantle cell lymphoma?
    A.   MEN1
    B.   WT1
    C.   IgH
    D.   Ig kappa
    E.   Ig lambda

129. Which of the following testing modalities offers the best sensitivity for detection of the t(11;14) associated with mantle cell lymphoma?
    A.   Southern blot
    B.   fluorescent *in situ* hybridization (FISH)
    C.   PCR
    D.   RT-PCR
    E.   immunohistochemistry

130. Which of the following neoplasms has the most aggressive clinical course?
    A.   CLL/SLL
    B.   marginal zone lymphoma
    C.   mantle cell lymphoma
    D.   follicular lymphoma
    E.   hairy cell leukemia

131. Grading of follicular lymphoma is based on the proportion of which of the following cells?
    A.   centroblasts
    B.   centrocytes
    C.   tingible body macrophages
    D.   mature T cells
    E.   mature NK cells

132. What is the most common translocation associated with follicular lymphoma?
    A.   t(2;14)
    B.   t(4;8)
    C.   t(14;18)
    D.   t(8;22)
    E.   t(11;18)

133. What other neoplasm shares the same translocation as follicular lymphoma?
    A.   mantle cell lymphoma
    B.   SLL/CLL
    C.   prolymphocytic lymphoma
    D.   diffuse large B cell lymphoma
    E.   pre B ALL

134. What is the most common pattern of follicular lymphoma involvement in the bone marrow?
    A.   diffuse
    B.   focal
    C.   follicular lymphoma doesn't involve the marrow
    D.   nodular
    E.   paratrabecular

135. In both nodal and extranodular marginal zone lymphoma what shape do B cells classically adopt?
    A.   monocytoid
    B.   plasmacytoid
    C.   giant cell
    D.   megaloblastic
    E.   small, cleaved

136. Which histological feature is most helpful in distinguishing the villous lymphocytes of splenic marginal zone lymphoma with villous lymphocytes from hairy cell leukemia?
    A.   the length of the hair-like processes
    B.   the presence or absence of nucleolus
    C.   indentation of nucleus
    D.   color of the cytoplasm
    E.   abundance or paucity of cytoplasm

137. What is the most common translocation found in extranodal marginal zone lymphoma of the stomach?
    A.   t(1;19)
    B.   t(1;14)
    C.   t(11;18)
    D.   t(14;18)
    E.   t(4;18)

4: Hematopathology Questions

138. All of the following are commonly involved by hairy cell leukemia, <u>except</u>:
    A. lymph nodes
    B. spleen
    C. bone marrow
    D. peripheral blood
    E. liver

139. What single cytopenia is most commonly associated hairy cell leukemia?
    A. neutropenia
    B. monocytopenia
    C. lymphopenia
    D. anemia
    E. thrombocytopenia

140. All of the following histological characteristics are consistently associated with hairy cell leukemia, <u>except</u>:
    A. large cells
    B. uniform cells
    C. flocculent pale cytoplasm
    D. hairy projections
    E. ground glass chromatin

141. All of the following disorders can be positive for tartrate-resistant acid phosphatase, <u>except</u>:
    A. hairy cell leukemia
    B. prolymphocytic leukemia
    C. mast cell disease
    D. extranodal marginal zone lymphoma
    E. Gaucher cells

142. All of the following markers are usually positive in hairy cell leukemia, <u>except</u>:
    A. CD11c
    B. CD5
    C. CD25
    D. CD103
    E. CD20

143. What percentage of prolymphocytes must be present for a diagnosis of prolymphocytic leukemia?
    A. >10%
    B. >25%
    C. >55%
    D. >75%
    E. >90%

144. What's the most common association with lymphoplasmacytic lymphoma?
    A. hypercalcemia
    B. macroglobulinemia
    C. hyperammonemia
    D. proteinuria
    E. mediastinal sclerosis

145. All of the following entities have been categorized under the rubric of diffuse large B cell lymphoma, except:
    A. anaplastic large cell lymphoma
    B. CD30+ B cell neoplasm with anaplasia
    C. centroblastic lymphoma
    D. immunoblastic lymphoma
    E. T cell-rich B cell lymphoma

146. What's the most common translocation associated with diffuse large B cell lymphoma?
    A. t(12;21)
    B. t(14;18)
    C. t(3;14)
    D. t(8:14)
    E. t(1;19)

147. Diffuse large B cell lymphoma, especially in AIDS patients is by far the most common primary lymphoma occurring in this organ:
    A. heart
    B. brain
    C. lung
    D. kidney
    E. skin

148. Of the three types of Burkitt lymphoma, which is most commonly associated with EBV?
    A. endemic
    B. sporadic
    C. immunodeficiency

149. Which of the following translocations is associated with Burkitt lymphoma?
    A. t(8;14)
    B. t(2;8)
    C. t(8;22)
    D. A & B
    E. A, B, C

150. All of the following entities are associated HHV-8, except:
    A. primary effusion lymphoma
    B. post-transplant lymphoproliferative disorder
    C. multicentric Castleman disease
    D. Kikuchi-Fujimoto lymphadenitis
    E. Kaposi sarcoma

151. What other disease entity is lymphomatoid granulomatosis most often confused with?
    A. tuberculosis
    B. primary vasculitis
    C. extranodal marginal zone lymphoma
    D. dermatitis herpetiformis
    E. sarcoidosis

152. Which of the following viruses is associated with post-transplant lymphoproliferative disorder?
    A. HIV
    B. HHV-8
    C. EBV
    D. HTLV-I
    E. BK virus

153. What percentage of acute lymphoblastic leukemia are of B cell lineage?
    A. <1%
    B. 10%
    C. 40%
    D. 80%
    E. 99%

154. What's the most common presentation of T-ALL?
    A. anterior mediastinal mass
    B. bone marrow involvement/cytopenias
    C. cervical lymphadenopathy
    D. dermal lymphatic infiltrates
    E. endocrine dysfunction

155. All of the following genetic alterations are associated unfavorable prognosis in pre-B-ALL, except:
    A. t(9;22)
    B. t(4;11)
    C. t(1;19)
    D. t(12;21)
    E. hypodiploidy

156. What marker is most sensitive for T-ALL, so much so that diagnosis of T-ALL should really not be made without it?
    A. CD19
    B. CD4
    C. CD7
    D. CD8
    E. HLA-DR

157. Which of the following markers is highly specific for AML?
    A. CD13
    B. CD2
    C. CD10
    D. CD117
    E. CD33

158. What is the most common Ig paraprotein present in multiple myeloma?
    A. IgG
    B. IgA
    C. light chains
    D. IgD
    E. IgE

4: Hematopathology Questions

159. What's the most common cause of an apparent lack of M-spike on serum protein electrophoresis in patients with multiple myeloma?
    A. IgA-producing tumor
    B. IgD-producing tumor
    C. IgE-producing tumor
    D. light chain only-myeloma
    E. nonsecretory myeloma

160. Which of the following statements accurately represents the requirements for the diagnosis of multiple myeloma?
    A. 2 major criteria
    B. 1 major + 1 minor criterion, or 3 minor (which must include the first two) criteria
    C. 2 major criteria + 1 minor criterion
    D. 1 major criterion + 2 minor (which must include the first two) criteria
    E. >20% marrow plasmacytosis + M component

161. All of the following translocations are commonly associated with multiple myeloma, except:
    A. t(14;18)
    B. t(14;16)
    C. t(4;14)
    D. t(11;14)
    E. del 17p13.1

162. What percentage of peripheral plasma cells is a prerequisite for a presumptive diagnosis of plasma cell leukemia?
    A. 0%; there's no such thing as plasma cell leukemia
    B. 5%
    C. 10%
    D. 20%
    E. 30%

163. What's the most common site of involvement for a solitary plasmacytoma?
    A. tibia
    B. vertebra
    C. pelvis
    D. ribs
    E. cranial bones

164. What feature separates smoldering myeloma from indolent myeloma?
    A. marrow plasmacytosis 10-30%
    B. renal failure
    C. lytic bone lesions
    D. hypercalcemia
    E. anemia

165. What percentage of people with monoclonal gammopathy of uncertain significance (MGUS) go on to develop myeloma (within 20 years)?
    A. <1%
    B. 10%
    C. 30%
    D. 70%
    E. >90%

4: Hematopathology Questions

166. All of the following are associated with POEMS syndrome, <u>except</u>:
    A. organomegaly
    B. polyneuropathy
    C. endocrinopathy
    D. syndrome of inappropriate diuretic hormone
    E. M-spike

167. What is the characteristic nuclear feature of peripheral T-cell lymphoma?
    A. multinucleation
    B. cloverleaf morphology
    C. prominent nucleoli
    D. cerebriform nuclei
    E. dark pyknotic nucleus

168. All of the following clinical features are associated with adult T-cell leukemia/lymphoma, <u>except</u>:
    A. hypocalcemia
    B. skin rash
    C. increased soluble IL-2 receptor
    D. lytic bone lesions
    E. splenomegaly

169. Which of the following cell surface markers is most consistently positive in cutaneous T-cell lymphomas?
    A. CD7
    B. CD4
    C. CD8
    D. CD25
    E. CD38

170. Which of the following findings is central to distinguishing angioimmunoblastic T-cell lymphoma from a reactive process?
    A. cortical proliferation
    B. prominent germinal centers
    C. angioinvasion/vasculitis
    D. absent follicles
    E. amyloid deposition

171. Which of the following presentations of anaplastic large cell lymphoma has the best prognosis?
    A. ALK (-) disease
    B. presentation of ALK (+) disease in children
    C. ALK (+) disease with a leukemic component
    D. ALK (+) disease in an older person
    E. older person with ALK (-) disease

172. All of the following translocations have been associated with anaplastic large cell lymphoma, <u>except</u>:
    A. t(2;5)
    B. t(2;13)
    C. t(1;2)
    D. t(2;3)
    E. inv(2)

4: Hematopathology Questions

173. In addition to a sustained large granular lymphocytosis, what additional finding in the peripheral smear is often seen with large granular lymphocytic leukemia?
    A. neutrophilia
    B. anemia
    C. thrombocytopenia
    D. monocytosis
    E. neutropenia

174. Which of the following disorders is most closely associated with enteropathy-type T cell lymphoma?
    A. *H. pylori* gastritis
    B. celiac sprue
    C. ulcerative colitis
    D. Crohn disease
    E. hereditary non-polyposis colon cancer

175. Which of the following is the most commonly associated with hepatosplenic T cell lymphoma?
    A. older man, alpha-beta T cells
    B. younger woman, alpha-beta T cells
    C. younger man, alpha-beta T cells
    D. older woman, gamma delta T cells
    E. young man, gamma delta T cells

176. Which of the following sites is blastic NK cell lymphoma most commonly seen?
    A. lymph nodes
    B. skin
    C. bone marrow
    D. peripheral blood
    E. nasal cavity

177. Extranodal NK/T cell lymphoma, nasal type is associated with which of the following viruses?
    A. EBV
    B. HIV
    C. HHV8
    D. HPV
    E. CMV

178. All of the following types of Hodgkin lymphoma are typically CD15+/CD30+/CD45-, except:
    A. lymphocyte-rich
    B. nodular lymphocyte-predominant
    C. lymphocyte-depleted
    D. nodular sclerosis
    E. mixed cellularity

179. What is the most common form of Hodgkin lymphoma among those with AIDS?
    A. lymphocyte-rich
    B. nodular lymphocyte-predominant
    C. lymphocyte-depleted
    D. nodular sclerosis
    E. mixed cellularity

4: Hematopathology Questions

180. What is the expected flow cytometric phenotype of a lymph node with classical Hodgkin lymphoma?
    A. CD15+/CD30+
    B. CD15-/CD30+
    C. CD15+/CD30-
    D. CD15-/CD30-
    E. CD3+/CD5+

181. What subtype of Hodgkin lymphoma most often presents as a mediastinal mass?
    A. lymphocyte-rich
    B. nodular lymphocyte-predominant
    C. lymphocyte-depleted
    D. nodular sclerosis
    E. mixed cellularity

182. All of the following are characteristics of the myelodysplastic syndromes, except:
    A. cytopenias
    B. splenomegaly
    C. dyshematopoietic cell morphology
    D. clonal stem cell disorder
    E. propensity to develop acute leukemia

183. All of the following are examples of myelodysplastic syndrome, except:
    A. chronic myelomonocytic leukemia (CMML)
    B. refractory anemia (RA)
    C. refractory anemia with excessive blasts (RAEB)
    D. 5q (-) syndrome
    E. refractory cytopenia with multilineage dysplasia (RCMD)

184. To what does the term "abnormal localization of immature precursors (ALIP)" refer?
    A. the presence of immature cells in soft tissue
    B. synonymous with extramedullary hematopoiesis
    C. immature cells in the peripheral smear
    D. clusters of immature cells between but not adjacent to marrow trabeculae or vessels
    E. the inability of stem cells to populate the bone marrow

185. All of the following cytogenetic abnormalities are associated with a good prognosis in myelodysplastic syndrome, except:
    A. single chromosomal abnormality
    B. del 5q
    C. loss of Y
    D. del 20q
    E. monosomy 7

186. In addition to blasts what other cell type is considered in the counting of blasts in acute monoblastic lymphoma?
    A. promyelocytes
    B. promonocytes
    C. monocytes
    D. pronormoblasts
    E. prolymphocytes

4: Hematopathology Questions

187. What translocation is most commonly associated with CMML with eosinophilia?
    A.   inv(16)
    B.   t(16;16)
    C.   t(5;12)
    D.   t(15;17)
    E.   t(9;22)

188. Which of the following disorders is characterized by anemia with increased hemoglobin F, frequent monosomy 7, and hypersensitivity of granulocytes and macrophages to GM-CSF?
    A.   chronic myelomonocytic leukemia (CMML)
    B.   atypical chronic myelogenous leukemia (aCML)
    C.   juvenile myelomonocytic leukemia (JMML)
    D.   refractory anemia with excessive blasts (RAEB)
    E.   chronic myelomonocytic leukemia with eosinophils (CMML with eos)

189. Which of the following features defines chronic myelogenous leukemia?
    A.   JAK2 mutation
    B.   myelocyte "bulge"
    C.   basophilia, eosinophilia, and thrombocytosis
    D.   chloroma
    E.   t(9;22)

190. What percentage of cases of chronic myelogenous leukemia (CML) will progress to AML within 3-7 years?
    A.   <1%
    B.   10%
    C.   25%
    D.   50%
    E.   95%

191. Myeloproliferative diseases all share a common platelet defect. What is the best characterization of that defect?
    A.   impaired binding to von Willebrand factor
    B.   dense granule defect
    C.   alpha granule defects
    D.   impaired aggregation with epinephrine
    E.   giant platelet with platelet clumping

192. All of the following have been shown to be associated with the accelerated phase of chronic myelogenous leukemia, except:
    A.   thrombocytopenia
    B.   leukocytosis
    C.   decreasing LAP score
    D.   increasing blasts (10-20%)
    E.   thrombocytosis

193. Which of the following mutations is often seen in addition to the Philadelphia chromosome in blast crisis chronic myelogenous leukemia?
    A.   i(17q)
    B.   t(4;11)
    C.   del (5q)
    D.   t(15;17)
    E.   t(2;22)

4: Hematopathology Questions

194. Which of the following conditions is an absolute requirement for the diagnosis of polycythemia vera?
    A. rule out secondary causes of erythrocytosis
    B. increased red blood cell mass or hemoglobin greater than or equal to 18.5 g/dL for men or 16.5 g/dL for women
    C. clonal cytogenetic abnormality
    D. A & B
    E. A, B, C

195. What's the most common cause of death in patients with polycythemia vera?
    A. thrombotic event
    B. acute leukemia
    C. bleeding secondary to thrombocytopenia
    D. sepsis
    E. bone marrow exhaustion/depletion

196. Which of the following conditions is most often associated with the V617F mutation of JAK2?
    A. chronic myelogenous leukemia
    B. essential thrombocytosis
    C. chronic idiopathic myelofibrosis
    D. polycythemia vera
    E. chronic neutrophilic leukemia

197. Which of the following myeloproliferative disease is mostly a diagnosis of exclusion of other types of myeloproliferative disease?
    A. chronic myelogenous leukemia
    B. essential thrombocytosis
    C. chronic idiopathic myelofibrosis
    D. polycythemia vera
    E. all myeloproliferative diseases are unique with characteristic phenotypic diagnostic features

198. Which phase of chronic idiopathic myelofibrosis is the most common stage for patients to present in?
    A. pre-fibrotic
    B. fibrotic
    C. indolent
    D. accelerated
    E. blast crisis

199. What feature distinguishes chronic eosinophilic leukemia from hypereosinophilic syndrome?
    A. the extent of the eosinophilia
    B. tissue destruction
    C. evidence of a cytogenetic anomaly or blasts up to 20%
    D. symptoms of hypereosinophilia
    E. etiology

200. Which of the following t(9;22) gene fusion products is associated with a form of chronic myelogenous leukemia that resembles chronic neutrophilic leukemia?
    A. p190 protein
    B. p210
    C. p230
    D. p272
    E. p300

4: Hematopathology Questions

201. All of the following are the main groups of acute myeloid leukemia (AML), <u>except</u>:
    A. AML with multilineage dysplasia
    B. AML with lymphoid differentiation
    C. AML with recurrent genetic abnormalities
    D. AML, NOS
    E. AML, therapy-related

202. What genes are translocated with t(8;21) acute myelogenous leukemia?
    A. PML-RARalpha
    B. AML1-ETO
    C. MYH11-CBFbeta
    D. MLL-AF9
    E. MLL-AF4

203. What type of extra-leukemic morphologically abnormal cells proliferate in acute myelogenous leukemia with inv(16)?
    A. monocytes
    B. macrophages
    C. erythrocytes
    D. platelets
    E. eosinophils

204. All of the following are true about acute myelogenous leukemia with t(15;17), <u>except</u>:
    A. most consistently demonstrates Auer rods
    B. patients often present with DIC
    C. most respond to all-trans retinoic acid
    D. strong expression of HLA-DR and CD34 in all subtypes
    E. the microgranular variant resembles acute monocytic leukemia

205. Which type of chemotherapeutic agent is most commonly associated with acute myelogenous leukemia with anomalies of 11q23?
    A. busulfan
    B. topoisomerase II inhibitors
    C. methotrexate
    D. microtubule inhibitors
    E. translation inhibitors

206. What defines acute myelogenous leukemia, minimally differentiated (FAB M0)?
    A. >20% blasts positive for Sudan black B
    B. positivity for Sudan black B, myeloperoxidase, or non-specific esterase in at least 50% of blasts
    C. positivity for Sudan black B, myeloperoxidase, or non-specific esterase in at least 100% of blasts
    D. >20% blasts lacking cytochemical evidence of myeloid differentiation
    E. >20% blasts with hypergranular cytoplasm

207. What developmental stage and percentage of total blasts must be seen for a diagnosis of acute myelogenous leukemia without maturation (FAB M1)?
    A. 20% blasts, of which 10% are myeloblasts
    B. 20% blasts, of which 90% are myeloblasts
    C. 30% blasts, of which 10% are myeloblasts
    D. 20% blasts, of which 10% are myeloblasts/promyelocytes
    E. 20% blasts, of which 90% are myeloblasts/promyelocytes

4: Hematopathology Questions

208. How does AML, M2 differ from AML, M1 in strictly diagnostic terms?
   A.   monocytes must compose a greater percentage of the marrow
   B.   there must be at least 20% monocytes in M1
   C.   there must be at least 20% promyelocytes in M1
   D.   M1 and M2 are the same but with different consistent genetic abnormalities
   E.   myeloblasts are greater than or equal to 90% in M1, less than 90% in M2

209. Which of the following best describes the criteria for the diagnosis of acute myelogenous leukemia, M4 (FAB)?
   A.   20% blasts, 20% monocytes, 20% neutrophilic precursors
   B.   20% blasts, 50% monocytes, 50% neutrophilic precursors
   C.   20% blasts, 90% monocytes, 10% neutrophilic precursors
   D.   30% blasts, 10% monocytes, 90% neutrophilic precursors
   E.   30% blasts, 90% monocytes, 10% neutrophilic precursors

210. What other entity is frequently confused with AML, M5?
   A.   AML, M0
   B.   T ALL
   C.   APL, microgranular variant
   D.   pre B ALL
   E.   AML, M8

211. Which of the following AML FAB subtypes commonly presents with gingival bleeding?
   A.   M0
   B.   M1
   C.   M3
   D.   M5
   E.   M7

212. What's the most common presentation of AML, M6?
   A.   >80% of nucleated marrow cells are erythroid precursors
   B.   >50% of nucleated marrow cells are erythroid precursors and >20% of non-erythroid cells are myeloblasts
   C.   >50% of nucleated marrow cells are erythroid precursors and <20% of non-erythroid cells are myeloblasts
   D.   80% blasts with 20% erythroid precursors, >20% myeloblasts
   E.   80% blasts with 20% erythroid precursors

213. Which of the following techniques can be used to enumerate megakaryoblasts for the purpose of diagnosing M7?
   A.   CD41 immunohistochemistry
   B.   CD61 immunohistochemistry
   C.   platelet peroxidase
   D.   A & B
   E.   A, B, C

214. Which of the following is associated with acute myelogenous leukemia, M7?
   A.   Down syndrome
   B.   mediastinal germ cell tumor
   C.   systemic mastocytosis
   D.   A & B
   E.   A, B, C

215. What's the most common type of congenital acute leukemia?
   A. AML, M0
   B. AML, M7
   C. AML, M4/M5
   D. T ALL
   E. pre-B ALL

216. All of the following are forms of mastocytosis, except:
   A. solitary mastocytosis
   B. anaphylactic reaction
   C. telangiectasia macularis eruptiva perstans
   D. urticaria pigmentosa
   E. diffuse erythrodermic mastocytosis

217. Which of the following markers correlates most closely with the presence of c-kit mutations in systemic mastocytosis?
   A. CD2
   B. IL-2 receptor
   C. CK7
   D. trk receptor
   E. CD25

218. Atypical lymphocytes are usually seen with which type of infection?
   A. bacterial
   B. viral
   C. fungal
   D. parasite
   E. amoebic

219. Which of the following borrelial spirochete organisms can be seen in the peripheral smear?
   A. *B. recurrentis*
   B. *B. afzelli*
   C. *B. anserina*
   D. *B. burgdorfei*
   E. *B. valasiana*

220. What is the WHO definition of hypoplastic AML subtype?
   A. <50% cellularity of marrow with >20% blasts
   B. <50% cellularity of marrow with >10% blasts
   C. <20% cellularity of marrow with >20% blasts
   D. <20% cellularity of marrow with >10% blasts
   E. you can't fool me; the WHO doesn't define a hypoplastic subtype

221. All of the following are characteristic of hematogones, except:
   A. immature features
   B. nuclear immaturity
   C. bone marrow aggregates
   D. TdT positivity
   E. CD34 positivity

4: Hematopathology Questions

222. How is the morphological remission of acute leukemia defined?
     A.   no PCR-amplifiable genetic anomalies
     B.   lack of CD34 staining
     C.   no IHC-demonstrable disease on bone marrow biopsy
     D.   <5% blasts in marrow
     E.   no demonstrable morphological disease but evidence of genetic disease by PCR

223. All of the following are potential causes of marrow fibrosis, except:
     A.   chronic idiopathic myelofibrosis
     B.   hairy cell leukemia
     C.   diffuse large B cell lymphoma
     D.   mastocytosis
     E.   Hodgkin lymphoma

224. What is the clinical definition of fever of unknown etiology?
     A.   an inpatient negative fever workup
     B.   a fever lasting one month or more
     C.   lymphoma, undiscovered
     D.   3 weeks of fevers >38.3°C without an obvious etiology
     E.   a fever in a patient with 3 consecutive negative cultures

225. Which malignancy is most often associated with sea-blue histiocytes?
     A.   acute lymphoblastic leukemia
     B.   chronic myelogenous leukemia
     C.   acute myelogenous leukemia
     D.   chronic lymphocytic lymphoma
     E.   multiple myeloma

226. Which of the following can be associated with a hemophagocytic syndrome?
     A.   T cell lymphoma
     B.   EBV infection
     C.   Hashimoto thyroiditis
     D.   A & B
     E.   A, B, C

227. What's the most common location of extranodal lymphoma?
     A.   esophagus
     B.   stomach
     C.   lungs
     D.   liver
     E.   CNS

4: Hematopathology Answers

1. D. SULFHEMOGLOBIN.

    The hemiglobin cyanide technique involves oxidizing hemoglobin and converting it to hemiglobin cyanide, which is measured at an absorbance of 540nm. Almost all forms of hemoglobin, with the notable exception of sulfhemoglobin, can be measured in this fashion.
    QCCP2, **Measurement of total hemoglobin,** p 242

2. B. HEMATOCRIT.

    Red cell counts are measured by the Coulter principle, which states the pulse in voltage that occurs when a cell passes through a current is proportional to the volume of the cell. The range of volumes is the RDW; the mean is the MCV. From the MCV and the RBC count, the hematocrit can be calculated (hematocrit = MCV × RBC).
    QCCP2, **Automated techniques,** p 242

3. B. LYSIS OF RED BLOOD CELLS.

    Because the volume of red blood cells and leukocytes is very similar, and the Coulter principle technique counts cells as a function of their volume, RBCs and WBCs are counted as one. In RBC counts, it's usually not a problem because there are a lot more red blood cells than white blood cells and red blood cells are lysed to count the white cells.
    QCCP2, **Leukocyte indices,** p 243

4. D. EOSINOPHILS.

    Side scatter is a measurement of cytoplasmic granularity or complexity. Eosinophils present with the highest level of side scatter due to the crystalline inclusions.
    QCCP2, **Flow cytometry,** p 247

5. B. 2-20 FL.

    Smaller than red blood cells and leukocytes, platelets can be quantitated by the Coulter method, too. From this it is evident why schistocytes (fragmented red blood cells) can present as an artefactually high platelet count and platelet clumping or large platelets can lead to a low platelet count.
    QCCP2, **Platelets,** p 243

6. D. RNA.

    Residual ribosomal RNA characterizes reticulocytes which can be demonstrated with supravital staining (crystal violet or methylene blue). Reticulocytes tend to be larger than mature red cells. However, this is not as dependable an index of reticulocytes as RNA.
    QCCP2, **Reticulocytes,** p 243

7. B. RNA CONTENT.

    Reticulocytes are non-nucleated. And while ribosomes, mitochondria, and Golgi bodies are often present in reticulocytes, it is the RNA content that best assists with determining its age.
    QCCP2, **Reticulocytes,** p 243

4: Hematopathology Answers

8.　C.　**15%.**

I don't even want to think of hematocrits of 5% or 2% - they are surely incompatible with life. The correction factor is a means of standardizing the reticulocyte count when calculating the proliferation index (RPI). As the hematocrit drops, younger reticulocytes with a longer maturation time are released, which could give an artefactually high RPI. As hematocrit drops, the correction factor increases, so that at a hematocrit of 15, the correction factor is 3.0, and at a hematocrit of 30, the correction factor is 2, and with a normal hematocrit, the correction factor is one.
QCCP2, **Reticulocytes,** p 244

9.　E.　**A, B, C.**

Almost any sickling hemoglobin in any combination can lead to a positive result - SS, SA, SC, etc - including C_{Harlem}. It is important to ensure there is sufficient HbS in order for the test to be positive.
QCCP2, **Detection of normal and variant hemoglobins,** p 244

10.　B.　PANCELLULAR.

This is true for the most part. Since almost all cells would be affected by persistence of fetal hemoglobin, it could be demonstrated to be present in almost all cells. Other conditions, such as sickle cell disease or thalassemia associated with increased hemoglobin F, have a heterocellular distribution of fetal hemoglobin.
QCCP2, **Detection of fetal hemoglobin,** p 244

11.　A.　HBS, HBD.

Alkaline electrophoresis is unable to distinguish (resolve) between HbS, HbD, and HbG. Electrophoresis under acidic conditions allows for the resolution of HbS from HbD and HbG (which are still not resolved between each other. I use an easy two-step method to read hemoglobin electrophoretic gels:

1.　align gels with positive electrodes together, alkaline on the left.

2.　utilize mnemonics to remember band migration:

Alkaline gel - from left, the bands: "$\underline{A}_2$ $\underline{CEO}$, $\underline{S}$ave me $\underline{D}$ear $\underline{G}$od $\underline{F}$rom $\underline{A}$nemia. $\underline{Bart}$ goes to the $\underline{NIH}$" HbA_2, HbC, E, O; HbS, D, G; HbF; HbA; HbBarts; HbN, I, H.

Acidic gel - from the left: "$\underline{C}$razy $\underline{S}$ick $\underline{AGED}$ $\underline{F}$ather" - HbC; HbS; HbA, G, E, D; HbF
QCCP2, **Hemoglobin electrophoresis, F4.2b,** p 244

12.　D.　**A & B.**

Due to a decrease in HbA (2 alpha and 2 beta chains) from making less beta globin, there is a relative increase in HbA_2. The other findings are considered "thalassemic indices," alpha thalassemia differs in that the HbA_2 is normal.
QCCP2, **Hemoglobin electrophoresis,** p 245

13.　C.　HBA_2.

　　E.　HBF.

They are the only hemoglobins that the FDA has approved for quantitation by HPLC.
QCCP2, **HPLC,** p 245

4: Hematopathology Answers

14. E. **A, B, C.**

Eosin stains the red blood cells. Nucleic acids are stained by the basic methylene blue. Stain tint varies with pH.
QCCP2, **Histochemical and cytochemical,** p 246

15. D. **A & B.**

While myeloperoxidase and chloracetate esterase (CAE) are fairly specific for granulocytes, Sudan black B can stain granulocytes and monocytes.
QCCP2, **Cytochemical stains for typing blasts,** p 246

16. A. MONOCYTES.

While all of the mentioned cell types can be stained to a variable extent by NSE, monocytes are the most consistently stained and the only cell type whose staining is inhibited by sodium fluoride.
QCCP2, **Cytochemical stains,** p 246

17. D. THE SUM OF SCORING OF 100 BANDS AND POLYMORPHONUCLEAR CELLS 0 TO 4+ BASED ON INTENSITY OF LAP STAINING.

The leukocyte alkaline phosphatase (LAP) score is a quantitative means of assessing the differential diagnosis of a high white blood cell count. Normal values fall in the 50-150 range. Low LAP scores are found in chronic myelogenous leukemia and paroxysmal nocturnal hemoglobinuria, while high LAP scores are seen with leukemoid (reactive) reaction, myeloproliferative disorders (other than CML), and steroid administration.
QCCP2, **LAP,** p 247

18. B. FOR SIMULTANEOUS ANALYSIS OF CELL SIZE AND COMPLEXITY.

As light passes through the single cell flow counter, it excites the fluorochrome while simultaneously being refracted to an extent based on the characteristics of the cells passing through. The refracted light information is at the original wavelength and, depending on the position of the detector, represents cell size (forward scatter) or cytoplasmic complexity (side scatter). At the same time, a third detector determines the intensity of fluorochrome emittance (at a different wavelength).
QCCP2, **Flow cytometry,** p 247

19. D. **A & B.**

The pro-B cell stage still retains some of the rudimentary stem cell markers while undergoing heavy chain rearrangement, the pre-B cells tend to lose TdT and CD34, but retain HLA-DR.
QCCP2, **Expected phenotypes of hematopoietic cells,** p 248

20. A. **CD19.**

CD19 is one of the most consistent B lymphocyte markers, present in all immature B cells and finally lost in the development of plasma cells.
QCCP2, **T4.2 B and T cell maturation stages,** p 248

4: Hematopathology Answers

21.　C.　**3-4:1.**

　　　The mantra "3-4:1" will support you through much of hematopathology. It is also the ratio of CD4 to CD8 T cells and the ratio of kappa:lambda in normal B cells.
　　　QCCP2, **B lymphocytes,** p 248

22.　D.　**T cell receptor.**

　　　CD3 expression in less mature T cells is restricted to the cytoplasm. With progressive maturation, cytoplasmic CD3 expression is lost while surface CD3 expression is seen. The appearance of CD3 on the surface is coincident with the expression of T cell receptor on the cell surface where it is noncovalently associated with CD3.
　　　QCCP2, **T lymphocytes,** p 248

23.　E.　**A, B, C.**

　　　While the vast majority of T cells are of the alpha beta subtype, there are significant numbers of gamma delta T cells found in the spleen, dermis, and intestine - which are also the most common sites of gamma delta T-cell lymphoma.
　　　QCCP2, **T lymphocytes,** p 248

24.　A.　**nodular sclerosis Hodgkin lymphoma.**

　　　The normal expression of bcl-6 is confined to normal germinal center B cells. It can also be expressed in a number of malignancies, aiding in diagnosis.
　　　QCCP2, **Immunophenotyping,** p 249

25.　B.　**Touton giant cells.**

　　　While CD1a expression is usually thought to be associated with Langerhans' cells, it is important to note that its expression is not limited to Langerhans cells. A common mistaken diagnosis for Langerhans histiocytosis is thymoma, due to the misinterpretation of a positive CD1a stain.
　　　QCCP2, **Immunophenotyping,** p 249

26.　D.　**CD4-/CD8-.**

　　　Choices A and B are the T cells we typically think of in the peripheral blood (remember "3-4:1" CD4+ to CD8+ cells). In the thymic cortex it is not unusual to have immature CD4+/CD8+ cells. CD4-/CD8- cells are abnormal and are most often associated with a neoplastic condition.
　　　QCCP2, **Immunophenotyping,** p 249

27.　E.　**A, B, C.**

　　　Benign polyclonal CD5+/CD19+/CD20+ B cells can be seen associated with several conditions, including rheumatoid arthritis. In addition, normal mature T-cells often express CD5, but it can be lost in T cell leukemia or lymphoma. Of course, several mature B cell neoplastic conditions, such as CLL/SLL and mantle cell lymphoma, are associated with CD5 expression.
　　　QCCP2, **Immunophenotyping,** p 249

4: Hematopathology Answers

28. C. **ANAPLASTIC LARGE CELL LYMPHOMA HALLMARK CELLS.**

Leu-M1 or CD15 is a widespread antigen expressed in a number of tissues. Classically, the differential diagnosis between Hodgkin lymphoma and ALCL, which are both usually CD30+, is resolved with CD15+ in Hodgkin lymphoma, but not ALCL.

QCCP2, **Immunophenotyping,** p 249

29. B. **DIM.**

Characteristically, the CD20 staining pattern is dim in CLL/SLL. A specific antigen on the CD20 cell surface marker is recognized by FMC-7. In cases of dim CD20, FMC-7 is typically negative, while other mature B cell neoplasms which have bright CD20 expression (and positive) FMC-7.

QCCP2, **Immunophenotyping,** p 250

30. D. **CD25.**

CD25 is a marker of activated T and B cells as well as certain neoplasms, such as hairy cell leukemia and adult T cell leukemia/lymphoma. Adult T cell leukemia is of particular interest because it is associated with elevated soluble IL-2 receptor. CD20 is a B cell marker, CD21 is the receptor for EBV, and CD23 is the IgE receptor. CD30 or Ki-1 is expressed on normal plasma cells and immunoblasts, as well as several neoplastic cells, such as Hodgkin Reed-Sternberg, anaplastic large cell lymphoma hallmark cells, embryonal carcinoma, and some subtypes of diffuse large B-cell lymphoma (particularly mediastinal).

QCCP2, **Immunophenotyping,** p 250

31. D. **CD38.**

Trisomy 12 and CD38 have been identified with a subset of cases of CLL/SLL with a more aggressive clinical course. DNA array studies have supported the findings of subtypes of CLL/SLL. Remember that CLL/SLL is typically associated with dim CD20 and consequent absent FMC-7.

QCCP2, **Immunophenotyping,** p 250

32. C. **CD59.**

CD59 (MIRL) and CD55 (DAF) are greatly reduced in cases of the acquired PIG-A mutation, which manifests as paroxysmal nocturnal hemoglobinuria.

QCCP2, **Immunophenotyping,** p 250

33. E. **CD99 IS EXPRESSED IN ALL OF THE ABOVE.**

CD99 was originally considered specific for Ewing/PNET, but as time has passed, it is now evident that many more tumors stain with CD99. In addition to the examples above, it is also expressed in some rhabdomyosarcomas and solitary fibrous tumors.

QCCP2, **Immunophenotyping,** p 251

34. E. **A, B, C.**

c-kit, or CD117, is found on the cell surface of a number of malignancies as well as non-malignant cells (junctional melanocytes and interstitial cells of Cajal).

QCCP2, **Immunophenotyping,** p 251

4: Hematopathology Answers

35. B. **B CELL ACUTE LYMPHOCYTIC LEUKEMIA.**

    HLA-DR is a type of MHC-Class II protein, expressed usually on the surface of antigen-presenting cells as a receptor for CD4+ T cells to recognize.
    QCCP2, **Immunophenotyping,** p 251

36. B. **D.**

    The first step in assembling heavy chains is D:J recombination followed by addition of the variable (V domain. On the kappa and lambda light chains there is no D (diversity domain), so only VJ segments compose the mature light chain.
    QCCP2, **Molecular technique,** p 251

37. A. **HEAVY CHAINS, KAPPA LIGHT CHAINS, LAMBDA LIGHT CHAIN.**

    It's alphabetical - H before K before L. First, heavy chain rearranges, which is followed by kappa rearrangement. Lambda chains will only form if kappa chains don't. This may explain why kappa chains outnumber lambda chains (3-4:1, right?).
    QCCP2, **Molecular techniques,** p 251

38. B. **CLONE COMPOSING >1-5% OF TOTAL CELLS.**

    With more than 1-5% of total cells represented by clonal cells, one can be fairly certain of a malignant process. Coincidentally, the gold standard for demonstration of clonal process is Southern blot, and the lower limit of detection by Southern blot is more than 1-5% cells.
    QCCP2, **Molecular techniques,** p 251

39. B. **DIGEST DNA WITH RESTRICTION ENDONUCLEASES.**

    The order of steps presented are E, B, A, C, D. After the probe hybridization and washing, the membrane is placed on film or a detector, then analyzed. A monoclonal process will display a band not present in the germline control.
    QCCP2, **Molecular techniques,** p 252

40. D. **T(11;14).**

    Mantle cell lymphoma and the t(11;14) translocation (IgH-cyclin D) are poorly suited for diagnosis by PCR. All of the other translocations can be sensitively diagnosed by PCR.
    QCCP2, **Molecular techniques,** p 252

41. C. **FLUORESCENT *IN SITU* HYBRIDIZATION (FISH).**

    FISH surpasses all other techniques with a sensitivity greater than 95%. That's followed (in order of decreasing sensitivity) by cytogenetics, Southern blot, and PCR. The decreased sensitivity of PCR is of particular note. Though the analytical sensitivity of PCR often exceeds that of all other techniques, the assay can also be far less sensitive than other modalities due to its requirement for defined amplifiable sequences, which is often limited by random translocation points and, to a lesser extent, overly long sequences too big to amplify.
    QCCP2, **T4.4 Detection of bcl-1 by various modalities,** p 252

4: Hematopathology Answers

42. B. **AUTOSOMAL DOMINANT.**

The majority of cases of hereditary spherocytosis are autosomal dominant, while a few are autosomal recessive. There are a number of proteins that can be affected leading to the phenotype, such as ankyrin, spectrin, and Band 3.
QCCP2, **Hereditary spherocytosis (HS)**, p 252

43. E. **MCHC.**

Even though clinically patients with HS experience chronic hemolysis, they often compensate well with an increased reticulocyte count. This accounts for the minimal change in hemoglobin, RBC count, and hematocrit. Also, due to the small spherocytes and the large reticulocytes, the MCV is fairly normal, though the RDW may be increased. Most often in HS, the MCHC is increased.
QCCP2, **Hereditary spherocytosis (HS)**, p 253

44. A. **OSMOTIC FRAGILITY TEST.**

To diagnose hereditary spherocytosis, one can use either the osmotic fragility test, which identifies spherocytes by their increased fragility with changes in NaCl concentration, or the autohemolysis test, which is similar but uses heat instead of salt to identify the spherocytes, which lyse more readily.
QCCP2, **Hereditary spherocytosis (HS)**, p 253-4

45. B. **SPECTRIN.**

Most often, HE is due to the inability to form spectrin tetramers, the main cytoskeletal stabilizing force in red blood cells. HE is inherited like HS, in a predominantly autosomal dominant fashion. HE is composed of a number of different diseases that share elliptocytes, including common HS, hereditary pyropoikilocytosis in African-Americans, spherocytic elliptocytosis in Europeans, and stomatocytic elliptocytosis. It is most common in S.E. Asia and conferring resistance to *Plasmodium vivax*.
QCCP2, **Hereditary elliptocytosis**, p 254

46. A. **ABNORMAL NA/K PERMEABILITY.**

There are two classes of hereditary stomatocytosis: those that have too much water in red blood cells and those with too little water. These water balance issues are due to abnormal Na/K permeability. Two important facts - splenomegaly is common in hereditary stomatocytosis, like most other chronic hemolytic disease, but splenectomy leads to increased risk of thrombosis in these patients, so it is not done. Also, the Rh$_{null}$ phenotype is associated with stomatocytosis.
QCCP2, **Hereditary stomatocytosis**, p 254

47. E. **HEINZ BODIES.**

While Heinz bodies representing precipitated hemoglobin are typically seen in G6PD deficiency, only supravital stains, such as crystal violet, are able to demonstrate the characteristic Heinz bodies.
QCCP2, **G6PD**, p 255

48. E. **3 MONTHS AFTER A HEMOLYTIC CRISIS.**

During a hemolytic crisis, the older cells with proportionally less G6PD are destroyed more readily than the younger cells, which have normal G6PD levels. Therefore, testing before the cells lose G6PD would give false negative results.
QCCP2, **G6PD**, p 255

4: Hematopathology Answers

49.   C.   ECHINOCYTES.

Echinocytes or "spiny cells" are classically seen in the post-splenectomy patient with pyruvate kinase deficiency.
QCCP2, **Pyruvate kinase deficiency,** p 255

50.   B.   CDA, TYPE II.

Congenital dyserythropoietic anemia, type II is the most common of CDAs and the only one that has a positive acidified serum test, hence the acronym HEMPAS, which stands for "hereditary erythroblastic multinuclearity with positive acidified serum test." The deficiency is CDA, type II is poorly understood but leads to decreased glycosylation of the red blood cell structural protein, Band 3 and increased i antigen on red blood cells.
QCCP2, **CDA,** p 255-256

51.   E.   IT'S NOT INHERITED; BUT RATHER SPORADIC.

Though PNH has features of an inherited disorder affecting multiple cell lines at fairly early stages of development, it is important to remember that it's due to a sporadic mutation of the phosphatidyl inositol glycan A (PIG-A) gene. The PIG-A mutation leads to decreased conjugation of particular proteins with a glycosyl phosphatidyl inositol (GPI cell surface anchor). The result is decreased cell surface expression of a number of protective proteins, such as membrane inhibitor of lysis (MIRL, CD59).
QCCP2, **Paroxysmal nocturnal hemoglobinuria,** p 256

52.   A.   DECREASED CONVERSION OF NADH TO NAD.

Decreased NAD is seen in pyruvate kinase deficiency. All of the other test results are consistent with the diagnosis of paroxysmal nocturnal hemoglobinuria. It is important to note that hemolysis in acid serum occurs with both homologous and heterologous serum, unlike in CDA, type II, where hemolysis occurs with heterologous serum - it's a complement thing.
QCCP2, **PNH, CDA,** p 255-6

53.   D.   PAPPENHEIMER BODIES.

In sideroblastic anemia, there is increased iron, which is typically deposited around the nucleus or erythroid precursor cells, the so-called ringed sideroblasts.
QCCP2, **Sideroblastic anemia,** p 256

54.   A.   CLONAL STEM CELL DEFECT.

Myelodysplastic syndromes, such as refractory anemia with ringed sideroblasts, where patients present with macrocytic hypochromic anemia and >15% ringed sideroblasts in the marrow, account for the majority of cases. All of the other choices presented are causes of sideroblastic anemia, but less so.
QCCP2, **Sideroblastic anemia,** p 257

55.   C.   PRONORMOBLAST.

Erythroid cells infected with parvovirus arrest at the pronormoblast developmental stage, which accounts for the characteristic giant pronormoblasts with glassy nuclear inclusions seen with infection.
QCCP2, **Pure red cell aplasia,** p 257

4: Hematopathology Answers

56.   D.   **LEUKOCYTES ARE ALSO DECREASED, PLATELETS ARE UNAFFECTED.**

Blackfan-Diamond syndrome is a pure red cell aplasia, meaning that other cell lines are unaffected - platelets and leukocytes are normal. All the other selections are true; patients (~75%) respond to steroid therapy.
QCCP2, **Pure red blood cell aplasia,** p 257

57.   C.   **AUTOSOMAL RECESSIVE CHROMOSOMAL BREAKAGE.**

Along with xeroderma pigmentosum, ataxia telangiectasia, Bloom syndrome, and Cockayne syndrome, Fanconi syndrome is a disorder characterized by increased chromosomal breakage, most likely due to defects in repair of DNA breaks.
QCCP2, **Fanconi anemia,** p 258

58.   D.   **ALL ARE APLASTIC DISORDERS OF A SINGLE CELL LINE.**

Each of the syndromes is associated with aplasia of a single hematopoietic line. Blackfan-Diamond has aplastic anemia, Kostmann has neutropenia, and with thrombocytopenia, absent radii syndrome is evident.
QCCP2, **Fanconi anemia,** p 257

59.   D.   **10%.**

Sickle cell disease is among the most common inherited diseases in the African-American population, with a carrier frequency over twice as high as the carrier frequency of hemochromatosis in Caucasians.
QCCP2, **HbS,** p 258

60.   B.   **17 DAYS.**

The red blood cells containing HbSS have a lifetime 1/10 of a normal RBCs due to the formation of destructive polymers of deoxygenated hemoglobin, which causes the RBCs to lose flexibility and sickle.
QCCP2, **Hb Sickle cell disease,** p 258

61.   E.   **A, B, C.**

Most patients with HbSS do not present at birth, but rather, most often at several months of age. Part of the reason is that HbF is at its highest *in utero* and immediately post-partum, affording babies many protective benefits.
QCCP2, **HbS,** p 258

62.   B.   **PARVOVIRUS B19.**

Just like in patients with HbS disease, parvovirus is the most common cause of aplastic anemia, accounting for at least 70% of cases. Patients with sickle cell disease have chronic thrombosis, which accounts for many of the other crises associated with sickle cell disease (acute chest, bone). Patients with HbSS are also at an increased risk for infections, especially *Salmonella.*
QCCP2, **HbS,** p 259

4: Hematopathology Answers

63.   C.   **LHERMITTE-DUCLOS.**

Lhermitte-Duclos is a rare cerebellar tumor associated with Cowden syndrome, not HbS disease. Patients with sickle cell disease are at an increased risk of increased risk of infection, especially with encapsulated bacteria due to autosplenectomy. There are several neurological manifestations of chronic thrombosis - TIAs, infarctions, and hearing loss as well as moyamoya disease. *Moyamoya* is Japanese for "puff of smoke," due to the characteristic diffuse expansion of contrast agent of cerebral angiography, due to the vast collateral vascular network that develops secondary to arterial stenosis.
QCCP2, **HbS**, p 259

64.   C.   **THIN BASEMENT MEMBRANE DISEASE.**

Thin basement membrane disease is a congenital disorders unrelated to sickle cell disease. There are 7 classic nephropathies of sickle cell disease, which, in addition to the above, include gross hematuria, isosthenuria, and nephrotic syndrome.
QCCP2, **HbS**, p 260

65.   E.   **PROLIFERATIVE RETINOPATHY.**

For some reason, proliferative retinopathy occurs more commonly in HbSC and HbS-beta thalassemia than in HbSS.
QCCP2, **HbS**, p 260

66.   C.   **ELEVATED.**

The proportion of HbS in patients with HbS/beta thalassemia is increased to >50%, unlike in HbS/alpha thalassemia, where there is a decreased percentage of HbS. The extent to which the HbS is decreased depends on the number of alpha globin genes detected.
QCCP2, **HbS**, p 260

67.   B.   **HBC.**

In addition to the rod-shaped crystals of hemoglobin, which results in the pencil cells of HbC, there are also abundant target cells, a nonspecific feature associated with many hemoglobinopathies.
QCCP2, **HbC**, p 261

68.   C.   **HB$_{\text{LEPORE}}$.**

The unusual proportion of little HbS is due to confusion in reading the alkaline cellulose acetate gel where Hb$_{\text{Lepore}}$ and HbS comigrate.
QCCP2, **Hb$_{\text{Lepore}}$,** p 261

69.   A.   **HB$_{\text{CHESAPEAKE}}$.**

Hb$_{\text{Chesapeake}}$ and Hb$_{\text{Denver}}$ are Hb mutants with increased oxygen affinity, which can be demonstrated on a Hb:O$_2$ dissociation graph. The remaining choices are all hemoglobin mutations with decreased stability, which can present with hemolysis following oxidative stress.
QCCP2, **Unstable and high oxygen affinity hemoglobin**, p 261-262

4: Hematopathology Answers

70.　B.　**FE^{+++}.**

Iron in its oxidized ferric form, Fe^{+++} is bound to hemoglobin in methemoglobin, also known as hemiglobin (Hi). Methemoglobin has three letters before hemoglobin just like the 3+ charge; ferric has an i in it like hemiglobin. Methemoglobin cannot bind oxygen like hemoglobin bound to the reduced ferrous form.

QCCP2, **Methemoglobin,** p 262

71.　A.　**METHYLENE BLUE.**

Methylene blue reduces the 3+ ferric to 2+ ferrous form, thus converting hemiglobin, which can't bind oxygen, to hemoglobin, which can bind oxygen. Hemiglobin can be used in the treatment of cyanide poisoning because hemiglobin binds cyanide with very high affinity. Desferroxamine and EDTA are chelating agents. Phenacetin can cause an acquired methemoglobinemia.

QCCP2, **Methemoglobin,** p 262

72.　C.　**ALPHA GLOBIN.**

The beta globin genes are clustered together as a number of genes and pseudogenes on chromosome 11. Alpha globin is present as 2 genes on chromosome 16.

QCCP2, **Thalassemia,** p 262

73.　A.　**NONSENSE MUTATIONS.**

Nonsense and frameshift mutations account for the majority of the mutations that lead to the loss of expression of beta-globin. beta° mutations produce no beta-globin, while beta$^+$ mutations lead to decreased beta-globin expression.

QCCP2, **Thalassemia,** p 263

74.　D.　**A & B.**

Alpha thalassemia trait manifests as 50% less HbA than wild type. It follows that the genotype of alpha thalassemia would show 1/2 the amount of alpha genes. There are several possibilities whose frequency depends on ethnicity. The -alpha/-alpha genotype is more common in the African-American population, while the --/alpha alpha genotype is seen more often in Asians. Hb$_{Constant Spring}$ is an alpha mutation in the 5' UTR that results in the loss of alpha expression, therefore the --/alpha^{CS}alpha phenotype is HbH.

QCCP2, **Thalassemia,** p 263

75.　A.　**DECREASED RBC COUNT.**

In fact, there is an increased RBC count perhaps responsive to the decreased hematocrit. All the other choices are recognized as consistent with thalassemia.

QCCP2, **Clinical features,** p 263

76.　D.　**IRON DEFICIENCY.**

The typical finding in beta thalassemia on hemoglobin electrophoresis is increased HbA$_2$ (>2.5%) with normal HbF. In the case of concomitant Fe deficiency with beta thalassemia in anemic patients, the HbA$_2$ percentage may be normal, giving the appearance of alpha thalassemia. In that case, it is important to note that electrophoresis should be repeated after ruling out iron deficiency and treatment if necessary.

QCCP2, **Thalassemia,** p 264

4: Hematopathology Answers

77.   E.   **NONE OF THE ABOVE.**

Admittedly, a trick question. Some of the genotypes above, most notably beta°/beta°, could be associated with beta thal major. However, the strict definition of beta thalassemia major is clinical - dependence on transfusion.
QCCP2, **Thalassemia,** p 264-5

78.   D.   **IgG ANTI-D.**

Broad specificity anti-Rh antibodies account for the majority of cases of warm autoimmune hemolytic anemia, while IgM anti-I is responsible for most cases of cold autoagglutinins.
QCCP2, **WAIHA,** p 265

79.   D.   **IgD.**

A subset of immunoglobulins are capable of binding to complement and lead to hemolysis. Of all the IgG subtypes, only IgG3 and IgG1 bind to complement. When IgG binds, it tends to lead to extravascular hemolysis in the spleen.
QCCP2, **WAIHA,** p 265

80.   D.   **ANTI-I.**

Anti-I is associated with atypical (mycoplasmic) pneumonia and is the most common cause of cold IgM autoagglutinins, which can be either pathological or non-pathological.
QCCP2, **Cold autoagglutinins,** p 265

81.   B.   **HEMOGLOBIN.**

Due to the potential for cold autoagglutinins to react at or near room temperature, there is a substantial risk of agglutination in automated counters leading to aberrant results for most CB indices. Since hemoglobin is directly measured and unaffected by clumping, it can be reliably measured.
QCCP2, **Cold autoagglutinins,** p 266

82.   A.   **TYPE O CORD BLOOD.**

Remember, little i is a more immature glycoprotein on red cells which matures with branching to form the big I antigen. The formation of little i antigen is associated with EBV mononucleosis.
QCCP2, **T4.10,** p 266

83.   B.   **IN CHILDREN FOLLOWING A VIRAL ILLNESS.**

Though originally described in syphilitics, the most common presentation nowadays is in children after viral (measles, mumps, VZV, EBV most commonly) infections.
QCCP2, **Paroxysmal cold hemoglobinuria,** p 267

84.   C.   **IgG BIPHASIC HEMOLYSIN.**

Donath-Landsteiner antibody is a biphasic anti-P IgG hemolysin described for its ability to bind to antigen and cold temperatures, such as at the periphery, but then to lyse when incubated at warm temperatures when the circulation brings the blood back to the central warmer areas.
QCCP2, **Paroxysmal cold hemoglobinuria,** p 267

4: Hematopathology Answers

85. D. **CLOT BLOOD AT 37°C, STORE SERUM 3 DAYS AT 4°C, COLLECT PRECIPITATE AND SUBJECT TO ELECTROPHORESIS.**

We need serum, not plasma, so choice E is out. Choice C wouldn't produce anything except native serum with a lot of IgM. Choices A and B also wouldn't be much different from normal serum. The cryoglobulins must be cold-precipitated from serum, then subjected to electrophoresis.
QCCP2, **Cryoglobulinemia,** p 267

86. A. **TYPE I.**

Type I is due to monoclonal cryoglobulins, which fits best with a monoclonal IgM gammopathy, such as Waldenstrom macroglobulinemia. Type II cryoglobulins are a mix of polyclonal and monoclonal (which is usually an IgM anti-IgG) and are the most common (mostly due to SLE and HCV). Type III is a mix of two different polyclonal processes.
QCCP2, **Cryoglobulins,** p 267

87. B. **PETECHIAE.**

Petechiae are a sign of microvascular bleeding due to either platelet or small vessel defects, not associated with cryoglobulinemia. The palpable purpura is very common and reflects an underlying leukocytoclastic vasculitis.
QCCP2, **Cryoglobulinemia,** p 267

88. E. **MEMBRANOPROLIFERATIVE GLOMERULONEPHRITIS, TYPE II.**

Renal disease commonly affects patients with cryoglobulinemia and usually presents several years after initial symptoms of disease. Clinically, it can manifest as a nephrotic or nephritic syndrome with severe hypocomplementemia. The dense deposits of type II MPGN have the ultrastructural feature of subendothelial immune complexes with a fibrillary pattern.
QCCP2, **Cryoglobulinemia,** p 268

89. B. **DECREASED FERRITIN.**

Usually, decreased ferritin is the most sensitive indication of a possible iron-deficiency anemia. This is followed by the rest of the choices presented, with a decrease in hemoglobin being a later manifestation of iron deficiency anemia. It is important to note that ferritin is an acute phase response protein and that, in patients with decreased hepatic clearance, the levels could be increased.
QCCP2, **Iron deficiency anemia,** p 268

90. A. **INCREASED SERUM SOLUBLE TRANSFERRIN RECEPTOR, ZINC PROTOPORPHYRIN, FREE ERYTHROCYTE PROTOPORPHYRIN, AND DECREASED FERRITIN.**

The pattern most consistent with iron-deficient anemia would be decreased serum Fe, ferritin, with increased TIBC, ZPP, FEP, and serum soluble transferrin receptor. It is important to note that many of the tests are nonspecific and false negative results are common due to confounding comorbidities, such as a chronic inflammatory state or hepatic insufficiency.
QCCP2, **Iron deficiency anemia,** p 268

4: Hematopathology Answers

91.　D.　**1.0 mg Fe/unit pRBCs.**

This is a good thing to remember for blood banking as well and very testable. The high iron content is why people with chronic hemolytic conditions, such as sickle cell disease, often develop very high Fe levels requiring chelation therapy.
QCCP2, **Iron deficiency anemia,** p 268

92.　C.　**decreased iron and increased lead independent of socioeconomic status.**

There is an inverse relationship between lead levels and iron levels, even when controlled for socioeconomic status. High lead levels inhibit intestinal absorption of iron, in addition to low iron facilitating lead uptake.
QCCP2, **Iron deficiency anemia,** p 268

93.　D.　**ileum.**

First, ingested B_{12} binds to a factor in the stomach where intrinsic factor is produced. It is not until the R Factor-B_{12} complex reaches the duodenum that R factor detaches and intrinsic factor binds, finally being absorbed in the ileum.
QCCP2, **B_{12} deficiency,** p 269

94.　E.　**jejunum.**

Unlike B_{12}, folate is not efficiently stored by the body and must be ingested regularly, usually from leafy greens. Once ingested, it is absorbed by enterocytes in the jejunum.
QCCP2, **Folate and B_{12},** p 269

95.　B.　**left-shifted leukocytosis.**

The WBC count is usually not elevated, much less left-shifted. There is a maturation arrest due to the lack of DNA precursors, which explains the hypersegmented neutrophils. This ineffective hematopoiesis leads to a bone marrow full of immature precursors. When these precursors lyse, there is an increase in LDH and bilirubin.
QCCP2, **Folate and B_{12},** p 269

96.　B.　**Cabot rings.**

Cabot rings and Howell-Jolly bodies are nuclear remnants that escaped extrusion. This accounts for their increased presence in post-splenectomy patients. Pappenheimer bodies are Fe-containing mitochondria, Heinz bodies are denatured hemoglobin, target cells are defective RBC with extraneous membrane, and basophilic stippling is due to ribosomes.
QCCP2, **T4.20,** p 270

97.　E.　**anemia of chronic disease.**

Anemia of chronic disease is more of a sign than a disease entity. The combination of decreased iron utilization and increased iron sequestration, as well as decreased erythropoietin secretion and response are responsible for the mild, usually normocytic anemia. ACD can accompany any of a number of chronic diseases, usually inflammatory in nature.
QCCP2, **Anemia of chronic disease,** p 271

98. B. **PENICILLIN-MEDIATED IMMUNE HEMOLYSIS.**

Penicillin-mediated immune hemolysis requires RBCs to be coated with antibodies rather than delivered to the reticuloendothelial system, where the red cells are destroyed. This is the definition of <u>extra</u>vascular hemolysis. All the other choices cause hemolysis on the spot and thus are causes of <u>intra</u>vascular hemolysis.
QCCP2, **Approach to the diagnosis of anemia,** p 271

99. B. **HEREDITARY SPHEROCYTOSIS.**

A microcytic anemia with a normal to low reticulocyte count indicates an inadequate response to the anemia by the marrow. An anemia with an increased reticulocyte count implies an inherent defect in the produced RBC or increased RBC destruction. Of all the choices above, only HS fits into this second category of hyperregenerative microcytic anemia.
QCCP2, **F4.5,** p 272

100. E. **SQUAMOUS CELL CARCINOMA OF THE LUNG.**

SCC of the lung is associated with hypercalcemia due to PTH production, not erythrocytosis and excess erythropoietin. All other tumors presented as choices have been shown to express erythropoietin.
QCCP2, **Erythrocytosis,** p 273

101. B. **UP TO 1% BLASTS.**

It is possible to see some cells less mature than metamyelocytes, but not blasts. Under normal circumstances, there should not be any blasts in the peripheral circulation.
QCCP2, **Nonneoplastic WBC disorders,** p 273

102. C. **NORMAL LAP SCORE.**

The LAP score is rarely unchanged in myeloproliferative disorders; usually it is elevated. But in CML it is <u>decreased</u>. The LAP score is not specific and can be elevated in reactive neutrophilia as well as myeloproliferative disease.
QCCP2, **Neutrophilia,** p 273

103. A. **HANTAVIRUS.**

The hantavirus pulmonary syndrome is characterized initially by thrombocytopenia followed by the rest of the signs mentioned above. Clinically, there is often extensive pulmonary edema. These signs together are very specific and sensitive for hantavirus.
QCCP2, **Neutrophilia,** p 273

104. C. **T CELLS.**

Atypical T cells are a frequent finding in cases of reactive lymphocytosis. A classic example is the reactive Downey cell of EBV. Although EBV infects B cells, the hallmark findings in the peripheral smear are the reactive atypical lymphocytes.
QCCP2, **Lymphocytosis,** p 273

4: Hematopathology Answers

105. **D.** **YOUNG FEMALE SMOKERS.**

The findings of bilobed small lymphocytes with abundant cytoplasm and a polyclonal IgM gammopathy in an otherwise healthy young female smoker is suggestive of the syndrome of persistent polyclonal B lymphocytes. In addition, most affected individuals are positive for HLA-DR7.
QCCP2, **Lymphocytosis,** p 273

106. **E.** **PERTUSSIS.**

A high WBC count of mature lymphocytes with clefted nuclei is most often seen with pertussis. These Reider cells are important because they can be confused with a mature B cell neoplasm. A helpful distinguishing feature is demography. Pertussis is more common in kids. Lymphocytosis in adults is much more suspicious for a neoplastic condition.
QCCP2, **Lymphocytosis,** p 274

107. **E.** **A, B, C.**

All of the above are suggestive of a neoplastic process rather than a reactive one. Serum lysozyme is elevated in both reactive and neoplastic monocytic proliferations and is therefore not helpful.
QCCP2, **Lymphocytosis,** p 274

108. **D.** **IL-5.**

Often seen in high levels with conditions that cause eosinophilia (parasitic infections, Hodgkin lymphoma, etc), IL-5 is the most specific stimulator of eosinophilic development.
QCCP2, **Eosinophilia,** p 274

109. **B.** **AUER RODS.**

Auer rods are the most specific morphological feature for blasts suggesting myeloid differentiation.
QCCP2, **Blasts,** p 274

110. **A.** **MEDICATIONS.**

A number of drugs can cause neutropenia, including antibiotics, anti-thyroid, anti-convulsants, and procainamide. Anti-thyroidals are of particular note because they can also cause a granulocytosis.
QCCP2, **Neutropenia,** p 275

111. **E.** **A, B, C.**

Felty syndrome is an alloimmune neutropenia seen in patients with rheumatoid arthritis.
QCCP2, **Neutropenia,** p 275

112. **D.** **KOSTMANN SYNDROME.**

Kostmann syndrome is a selective disorder of neutrophils presenting as neutropenia with affecting lymphocyte production or development. In addition to Kostmann syndrome, there are a number of syndromic conditions with selective neutropenia such as cyclic neutropenia and Chediak-Higashi. Other syndromes may have neutropenia but may also present with additional cytopenias, including Schwachman-Diamond and Fanconi anemia.
QCCP2, **Lymphopenia,** T4.22, p 276

4: Hematopathology Answers

113.   B.   MANTLE ZONE.

Reactive follicular pattern expansion of lymph nodes maintains normal gene expression patterns, such as bcl-2 in the mantle zone. Mantle cell lymphoma often has aberrant cyclin D1 expression and bcl-2 overexpression in the follicle center is often abnormal.

QCCP2, **Non-neoplastic lymph node proliferations,** p 276

114.   B.   HIV.

HIV infection in lymph nodes follows a predictable pattern of first a reactive florid expansion of follicles often with abnormal shapes, followed by follicle lysis and involution regressively transformed germinal centers, and finally lymphocyte depletion.

QCCP2, **Non-neoplastic lymph node proliferations,** p 276

115.   D.   HHV8 INFECTION.

The two types of Castleman disease are very different both symptomatically and etiologically. The hyaline-vascular type is much more common and characterized by the choices presented in the question, except for the HHV8 association. HHV8, however, is associated with the other less common type of Castleman disease, multicentric or plasma cell variant. The salient features of plasma cell Castleman disease are an association with POEMS syndrome and dissolution of the follicle/mantle cell boundary.

QCCP2, **Castleman disease,** p 277

116.   A.   YOUNG ASIAN MAN WITH SOFT TISSUE HEAD/NECK MASS, CERVICAL LYMPHADENOPATHY, PERIPHERAL EOSINOPHILIA, AND INCREASED IgE.

Kimura disease is similar to but distinct from angiolymphoid hyperplasia with eosinophilia. Kimura disease has different demographics, eosinophilia, soft tissue mass, and the characteristic lymph node findings of follicular hyperplasia, eosinophilic deposits, and increased vascularity. Choice C describes Kawasaki disease; choice E describes Whipple disease.

QCCP2, **Interfollicular pattern,** p 277

117.   A.   HEMOPHAGOCYTOSIS.

Emperipolesis, while resembling hemophagocytosis, actually represents cells "passing through" histiocytes unharmed rather than being actually ingested and finally destroyed by histiocytes.

QCCP2, **Sinus pattern,** p 277

118.   E.   A, B, C.

Suppurative granulomas should be differentiated from necrotizing granulomas with suppuration. The former is caused by the listed entities while the latter is due to mycobacterium, several fungi, brucellosis, or yersinial infections. An additional granulomatous condition is necrotizing granulomas without suppuration most commonly associated with Kikuchi-Fujimoto disease.

QCCP2, **Granulomatous lymphadenitis,** p 278

119.   B.   HODGKIN LYMPHOMA.

A number of different viruses can cause the diffuse pattern of nodal expansion, including EBV, CMV, HSV, and measles. Look for the characteristic features of each nuclear inclusions, etc to help differentiate them.

QCCP2, **Diffuse pattern,** p 278

4: Hematopathology Answers

120. **D.** **CD5+/CD23+.**

Mature B-cell neoplasms all look very similar and immunohistochemistry or flow cytometry are often required to further characterize. This is especially the case in distinguishing SLL from mantle cell lymphoma, both of which can appear somewhat nodular, and are positive for CD5. What helps is that while SLL is often positive for CD23, it's not the case for mantle cell lymphoma. In addition, there is often the characteristic dim CD20 positivity and "cloudy sky" appearance with SLL.
QCCP2, **SLL/CLL,** p 279

121. **B.** ARTIFACT DUE TO EDTA.

Smudge cells and basket cells of CLL are lysed cells with smeared or spindled nuclear material. They are formed artefactually when EDTA-preserved blood is used for peripheral smears. If the blood is prepared with heparin, the artifact is not present.
QCCP2, **CLL/SLL,** p 279, col I0

122. **A.** DIFFUSE.

The diffuse pattern has the worst prognosis, with slightly better prognosis for interstitial or nodular.
QCCP2, **SLL/CLL,** p 279

123. **D.** **A & B.**

A subset of CLL/SLL expresses B cell markers and is associated with a worse prognosis. This poor prognostic subset is associated with trisomy 12.
QCCP2, **CLL/SLL,** p 279

124. **B.** INCREASED CD5.

The loss of the more characteristic SLL/CLL markers, such as CD5 and CD23, along with the increase in markers that are typically not strongly expressed in SLL/CLL portends a transformation to prolymphocytic leukemia, defined by 11-55% prolymphocytes.
QCCP2, **SLL/CLL,** p 280

125. **A.** ANEMIA.

Both anemia (hemoglobin less than 11 g/dL) and thrombocytopenia (platelets less than 100,000/mL) are sufficient to place a patient in a high risk stage (RAI III or IV ir Binet C) that carries with it a 2-3 year survival. Lymphadenopathy and splenomegaly also affect the prognosis, but not as much as anemia and thrombocytopenia.
QCCP2, **SLL/CLL,** p 281 **and T4.23**

126. **D.** **A & B.**

Both ZAP-70 and CD38 are associated with a poor prognostic subgroup and unmutated Ig heavy chain gene. This subset probably arises from pregerminal center B cells. Another subtype that is likely post-germinal center is associated with hypermutation of the Ig heavy chain variable region and prolonged survival.
QCCP2, **SLL/CLL,** p 281

4: Hematopathology Answers

127. D. **A & B.**

Lymphoblastic leukemia/lymphoma may resemble blastic mantle cell lymphoma. However, it will not express CD5 and increased cyclin D1 (bcl-1). Instead, lymphoblastic leukemia expresses CD99 and TdT, which are not usually found in blastic mantle cell lymphoma.
QCCP2, **Mantle cell lymphoma,** p 281

128. C. **IgH.**

The immunoglobulin heavy chain promoter induces the expression of cyclin D1, whose gene product stimulates the entry of cells into the G1 phase of the cell cycle, promoting growth. Both WT1 and MEN1 are also located on chromosome 11, but have nothing to do with mantle cell lymphoma.
QCCP2, **Mantle cell lymphoma,** p 282

129. B. **FLUORESCENT *IN SITU* HYBRIDIZATION.**

The mechanistic details behind the t(11;14) make Southern blot and PCR difficult to perform. There are multiple breakpoints, some quite far from the fusion partner. At best, due to these limitations, Southern blot and PCR will only detect 1/2 of all translocations. IHC will detect 3/4 of all cases, slightly less than RT-PCR. FISH has a nearly 100% sensitivity for t(11;14).
QCCP2, **Mantle cell lymphoma,** p 282

130. C. **MANTLE CELL LYMPHOMA.**

For the most part, the mature B cell neoplasms are an indolent lot of neoplasms both appearing and behaving in a non-aggressive fashion. Mantle cell lymphoma, despite its benign appearance has an aggressive clinical course, presenting with disseminated disease often and a survival of only 3-4 years.
QCCP2, **Mantle cell lymphoma,** p 283

131. A. **CENTROBLASTS.**

Centroblasts are the large non-cleaved cells found in the follicle. Compare these with the more numerous smaller, cleaved cells, the centrocytes that surround them. Grade I follicular lymphoma is defined as 0-5 centroblasts per high powered field. Grade II is defined as 6-15/HPF, and Grade III as more than 15 centroblasts/HPF.
QCCP2, **Follicular lymphoma,** p 283

132. C. **T(14;18).**

t(14;18) transposes the immunoglobulin heavy chain regulatory region on chromosome 14 adjacent to the anti-apoptotic gene, bcl-2. Since the majority of translocations occur within a small region (the major breakpoint region), the diagnosis is best made with PCR or FISH.
QCCP2, **Follicular lymphoma,** p 283

133. D. **DIFFUSE LARGE B CELL LYMPHOMA.**

While the vast majority of follicular lymphomas are associated with t(14;18), a substantial number of DLBCL are too. The subset of DLBCL with the t(14;18) translocation has a favorable prognosis.
QCCP2, **Follicular lymphoma,** p 283

4: Hematopathology Answers

134. **E.** **PARATRABECULAR.**

When follicular lymphoma involves the bone marrow, it usually does so in a focal trabecular pattern. It is a fairly unique pattern and very characteristic of follicular lymphoma.
QCCP2, **Follicular lymphoma,** p 283

135. **A.** **MONOCYTOID.**

The monocytoid (abundant cytoplasm with indented nuclei) B cells of marginal zone lymphoma can be found in both nodal and extranodal forms of the disease. They are usually accompanied by hypersecretory plasma cells containing Dutcher bodies.
QCCP2, **Marginal zone lymphoma,** p 284

136. **B.** **THE PRESENCE OR ABSENCE OF A NUCLEOLUS.**

It is fairly often that one can observe a nucleolus within the nucleus of the peripheral villous lymphocyte, but not the hairy cells. The immunophenotype (not one of the choices) is the most reliable means of distinguishing the two.
QCCP2, **Marginal zone lymphoma,** p 284

137. **C.** **T(11;18).**

The t(11;18) translocation juxtaposes the MALT1 scaffold, signaling proteins with the API2 gene. In addition to stomach tumors, t(11;18) is commonly seen in pulmonary tumors. The t(1;14) translocation involves the fusion of the bcl-10 gene on chromosome 1 with the IgH promoter on chromosome 14 and can also be seen in a subset of extranodal marginal zone lymphomas.
QCCP2, **Marginal zone lymphoma,** p 284

138. **A.** **LYMPH NODES.**

Hairy cell leukemia is not commonly found in lymph nodes. The other sites listed are much more commonly involved.
QCCP2, **Hairy cell lymphoma,** p 285

139. **B.** **MONOCYTOPENIA.**

Pancytopenia is the norm with hairy cell leukemia, but the out of proportion monocytopenia is fairly specific for hairy cell leukemia. A confounding problem is that often the neoplastic hairy cells are counted in an automated counter as monocytes, potentially artificially raising the monocyte count while underestimating hairy cells.
QCCP2, **Hairy cell leukemia,** p 285

140. **D.** **HAIRY PROJECTIONS.**

You knew that it had to be a trick, right? While all the other choices are very consistent in hairy cell, the actual projections that give the disease its name are not really that consistent. It is more often that the cytoplasmic borders are uneven and ill-defined.
QCCP2, **Hairy cell leukemia,** p 285

141.   D.   **EXTRANODAL MARGINAL ZONE LYMPHOMA.**

There are several varieties of acid phosphatase, such as the prostatic acid phosphatase expressed in adenocarcinoma of prostatic origin. Tartrate-resistant acid phosphatase is often associated with hairy cell leukemia, but it's important to know that TRAP is not specific for hairy cell leukemia and is in fact associated with several other conditions.
QCCP2, **Hairy cell leukemia,** p 286

142.   B.   **CD5.**

It helps that hairy cell leukemia is negative for CD10 (90%), CD5, and CD23, differentiating it from follicular lymphoma, mantle cell lymphoma, and SLL/CLL. The characteristic CD11c, CD25, and CD103 positivity should be committed to memory. While CD11c and CD25 can be expressed in SLL/CLL also, the expression is usually stronger in hairy cell leukemia, while CD103 is very specific for hairy cell leukemia.
QCCP2, **Hairy cell leukemia,** p 286

143.   C.   **>55%.**

PLL can arise both *de novo* or from a previous CLL. When the number of prolymphocytes get into the 11-55% range, the neoplasm is categorized as CLL/SLL; above that is PLL. In addition, expression of CD5 is lost and CD11c gained.
QCCP2, **PLL,** p 286

144.   B.   **MACROGLOBULINEMIA.**

LPL is most commonly associated with Waldenstrom macroglobulinemia, a hyper-IgM syndrome that can lead to hyperviscosity and "sludging" of the blood. There is usually numerous plasma cells with Dutcher bodies and an M-spike on SPEP
QCCP2, **LPL,** p 287

145.   A.   **ANAPLASTIC LARGE CELL LYMPHOMA.**

A number of entities presenting with diffuse effacement of the lymph node by large cells can be categorized as DLBCL. Even CD30+ neoplasms, usually associated with anaplastic large cell lymphoma, can be categorized as DLBCL if there are B cell markers (CD19, CD20, etc) and anaplasia.
QCCP2, **DLBCL,** p 287

146.   C.   **T(3;14).**

t(3;14) translocation puts the IgH locus with bcl-6. Bcl-6 overexpression is not specific for DLBCL and can be found in follicular lymphoma and Burkitt lymphoma. The subset of follicular lymphoma associated with bcl-6 has a worse prognosis.
QCCP2, **DLBCL,** p 288

147.   B.   **BRAIN.**

Primary CNS lymphoma is a rare neoplasm that occurs most commonly in AIDS patients and is almost always a form of DLBCL.
QCCP2, **DLBCL,** p 288

4: Hematopathology Answers

148.   A.   **ENDEMIC.**

The endemic form of Burkitt lymphoma is found most commonly in Africa, presenting as a large jaw mass. The sporadic form more often presents as an abdominal mass and has a less strong association with EBV than the endemic form. The immunodeficiency-associated, or Burkitt-like, lymphoma is the least associated with EBV and presents in lymph nodes. In almost all cases of Burkitt lymphoma, independent of subtype, there is deranged expression of c-myc.

QCCP2, **Burkitt lymphoma,** p 288

149.   E.   **A, B, C.**

c-myc on chromosome 8 is almost always overexpressed in Burkitt lymphoma, as previously mentioned. The translocations of the Ig heavy chain regulatory region on chromosome 14 and both of the Ig light chain regulatory regions QCCP2, on chromosome 2 for kappa, 22 for lambda have been demonstrated to be fusion partners with c-myc in Burkitt lymphoma.

QCCP2, **Burkitt lymphoma,** p 288

150.   B.   **POST-TRANSPLANT LYMPHOPROLIFERATIVE DISORDER.**

PTLD is associated with EBV, not HHV8. The presence of HHV8 has been documented in a small percentage of cases of Kikuchi lymphadenitis. In addition to HHV8, EBV has been found in a majority of cases of primary effusion lymphoma, a rare disease that is even more rare outside of coexistent HIV infection.

QCCP2, **Intravascular large B-cell lymphoma,** p 289

151.   B.   **PRIMARY VASCULITIS.**

The destruction of vascular walls by neoplastic B cells resembles a primary vasculitis, but lacks the neutrophils. Lymphomatoid granulomatosis also can resemble extranodal NK/T cell lymphoma, nasal type when it affects the nasopharynx. LG is associated with EBV, like several other lymphomas.

QCCP2, **Intravascular large B-cell lymphoma,** p 289

152.   C.   **EBV.**

Almost all cases of posttransplant lymphoproliferative disorder (PTLD) have demonstrated EBV infection present.

QCCP2, **Invascular large B-cell lymphoma,** p 289

153.   D.   **80%.**

Another example of the 3-4:1 rule previously mentioned. In medical school, we also called it the 80:20 rule. If something was common, guess 80%; uncommon, 20%. B cell lymphoblastic leukemias account for ~80% of the lymphoblastic leukemias. The opposite holds true for lymphoblastic lymphoma, where B-cell lineage cases account for 20% of the total.

QCCP2, **Acute lymphoblastic leukemia/lymphoma,** p 289

154.   A.   **ANTERIOR MEDIASTINAL MASS.**

Part of the 5T mnemonic learned in medical school for the clinical differential diagnosis on chest x-ray, T-ALL most often presents as an anterior mediastinal mass and may be clinically associated with hypercalcemia.

QCCP2, **Acute lymphoblastic leukemia and lymphoma,** p 289

4: Hematopathology Answers

155. D. T(12;21).

A number of translocations are associated with pre-B-ALL, but of all of them, the only one uniformly associated with a better prognosis is t(12;21); in addition, hyperdiploidy is associated with a favorable prognosis.
QCCP2, **Acute lymphoblastic leukemia and lymphoma,** p 291

156. C. CD7.

CD19 is predominantly a B cell lineage marker. CD4 and CD8 are either both coexpressed or neither expressed, while HLA-DR is usually not expressed T ALL. Like CD19 in B ALL, CD7 is the most sensitive marker of T ALL.
QCCP2, **Precursor T ALL,** p 290

157. D. CD117.

CD13 and CD33 are mostly myeloid-specific, but not as much as CD117, whose specificity approaches 100%. CD2 and CD10 are not myeloid markers and are almost never seen in AML.
QCCP2, **Acute leukemia with mixed immunophenotypes,** p 291

158. A. IgG.

The selections in the question are listed in order of prevalence in multiple myeloma, with IgG accounting for more than 1/2 of the cases. It is important to note that IgM-secreting multiple myeloma doesn't exist because those cases are classified as non-myelomas, such as lymphoplasmacytic lymphoma with its associated Waldenstrom macroglobulinemia.
QCCP2, **Plasma cell myeloma, or multiple myeloma,** p 291-2

159. D. LIGHT CHAIN ONLY-MYELOMA.

The vast majority (90%) of cases lacking an apparent paraproteinemia will be due to light chain-only expression. Interestingly, IgD myelomas, which are the second most common cause of an apparent lack of paraproteinemia, almost always (90%) express lambda light chains. Most other cases overexpress kappa light chains.
QCCP2, **Plasma cell myeloma or multiple myeloma,** p 292

160. B. 1 MAJOR + 1 MINOR CRITERION, OR 3 MINOR (WHICH MUST INCLUDE THE FIRST TWO CRITERIA).

While choice E would fulfill the requirements, it is very specific and would greatly limit the diagnosis. The major criteria are: 1. marrow plasmacytosis >30%, 2. plasmacytoma on biopsy and significant M spike (either by >3.5 g/dL in serum for IgG or >1g/24hr from urine). The first two minor criteria are similar to the major but with decreased levels: 1. plasmacytosis of 10-30%, 2. M spike present but less than in major criteria. Also: 3. lytic bone lesions, 4. Ig reduced to <50% normal.
QCCP2, **Diagnostic criteria for multiple myeloma, T4.26,** p 292

161. A. T(14;18).

Ultimate trivia! There are numerous chromosomal anomalies associated with multiple myleoma, some associated with a mild longer median survival, such as t(11;14), different breakpoint from mantle cell lymphoma, and some with shorter survival, such as t(4;14). The unifying factor and take-away message is that most of them involve the IgH locus on chromosome 14q32.
QCCP2, **Multiple myeloma,** p 292

4: Hematopathology Answers

162. D. **20%.**

While the cutoff value for the diagnosis of multiple myeloma in the marrow is 30% (major criterion), the cutoff for plasma cell leukemia in the peripheral blood is 20% or an absolute plasma cell count $>2.0 \times 10^9$ prolymphocytes/mL.

QCCP2, **Plasma cell leukemia,** p 292

163. B. **VERTEBRA.**

The vertebrae are the most commonly involved, followed by the ribs and pelvis. A solitary medullary plasmacytoma is most often (75%) a herald lesion portending multiple myeloma. This is unlike extramedullary plasmacytoma, such as in the nasal cavity, which is not associated with progression to multiple myeloma.

QCCP2, **Solitary plasmacytoma,** p 293

164. C. **LYTIC BONE LESIONS.**

For a diagnosis of smoldering myeloma, there must be a marrow plasmacytosis of 10-30% and no evidence of the renal failure, anemia, or hypercalcemia that are associated with active myeloma. The same criteria apply to indolent myeloma, except these can be up to 3 radiologically documented osteolytic lesions.

QCCP2, **Smoldering myeloma,** p 293

165. C. **30%.**

While not a certainty, there is a 1/3 chance that an individual with MGUS will develop myeloma within 20 years of the diagnosis. This is of particular importance because almost 3% of people over 70 meet the criteria for the diagnosis of MGUS. As people live longer, that means that 1% of all 90-year-olds will have myeloma!

QCCP2, **Monoclonal gammopathy of unknown significance (MGUS),** p 293

166. D. **SYNDROME OF INAPPROPRIATE DIURETIC HORMONE.**

The "S" in POEMS stands for skin changes, not SIADH. Crow-Fukase or POEMS syndrome is a constellation of symptoms in a patient with a plasmacytoma. In addition to the numerous symptoms of POEMS, there is a significant association with the plasma cell variant of Castleman disease.

QCCP2, **Osteosclerotic myeloma (POEMS syndrome),** p 294

167. B. **CLOVERLEAF MORPHOLOGY.**

The morphology of the PTCLs is considerably varied with both large and small cells, but fairly consistent is the cloverleaf morphology. A similar morphology is seen with adult T cell leukemia, but unlike ATCL, there is no association with HTLV-I.

QCCP2, **Peripheral T-cell lymphoma (PTCL),** p 294

168. A. **HYPOCALCEMIA.**

There is a very significant hypercalcemia associated with ATCL, partly due to the expression of osteoclast-activating factor. There are several important take-away principles with ATCL: 1. HTLV-I association. 2. hypercalcemia. 3. cloverleaf nuclei. 4. CD4+/CD8-.

QCCP2, **Adult T-cell lymphoma (ATCL),** p 294

...

4: Hematopathology Answers

169. **B. CD4.**

Cutaneous T-cell lymphoma, mycosis fungiodes, and Sezary syndrome are all related entities of similar origin. Sezary syndrome refers to the finding of circulating MF cells (Sezary cells) with their characteristic cerebriform nuclei in the peripheral blood. All are consistently CD4+.

QCCP2, **Cutaneous T-cell lymphoma (CTCL),** p 295

170. **D. ABSENT FOLLICLES.**

Normal reactive lymph nodes tend to have large expanded follicles with prominent germinal centers. In AITCL, there is a lack of follicles and germinal centers that helps to distinguish it from reactive lymphadenopathy.

QCCP2, **Angioimmunoblastic T-cell lymphoma (AITCL),** p 295

171. **B. PRESENTATION OF ALK (+) DISEASE IN CHILDREN.**

A few things are associated with better prognosis in ALCL, while some others are associated with worse prognosis. With ALCL, it is better to be young, and with ALK (+) than to be older, ALK (-), or have a leukemic presentation.

QCCP2, **Anaplastic large cell lymphoma (ALCL),** p 296

172. **B. T(2;13).**

The anaplastic lymphoma kinase (ALK) gene is overexpressed in the majority of cases of ALCL. The most common translocation, t(2;5) fuses the nucleophosmin nuclear localization signal to the ALK gene, resulting in the characteristic nuclear staining pattern. All the other translocations involve relocation of the ALK gene on chromosome 2. t(2;13) created as PAX3-FKHR fusion protein is most often associated with alveolar rhabdomyosarcoma.

QCCP2, **Angioplastic large cell lymphoma (ALCL),** p 286

173. **E. NEUTROPENIA.**

Normal LGLs circulate as NK or cytotoxic T cells that are combatting virus infections. Disorders involving LGLs include numerous autoimmune conditions, most notably rheumatoid arthritis, when LGLs are greater than 2×10^9/L. For a sustained period, the differential diagnosis should be less suggestive of a reactive process and more of a neoplastic one.

QCCP2, **Large granular lymphocytic leukemia (LGL),** p 296

174. **B. CELIAC SPRUE.**

Enteropathy-type T cell lymphoma (ETTCL) is a lymphoma usually associated with celiac disease and most often refractory sprue. Most patients have adult-onset sprue and often a prodromal ulcerative jejunoileitis.

QCCP2, **Enteropathy-associated T-cell lymphoma (EATCL),** p 297

175. **E. YOUNG MAN, GAMMA DELTA T CELLS.**

Hepatosplenic T cell lymphoma is predominantly a disease of adolescent and young adult men and carries a gamma delta TCR T cell predominance. There is also almost always an isochromosome 7q. There have been cases of alpha beta, but they are much less common and considered a variant of the more common gamma delta.

QCCP2, **Hepatosplenic T-cell lymphoma (HTCL),** p 297

176. **B.** **SKIN.**

Most often, the disease is found in the skin, though cases of it have been found in all the other sites listed. For the most part, the extradermal cases may be seen in the context of coinvolvement with the skin.

QCCP2, **Blastic NK cell lymphoma,** p 297

177. **A.** **EBV.**

While the CD56 can be either positive (NK cell) or negative (T cell), almost all cases are positive for EBV. It is the cause of the so-called "lethal midline granuloma" due to the extensive destruction of the nasal area, not because it appears granulomatous. It is similar to another EBV-associated lesion, lymphatoid granulomatosis, which is a T cell-rich, B cell lymphoma.

QCCP2, **Extranodal NK/T cell lymphoma,** p 297

178. **B.** **NODULAR LYMPHOCYTE-PREDOMINANT.**

NLPHD is an "non-classical" type of Hodgkin lymphoma characterized by the staining pattern CD15-/CD30-, but positive for CD45. Lymphocyte-rich Hodgkin lymphoma morphologically resembles NLPHD (nodules of small lymphocytes) with scattered L- and H-like cells but stains similarly to classic Hodgkin lymphoma.

QCCP2, **Nodular lymphocyte predominant Hodgkin lymphoma (NLPHD),** p 297

179. **E.** **MIXED CELLULARITY.**

Each of the subtypes of classic Hodgkin lymphoma has a unique demographic feature - NS is overall most common, LD is in older patients, and MC is most common in underdeveloped areas and among patients with AIDS.

QCCP2, **Classic Hodgkin lymphoma,** p 297-8

180. **E.** **CD3+/CD5+.**

Overall, the predominant cell in lymph nodes with classic Hodgkin lymphoma is a reactive T cell, making flow cytometry most often a fruitless endeavor. Diagnosis of classic Hodgkin lymphoma is not made with flow cytometry but rather with morphology and immunohistochemistry.

QCCP2, **Classic Hodgkin lymphoma,** p 298

181. **D.** **NODULAR SCLEROSIS.**

The most common Hodgkin lymphoma of the mediastinum is nodular sclerosis. It is overall most common, too. Abdominal Hodgkin lymphoma is most often mixed cellularity (MC), while lymphocyte-depleted (LD) can spread to noncontiguous lymph node, most often unlike Hodgkin lymphoma.

QCCP2, **Hodgkin lymphoma,** p 298

182. **B.** **SPLENOMEGALY.**

Unlike many of the lymphoid disorders, the myeloid disorders tend to not present with splenomegaly. Characteristic dyspoietic features vary with each disorder but are fairly consistently present. It follows, too, that cytopenias would follow. All are clonal stem cell disorders, too.

QCCP2, **Myelodysplastic syndromes,** p 298

183. A. **CHRONIC MYELOMONOCYTIC LEUKEMIA (CMML).**

The preleukemic conditions as classified by the WHO fall into 3 distinct categories: the myeloproliferative, where there is too much of one cell type or another usually at the expense of the others; the myelodysplastic, where development goes away, leading to ugly cells and cytopenias; and the combination of the two, the myelodysplastic/myeloproliferative, with features of each but insufficient features to be called lymphoma or leukemia. CMML is in the overlap category.

QCCP2, **Myelodysplastic syndromes**, p 299-300

184. D. **CLUSTERS OF IMMATURE CELLS BETWEEN BUT NOT ADJACENT TO MARROW TRABECULAE OR VESSELS.**

In normal marrow, the most immature cells are located immediately adjacent to the perforating bony trabeculae and then, as they mature, grow into the intertrabecular space. ALIP refers to the process where, instead of immature cells being found at the trabeculae, they are in the region between. There is a strong propensity for progression to leukemia.

QCCP2, **Myelodysplastic syndrome**, p 300

185. E. **MONOSOMY 7.**

Complex chromosomal abnormalities of more than one clone are the most common and are associated with a poor prognosis. The other chromosomal changes are associated with good prognosis, especially 5q- QCCP2, if isolated.

QCCP2, **Myelodysplastic syndrome**, p 300

186. B. **PROMONOCYTES.**

It is important to note that, in addition to blasts, "blast equivalents" are also considered in the accounting. The total number of blasts and promonocytes must be less than 20%.

QCCP2, **Myeloproliferative and myelodysplastic syndrome**, p 399

187. C. **T(5;12).**

The t(5;12) translocation involves the TEL gene on chromosome 5. CMML with eosinophilia is known for its high eosinophil count ($>1.5 \times 10^9$/L) and its tissue-invasive nature.

QCCP2, **Chronic myelomonocytic leukemia (CMML)**, p 300

188. C. **JUVENILE MYELOMONOCYTIC LEUKEMIA (JMML).**

As the name would suggest, JMML presents in children, often with both monocytosis and granulocytosis. There are usually clonal abnormalities like monosomy 7 as well as anemia and thrombocytopenia. Interestingly, there is a small, but significant association with NF1.

QCCP2, **Juvenile myelomonocytic leukemia (JMML)**, p 300

189. E. **T(9;22).**

The chimeric bcr-abl tyrosine kinase is formed by the fusion of the breakpoint cluster region on chromosome 22 with the abl tyrosine kinase on chromosome 9. t(9;22) and bcr-abl are the *sine qua non* of CML. Notably, unlike many of the other myeloproliferative disorders, there is no JAK2 mutation.

QCCP2, **Myeloproliferative disease, (CML)**, p 301

190. E. **95%.**

By far, CML is the most progressive MPD with ~95% of cases undergoing transformation to AML. Other MPDs only progress around 10% of the time within the same time frame.
QCCP2, **Chronic myelogenous leukemia (CML)**, p 301

191. D. **IMPAIRED AGGREGATION WITH EPINEPHRINE.**

There are a few unusual features of the myeloproliferative disorders that are trivial enough to remember for testing purposes. One is the impaired platelet aggregation response to epinephrine. The other is that CML can be a cause of elevated vitamin B$_{12}$ levels (unlike *Diphyllobothrium latum* infection).
QCCP2, **Chronic myelogenous leukemia (CML)**, p 301

192. C. **DECREASING LAP SCORE.**

Testmanship would have steered you wrong on this one. When you have two choices that are the opposite, usually that means that one of them has to be the choice. In this case, however, both increases and decreases in the platelet count have been demonstrated. One thing is not true - the already low LAP score seen with the chronic phase of CML does not decrease further, but actually may rise with the accelerated phase.
QCCP2, **Chronic myelogenous leukemia (CML)**, p 301

193. A. **I(17Q).**

Both i(17q) and trisomy 8 are often accumulated as CML begins its inevitable march towards acute leukemia. Interestingly, the phenotype of the leukemia is myeloid in only 2/3 of cases. Of the remaining 1/3, most are ALL, usually of the pre B type.
QCCP2, **Chronic myelogenous leukemia (CML)**, p 301

194. D. **A & B.**

A bit of a tricky question. A presumptive diagnosis of polycythemia vera could be made if the patient fulfilled all three of the choices presented. However, the diagnosis of PV can be made with an absolute requirement for the first two criteria (increased RBC count) and ruled out secondary causes and any of a series of additional criteria.
QCCP2, **Criteria for PV, T4.28,** p 302

195. A. **THROMBOTIC EVENT.**

1/3 of patients with PV die due to thrombotic events such as myocardial infarction, cerebrovascular accident, or pulmonary embolus. 1/5 of PV patients die from acute leukemia. The rest of the choices have not been shown to be associated with PV.
QCCP2, **Polycythemia vera (PV)**, p 302

196. D. **POLYCYTHEMIA VERA.**

Over 80% of cases of PV have an associated V617F JAK2 mutation, much more than in other MPD or myeloid disorders for that matter. JAK-STAT signaling is involved with transducing cytokine signals into changes in gene expression within the nucleus. The mutation of JAK2 leads to activation in the absence of cytokine signaling.
QCCP2, **Polycythemia vera (PV)**, p 302

4: Hematopathology Answers

197. B. **ESSENTIAL THROMBOCYTOPENIA.**

The basis of ET diagnosis is high platelets without any other obvious cause, such as reactive changes, other myeloproliferative disorders, or myelodysplastic syndromes.
QCCP2, **Essential thrombocythemia (ET)**, p 302

198. B. **FIBROTIC.**

There is usually a delay in diagnosis due to the difficulty of classifying prefibrotic patients due to the fairly non-specific nature of the symptoms. The majority of patients present once marrow fibrosis has begun (fibrotic phase) and they have features suggesting a crowding of the marrow - peripheral immature cells (nucleated red blood cells, dacrocytes), and a dry marrow tap.
QCCP2, **Chronic idiopathic myelofibrosis (CIMF)**, p 303

199. C. **EVIDENCE OF A CYTOGENETIC ANOMALY OR BLASTS UP TO 20%.**

For the most part, chronic eosinophilic leukemia is the same as hypereosinophilic syndrome, except either increased blasts or evidence of chromosome tinkering is present. The diagnosis also requires the exclusion of other potential causes of secondary eosinophilia.
QCCP2, **Chronic eosinophilic leukemia**, p 303

200. C. **P230.**

The 3 characteristic bcr-abl gene fusion translocations of t(9;22) are a 190kDa product associated with poor prognosis in ALL, the standard p210 seen in CML, and the largest, p230, which is associated with neutrophil-rich CML as described.
QCCP2, **Chronic neutrophilic leukemia (CNL)**, p 303

201. B. **AML WITH LYMPHOID DIFFERENTIATION.**

While some AMLs can express some lymphoid markers, such as CD7, it is not a significant enough occurrence (or etiological reason) for a separate category of AML.
QCCP2, **Acute myeloid leukemia (AML)**, p 304

202. B. **AML1-ETO.**

The name itself gives it away. The ETO gene was named to correspond to the common translocation with which it was involved, Eight:Twenty-One.
QCCP2, **Acute myeloid leukemia (AML)**, p 304

203. E. **EOSINOPHILS.**

Reflecting the FAB classification, M4Eo demonstrates a significant eosinophilia. The leukemic cells themselves display a myelomonocytic morphology.
QCCP2, **Acute myeloid leukemia (AML) with inv(16)**, p 305

204. D. **STRONG EXPRESSION OF HLA-DR AND CD34 IN ALL SUBTYPES.**

Both the standard type, which accounts for the majority of cases, and the microgranular variant expresses neither HLA-DR, nor CD34. Only the M3 variant shows a small amount of CD34 and HLA-DR.
QCCP2, **Acute myeloid leukemia (AML) with t(15;17)**, p 305

4: Hematopathology Answers

205. **B.** **TOPOISOMERASE II INHIBITORS.**

   There is an increased incidence of AML with 11q23 mutations in young adults with a history of topoisomerase II inhibitor therapy. The MLL gene is thought to be the causative agent localized to 11q23.
   QCCP2, **Acute myeloid leukemia (AML) with anomalies of 11q23 (MLL),** p 305

206. **D.** **>20% BLASTS LACKING CYTOCHEMICAL EVIDENCE OF MYELOID DIFFERENTIATION.**

   M0, or minimally differentiated AML, falls into the general category of AML, NOS. Since it is minimally differentiated, there should be a lack of differentiation in <3% of blasts as defined by lack of staining with Sudan black, myeloperoxidase, or non-specific esterase. Also, at least 20% of marrow nucleated cells should be these agranular cytoplasmic cells.
   QCCP2, **Acute myeloid leukemia (AML), M0,** p 306

207. **B.** **20% BLASTS, OF WHICH 90% ARE MYELOBLASTS.**

   In order to be categorized as acute leukemia, there should be 20% blasts. Of these blasts at least 90% must be no more mature than the myeloblast stage. Furthermore, 3% of the blasts should stain with myeloid stains, such as myeloperoxidase.
   QCCP2, **Acute myeloid leukemia (AML) without maturation,** p 307

208. **E.** **MYELOBLASTS ARE GREATER THAN OR EQUAL TO 90% IN M1, LESS THAN 90% IN M2.**

   AML, M1 has to have greater than or equal to 90% of blasts to be myeloid, M2 calls for less blasts and more mature cells (promyelocytes, etc). Also important is to not have more than 20% monocytes or else a myelomonocytic (M4) or monocytic (M5) leukemia would have to be considered.
   QCCP2, **Acute myeloid leukemia (AML), M2,** p 307

209. **A.** **20% BLASTS, 20% MONOCYTES, 20% NEUTROPHILIC PRECURSORS.**

   A significant portion of the blasts must be both myeloid and monocytic in order to be classified as AML, M4 (myelomonocytic). The FAB AML system is easily broken down as progressing from undifferentiated/minimally differentiated (M0) to myeloblastic (M1, M2) to myelomonocytic (M4) to monocytic (M5). The leftover myeloid origin cells are red blood cells (M6) erythroid and platelets (M7) megakaryocytic.
   QCCP2, **Acute myeloid leukemia (AML), M4,** p 307

210. **C.** **APL, MICROGRANULAR VARIANT.**

   The microgranular variant of promyelocytic leukemia can resemble AML, M5 with the lack of granularity, lobulated nucleus, and a lack of Auer rods. The immunohistochemical and flow cytometric as well as genetic profiles are very different, allowing for distinguishing them.
   QCCP2, **Acute myeloid leukemia (AML), M5,** p 307

211. **D.** **M5.**

   The unusual gingival involvement pattern is remarkable in AML, M5. There is often gingival and soft tissue infiltration with bleeding disorders. There is also a predilection for younger patients.
   QCCP2, **Acute myeloid leukemia (AML), M5,** p 307

212. B. **>50% OF NUCLEATED MARROW CELLS ARE ERYTHROID PRECURSORS AND >20% OF NON-ERYTHROID CELLS ARE MYELOBLASTIC.**

There are two varieties of acute erythroid leukemia, FAB M6. Less common is a pure erythroid where there is >50% erythroid precursors but less than 20% myeloblasts. This can also be classified as refractory anemia with excessive blasts, a myelodysplastic syndrome. More often there is also an excess of myeloblasts.
QCCP2, **Acute myeloid leukemia (AML), M6,** p 307-8

213. E. **A, B, C.**

The diagnosis of greater than 50% megakaryocytic blasts (of course >20% blasts overall, of which >50% must be of megakaryocytic origin) is most often made by counting the precursors in bone marrows stained with CD41/CD61. Platelet peroxidase is very infrequently used.
QCCP2, **Acute myeloid leukemia (AML), M7,** p 308

214. D. **A & B.**

Anomalies of chromosomes 21 (trisomy) and 12 i(12p) are associated with M7 AML. Down syndrome can present with both a transient myeloproliferative disorder, which usually resembles M7, as well as a sustained acute leukemia, also usually M7. About 1/2 of the time acute leukemia in Down syndrome is lymphocytic.
QCCP2, **Acute myeloid leukemia (AML), M7,** p 308

215. C. **AML, M4/M5.**

Congenital acute leukemia is defined as occurring within one month of birth. The most common differential diagnosis is a leukemoid reaction secondary to sepsis. Most often the leukemia is myeloid (~2/3) with 1/3 ALL. Of the myeloid subtypes a myelomonocytic (M4) or monoblastic (M5).
QCCP2, **Congenital acute leukemia,** p 308

216. B. **ANAPHYLACTIC REACTION.**

Mastocytosis is a broad-ranging term that covers both neoplastic and non-neoplastic mast cell disorders. Of all of the disorders, the most common is urticaria pigmentosum, which presents clinically with diffuse pruritis and the characteristic Darier sign (dermatographism).
QCCP2, **Mastocytosis,** p 309

217. E. **CD25.**

Neoplastic mast cell processes differ from non-neoplastic with the presence of frequent c-kit mutations. The expression of cell surface marker CD25 is associated with c-kit mutations. Aberrant CD2 expression is also associated with malignant mast cells.
QCCP2, **Systemic mastocytosis,** p 309

218. B. **VIRAL.**

The atypical Downey lymphocytes are often associated with by viral infections, most notably the reactive T lymphocyte changes in response to EBV infections of B cells. They are not specific for viral infection and can also be seen in collagen vascular disease.
QCCP2, **Hematopathology take home points,** p 309

4: Hematopathology Answers

219. A. **BORRELIA RECURRENTIS.**

    The cause of relapsing fever is the only borrelial species that can be seen in the peripheral blood and only during one of the fevers.
    QCCP2, **Hematopathology take home points**, p 309

220. E. **YOU CAN'T FOOL ME; THE WHO DOESN'T DEFINE A HYPOPLASTIC SUBTYPE.**

    There is no WHO-recognized hypoplastic AML subtype. However, hypoplastic features can be described if there is less than 20% overall cellularity. Of course, to be classified as an acute leukemia, there must still be at least 20% blasts in the hypocellular marrow.
    QCCP2, **Hematopathology take home points**, p 310

221. C. **BONE MARROW AGGREGATES.**

    The finding of aggregates of immature CD34/TdT+ cells and nuclear immaturity should suggest an abnormal process, as would mature-appearing clumped cells with abnormal features, such as B>T cells. Hematogones should be dispersed among the remaining marrow elements.
    QCCP2, **Hematopathology take home points**, p 310

222. D. **<5% BLASTS IN MARROW.**

    Remission is defined as <5% blasts in marrow, while below that is the realm of minimal residual disease, a diagnosis made on the basis of either PCR or multiparametric flow cytometry.
    QCCP2, **Hematopathology take home points**, p 310

223. C. **DIFFUSE LARGE B CELL LYMPHOMA.**

    There is a panoply of disorders that can lead to marrow fibrosis, some obvious (CIMF), hairy cell leukemia, some less so (Hodgkin lymphoma).
    QCCP2, **Hematopathology take home points**, p 311

224. D. **3 WEEKS OF FEVER >38.3°C WITHOUT OBVIOUS ETIOLOGY.**

    A fever of unknown origin requires an appropriate workup for a patient with at least 3 weeks of documented fevers over 38.3°C (100.9°F). Most often, the cause is infectious, with undetermined malignancy second (especially lymphoma).
    QCCP2, **Hematopathology take home points**, p 311

225. B. **CHRONIC MYELOGENOUS LEUKEMIA.**

    Abundant pale green-blue cytoplasm with Wright-Giemsa staining and histiocyte nuclear features define the sea-blue histiocytes that can be seen in several of the myeloproliferative syndromes, most notably CML. A glycogen storage disease with a defect associated with ApoE and sphingomyelin accumulation may have numerous sea-blue histiocytes.
    QCCP2, **Hematopathology take home points**, p 311

4: Hematopathology Answers

226. E. **A, B, C.**

HPS can be associated with a broad array of disease entities which can be categorized as either neoplastic, infectious, or autoimmune. Cases of HPS in each of the named choices have been described.

QCCP2, **Hematopathology take home points,** p 311

227. B. **STOMACH.**

The GI tract holds the most extranodal lymphomas with the stomach comprising the majority of those cases, mostly due to *Helicobacter pylori*.

QCCP2, **Hematopathology take home points,** p 312

Chapter 5

Coagulation and Thrombosis

1. Which of the following best represents the three steps of normal hemostasis?
    A. decreased heart rate, adhesion of platelets, plug formation
    B. fibrin plug, inflammation, hypotension
    C. heat, redness, swelling
    D. vasoconstriction, platelet aggregation, fibrin formation
    E. vascular damage, stasis, endothelial injury

2. All of the following are components of platelet alpha granules, <u>except</u>:
    A. von Willebrand Factor
    B. platelet-derived growth factor
    C. serotonin
    D. platelet factor-4
    E. P-selectin

3. What do most of the molecules in the platelet dense granules have in common?
    A. they are very complex molecules
    B. they are all proteins
    C. they are all positively charged
    D. they are small
    E. they are all exclusively produced in dense granules

4. Which platelet surface antigen acts as the receptor for fibrinogen?
    A. GPIb/V/IX
    B. ADP receptor
    C. GPIIb/IIIa
    D. GPIa/IIa
    E. GPIc/IIa

5. How does GPIb become activated *in vivo* and *in vitro,* respectively?
    A. shear force, ristocetin
    B. ristocetin, compression
    C. activation of ADP receptor, ristocetin
    D. binding vWF, epinephrine
    E. fibrin, fibrin

6. Which protein crosslinks platelets through GPIIb/IIIa?
    A. collagen
    B. fibrin
    C. Factor XIII
    D. Factor IIa
    E. antithrombin

5: Coagulation and Thrombosis Questions

7. Which factor is unique to the extrinsic pathway of coagulation?
   A. II
   B. V
   C. VII
   D. IX
   E. X

8. All of the following are required to activate Factor X *in vivo*, except:
   A. Ca^{++}
   B. ATP
   C. platelet surface
   D. Factor VIIIa
   E. Factor IXa

9. How does tissue factor pathway inhibitor inhibit coagulation?
   A. inhibition of tissue factor-Factor VIIa-Factor Xa complex
   B. conversion of thrombin to prothrombin
   C. uncoupling Factor XII-dependent crosslinking of fibrin
   D. binding and hiding tissue factor on the endothelial surface
   E. consumption of activating ATP

10. All of the following factors are inhibited by antithrombin, except:
    A. thrombin
    B. Factor IXa
    C. Factor Xa
    D. Factor XIIa
    E. Factor Va

11. All of the following are routinely used in assaying platelet function by aggregometry, except:
    A. ATP
    B. collagen
    C. epinephrine
    D. ristocetin
    E. arachidonate

12. What does the secondary wave of platelet aggregation seen with the biphasic low-dose ADP and epinephrine response represent?
    A. increased binding to collagen
    B. platelet degranulation
    C. increased activation by collagen
    D. costimulation by coagulation
    E. formation of fibrin dimers

13. Which of the following disorders is associated with normal platelet aggregation with all agonists except ristocetin?
    A. von Willebrand disease
    B. Bernard-Soulier syndrome
    C. Glanzmann thrombasthenia
    D. A & B
    E. A, B, C

5: Coagulation and Thrombosis Questions

14. Which disorder is associated with diminished clot retraction?
    A. grey platelet syndrome
    B. Glanzmann thrombasthenia
    C. storage pool defect
    D. Bernard-Soulier syndrome
    E. von Willebrand disease

15. What is the primary use of the point of care clotting time assay?
    A. monitoring dialysis effectiveness
    B. monitoring coumadin therapy
    C. monitoring heparin therapy
    D. screening test for von Willebrand disease
    E. screening test for activated protein C resistance

16. What is the usual effect on coagulation testing in the presence of elevated Factor VIII levels?
    A. prolong PT
    B. shorten PT
    C. prolong PTT
    D. shorten PTT
    E. no change in either PT or PTT

17. All of the following can cause prolongation of both PTT and PT, except:
    A. deficiencies of Factors X, V, and II
    B. disseminated intravascular coagulation
    C. liver disease
    D. anti-Factor VIII antibodies
    E. vitamin K deficiency

18. What ratio of patient plasma to normal plasma is recommended for the detection of weak inhibitors of coagulation?
    A. 1:1
    B. 2:1
    C. 4:1
    D. 1:2
    E. 1:4

19. A mutation in this coagulation factor accounts for activated protein C (APC) resistance:
    A. thrombin
    B. Factor V
    C. Factor VIII
    D. Factor X
    E. Protein C

20. What's the most common cause of antiphospholipid syndrome?
    A. lupus anticoagulant
    B. anti-phospholipase antibody
    C. anti-Factor Xa antibody
    D. anti-cardiolipin antibody
    E. Factor V Leiden

5: Coagulation and Thrombosis Questions

21. What is the purpose of the anti-Factor Xa assay?
    A. routine workup of elevated aPTT
    B. routine workup of elevated PT
    C. monitoring low molecular weight heparin
    D. alternative to PT for monitoring coumadin
    E. indirect assay of protein C levels

22. What is the essentially normal cutoff value for antithrombin in patients over 6 months of age?
    A. 10%
    B. 30%
    C. 60%
    D. 75%
    E. 100%

23. What's the most common coagulation factor to which antibodies arise?
    A. Factor II
    B. Factor VIII
    C. Factor IX
    D. Factor X
    E. Protein C

24. What factor is assayed with the clot stability test?
    A. Factor II
    B. Factor V
    C. Factor IX
    D. Factor X
    E. Factor XIII

25. What are D-dimers?
    A. products of plasmin-mediated degradation of fibrin
    B. crosslinked fibrin polymers of 20-30 units
    C. fibrinogen degradation products
    D. functionally active plasmin
    E. Factor XIII inactive enzyme

26. What's the most common factor deficiency leading to a normal PTT, but prolonged PT?
    A. Factor II
    B. Factor V
    C. Factor VII
    D. Factor X
    E. Factor XIII

27. What is the preferred interval post-cessation of anticoagulants and post-thrombosis, respectively, for testing of protein C deficiency?
    A. 1 month, 1 week
    B. 1 week, 1 month
    C. 6 weeks, 6 months
    D. 1 week, 6 months
    E. 1 month, 6 months

5: Coagulation and Thrombosis Questions

28. All of the following are required to perform the prothrombin time assay, <u>except</u>:
    A.   tissue factor
    B.   phospholipid
    C.   citrated plasma
    D.   calcium
    E.   thrombin

29. What product is compared directly with the international normalized ratio?
    A.   thromboplastin
    B.   calcium
    C.   thrombin
    D.   phospholipid
    E.   citrate

30. What is the <u>most</u> common cause of a prolonged thrombin time?
    A.   fibrinogen deficiency
    B.   dysfibrinogenemia
    C.   heparin
    D.   coumadin
    E.   platelet dysfunction

31. What is the purpose of the low-dose ristocetin cofactor assay?
    A.   workup of a suspected Bernard-Soulier syndrome
    B.   workup of a suspected von Willebrand disease, type 2B
    C.   workup of a suspected Glanzmann thrombasthenia
    D.   workup of a suspected platelet storage pool defect
    E.   workup of suspected hypercoagulability

32. What test is the primary means of subclassifying von Willebrand disease?
    A.   low-dose ristocetin cofactor assay
    B.   multimer assays
    C.   high-dose ristocetin assay
    D.   Factor VIII levels
    E.   D-dimers

33. Which ABO blood type has the mean lowest levels of von Willebrand Factor?
    A.   O
    B.   A
    C.   B
    D.   AB

34. All of the following are commonly seen with coagulation-type bleeding disorders, <u>except</u>:
    A.   mucosal bleeding
    B.   hemarthrosis
    C.   delayed bleeding
    D.   deep hematomas
    E.   male predominance

5: Coagulation and Thrombosis Questions

35. Which characteristic of Bernard-Soulier syndrome helps distinguish it from von Willebrand disease?
    A. concomitant storage pool defects in platelets
    B. giant platelets
    C. thrombocytosis
    D. thrombocytopenia
    E. absolute lymphocytosis

36. Which of the following characteristics are common between Hermansky-Pudlak and Chediak-Higashi syndromes?
    A. giant inclusion granules in platelets
    B. alpha granule storage pool defects
    C. ceroid-like inclusions in macrophages
    D. oculocutaneous albinism
    E. giant inclusion granules in granulocytes

37. Which of the following patients is more likely to have Hermansky-Pudlak syndrome?
    A. an Aleutian Islander
    B. a Puerto Rican Islander
    C. a Southeast Asian immigrant
    D. an Eastern African
    E. a Pacific Islander

38. All of the following are associated with Wiskott-Aldrich syndrome, except:
    A. thrombocytopenia
    B. eczema
    C. absent radii
    D. small platelets
    E. immunodeficiency

39. Which platelet cell surface marker is aberrantly unstimulated with high-dose thrombin in patients with grey platelet syndrome?
    A. CD15
    B. CD23
    C. CD30
    D. CD42
    E. CD62

40. Which of the following disorders presents as both a defect in clotting as well as coagulation?
    A. von Willebrand disease
    B. Bernard-Soulier syndrome
    C. Glanzmann thrombasthenia
    D. Chediak-Higashi syndrome
    E. Hermansky-Pudlak syndrome

41. Which subtype of von Willebrand disease is the most common?
    A. type 1
    B. type 2a
    C. type 2b
    D. type 2M
    E. type 3

5: Coagulation and Thrombosis Questions

42. Which of the following types of von Willebrand disease should not be treated with DDAVP?
    A. type 2B
    B. type 3
    C. type 1
    D. A & B
    E. A, B, C

43. Which inheritance pattern characteristic of type 2N von Willebrand disease helps to distinguish it from hemophilia A?
    A. autosomal recessive
    B. autosomal dominant
    C. X-linked recessive
    D. X-linked dominant
    E. mitochondrial

44. What advantage does Humate-P provide over cryoprecipitate in the treatment of von Willebrand disease?
    A. virus inactivation
    B. less expensive
    C. more concentrated
    D. smaller volume
    E. presence of additional clotting factors

45. Which of the following is a product of COX-1, exerting a direct stimulatory effect on platelets?
    A. platelet-derived growth factor
    B. arachidonic acid
    C. prostacyclin
    D. thromboxane A_2
    E. inositol-3-phosphate

46. How do ticlopidine and clopidogrel inhibit platelets?
    A. bind von Willebrand Factor
    B. degrade GPIa
    C. inhibit ADP-mediated platelet aggregation
    D. inhibit GPIIb/IIIa
    E. depletion of platelet alpha granule content

47. Which of the following is an effective therapy for uremia-induced platelet dysfunction?
    A. dialysis
    B. DDAVP
    C. estrogen
    D. A & B
    E. A, B, C

48. Overall, what's the most common cause of thrombocytopenia?
    A. ITP
    B. TTP
    C. myelodysplastic syndromes
    D. lymphoma
    E. nutritional deficiency

5: Coagulation and Thrombosis Questions

49. All of the following have thrombocytopenia often accompanied by schistocytes, <u>except</u>:
     A. TTP
     B. HUS
     C. HELLP
     D. DIC
     E. ITP

50. What is the preferred <u>initial</u> therapy for idiopathic thrombocytopenic purpura?
     A. splenectomy
     B. methylprednisolone and IVIg
     C. gamma globulin
     D. antibiotics
     E. plasma exchange

51. What do post-transfusion purpura and neonatal alloimmune thrombocytopenia have in common?
     A. antibodies against GPIIb/IIIa
     B. antibodies directed against PLA-1 antigens
     C. immature micromegakaryocytes
     D. myelophthstic pancytopenia
     E. giant platelets

52. Which of the following causes of thrombocytopenia is a contraindication for future heparin use?
     A. neonatal alloimmune thrombocytopenic purpura
     B. post-transfusion purpura
     C. heparin-induced thrombocytopenia, type I
     D. heparin-induced thrombocytopenia, type II
     E. thrombotic thrombocytopenic purpura

53. Which of the following tests provides an appropriate laboratory confirmation of immune-mediated heparin-induced thrombocytopenia?
     A. anti-PF4 antibody
     B. serotonin release assay
     C. heparin-induced platelet aggregation assay
     D. A & B
     E. A, B, C

54. Which serum protein can be elevated in TTP?
     A. gamma globulin
     B. lactate dehydrogenase
     C. ALT
     D. albumin
     E. thyroglobulin

55. All of the following are diagnostic criteria for TTP, <u>except</u>:
     A. fever
     B. anemia
     C. thrombocytopenia
     D. liver failure
     E. neurological changes

5: Coagulation and Thrombosis Questions

56. What therapeutic modality has significantly changed the prognosis for TTP?
     A.   full-body irradiation
     B.   intrathecal chemotherapy
     C.   broad-spectrum antibiotics
     D.   liver transplant
     E.   daily plasma exchange

57. All of the following present with giant platelets and thrombocytopenia, except:
     A.   Bernard-Soulier syndrome
     B.   Wiskott-Aldrich syndrome
     C.   Grey Platelet syndrome
     D.   May-Hegglin syndrome
     E.   Sebastian syndrome

58. What is usually the Factor VIII level in a hemophiliac patient with spontaneous bleeding?
     A.   <1%
     B.   5-10%
     C.   20-30%
     D.   50-60%
     E.   70%

59. What type of Factor VIII mutation accounts for more cases of hemophilia than any other type of mutation?
     A.   a conserved point mutation
     B.   a splice site mutation
     C.   an inversion mutation
     D.   a nonsense mutation
     E.   a missense mutation

60. Approximately what percentage of patients with hemophilia A who receive Factor VIII replacement therapy develop anti-Factor VIII antibodies?
     A.   <1%
     B.   ~5%
     C.   10-25%
     D.   50-75%
     E.   >90%

61. What is the primary difference in the treatment of hemophilia A and B?
     A.   there is less than 50% recovery of Factor VIII due to distribution into intra- and extravascular spaces
     B.   there is less than 50% recovery of Factor IX due to distribution into intra- and extravascular spaces
     C.   the half-life of Factor VIII is considerably shorter than Factor IX and must be dosed with greater frequency
     D.   the half-life of Factor VIII is considerably longer than Factor IX and must be dosed with lesser frequency
     E.   DDAVP can be used to treat hemophilia B

62. Deficiency of this coagulation factor may be the only congenital cause of an isolated prolonged PT:
     A.   Factor VIII
     B.   Factor IX
     C.   Factor V
     D.   Factor VII
     E.   Factor XIII

5: Coagulation and Thrombosis Questions

63. Which of the following factors is directly activated by dilute Russell viper venom?
    A. Factor II
    B. Factor VII
    C. Factor IX
    D. Factor X
    E. Factor XIII

64. What's the most common presentation of Factor XIII deficiency?
    A. clinically inapparent
    B. delayed bleeding tendency
    C. severe bleeding responsive to DDAVP
    D. severe bleeding not responsive to DDAVP
    E. not seen due to its incompatibility with life

65. Deficiencies of which pair of factors accounts for the most common inherited combined deficiency?
    A. Factor II and Factor V
    B. Factor V and Factor VIII
    C. Factor VIII and Factor IX
    D. Factor II and Factor XIII
    E. Factor VII and Factor X

66. What is the most common comorbidity in patients with hypofibrinogenemia due to defects in secretion of fibrinogen from the liver?
    A. cirrhosis
    B. alpha-1-antitrypsin disease
    C. hepatocellular carcinoma
    D. cholangiocarcinoma
    E. primary biliary cirrhosis

67. Deficiency of which of the following factors is associated with amyloidosis?
    A. Factor II
    B. Factor V
    C. Factor VII
    D. Factor VIII
    E. Factor X

68. While Factor VII has the shortest half-life of all the vitamin K-dependent coagulation factors, what vitamin K-dependent factor has the second shortest half-life?
    A. Factor II
    B. Protein C
    C. Factor VI
    D. Factor IX
    E. Factor V

69. All of the following tests are the most helpful in the diagnosis of disseminated intravascular coagulation, except:
    A. PT
    B. D-dimer levels
    C. antithrombin levels
    D. prothrombin fragment 1+2 levels
    E. fibrinopeptide levels

70. What's the most common presentation of arterial thrombosis?
    A.   deep femoral thrombosis
    B.   gangrenous digits
    C.   stroke
    D.   myocardial infarction in a young person
    E.   hepatic artery thrombosis

71. Which of the following are common causes of <u>both</u> arterial and venous thromboses?
    A.   antiphospholipid syndrome
    B.   prothrombin G20210A mutation
    C.   antithrombin deficiency
    D.   A & B
    E.   A, B, C

72. What's the most common cause of inherited thrombophilia?
    A.   antiphospholipid syndrome
    B.   prothrombin G20210A mutation
    C.   Factor V Leiden
    D.   hyperhomocysteinemia
    E.   Factor XII deficiency

73. Which of the following is associated with the highest incidence of prothrombin G20210A mutation?
    A.   antiphospholipid syndrome
    B.   Factor V Leiden
    C.   antithrombin deficiency
    D.   European ancestry
    E.   Protein C deficiency

74. Which of the following causes of thrombophilia most often presents as thrombotic episodes with resistance to heparin?
    A.   Protein C deficiency
    B.   antithrombin deficiency
    C.   prothrombin G20210A mutation
    D.   Factor V Leiden
    E.   antiphospholipid syndrome

75. Which of the following coagulation factors is inactivated by Protein C?
    A.   Factor V
    B.   Factor VIII
    C.   Factor IX
    D.   A & B
    E.   A, B, C

76. What are patients with homozygous Protein C deficiency particularly at an increased risk of developing?
    A.   post-transfusion purpura
    B.   warfarin skin necrosis
    C.   purpura fulminans
    D.   thrombocytophilia
    E.   Bernard-Soulier syndrome

5: Coagulation and Thrombosis Questions

77. Provocative testing with ingestion of this amino acid is used to diagnose hyperhomocysteinemia:
    A. tryptophan
    B. methionine
    C. cysteine
    D. tyrosine
    E. phenylalanine

78. Deficiency of this factor produces a prolonged PTT without obvious increased clinical risk of bleeding:
    A. Factor XIII
    B. Factor XII
    C. Factor X
    D. Factor VII
    E. Factor V

79. All of the following are commonly seen with both anti-cardiolipin antibody and lupus anticoagulant, except:
    A. arterial thrombosis
    B. fetal demise
    C. patients otherwise healthy
    D. antiphospholipid syndrome
    E. thrombocytopenia

80. Which pulmonary disorder is associated with anti-phospholipid antibodies?
    A. desquamative interstitial pneumonia
    B. primary pulmonary hypertension
    C. organizing pneumonia
    D. respiratory bronchiolitis
    E. non-specific interstitial pneumonia

81. Which of the following reagents can be used to correct prolongation of the PTT seen in patients with lupus anticoagulant?
    A. platelet membrane phospholipids
    B. Tween 20
    C. hirudin
    D. Factor X
    E. excess calcium + tissue factor

82. This disorder presents with strokes in young people and is characterized by hyperaggregation of platelets with ADP and/or epinephrine:
    A. grey platelet syndrome
    B. Wein-Penzing defect
    C. lupus anticoagulant
    D. sticky platelet syndrome
    E. Kawasaki disease

83. Which of the following can be used to distinguish a reactive thrombocytosis from a neoplastic one?
    A. C-reactive protein levels
    B. erythrocyte sedimentation rate
    C. iron studies
    D. A & B
    E. A, B, C

5: Coagulation and Thrombosis Questions

84. What is the most common cause of pediatric thrombocytosis?
    A. Kawasaki disease
    B. infection
    C. acute lymphocytic leukemia
    D. iron deficiency
    E. juvenile arthritis

85. What is the likelihood of an adult having a myeloproliferative disorder when their platelet count is greater than 2 million platelets/dL?
    A. <0.1%
    B. 1%
    C. 10%
    D. 50%
    E. 90%

86. All of the following agents have shown to be capable of enhancing the action of coumadin, except:
    A. metronidazole
    B. cholestyramine
    C. cimetidine
    D. sulfamethoxazole-trimethoprim
    E. omeprazole

87. Concurrent therapy with this drug when starting coumadin can help prevent a transient hypercoagulability in patients with Protein C deficiency:
    A. argatroban
    B. vitamin K
    C. heparin
    D. lecithin
    E. omeprazole

88. What time frame is needed to discontinue coumadin before an invasive surgical procedure?
    A. 2 hours
    B. 1 day
    C. 1 week
    D. 2 weeks
    E. 1 month

5: Coagulation and Thrombosis Answers

1. D. **VASOCONSTRICTION, PLATELET AGGREGATION, FIBRIN FORMATION.**

    Initially, vascular damage is met with the body's reaction of "clamping down" to avoid further blood loss. This usually takes the form of vasoconstriction. In response, platelets adhere to vessels, then aggregate with each other. The primitive platelet plug (alliteration!) is then replaced by the fibrin clot produced through the action of the clotting cascade.

    QCCP2, **Normal hemostasis,** p 322

2. C. **SEROTONIN.**

    The P compounds (PDGF, P-selectin, PF4) and vWF, along with a number of other proteins, such as IGF-1 and TGF beta, are all found in the alpha granules of platelets. These granules give the platelets their distinctive purple color with Wright-Giemsa staining. Deficiencies of alpha granules lead to grey platelet syndrome.

    QCCP2, **Normal platelet function,** p 322

3. D. **THEY ARE SMALL.**

    The dense granule molecules, unlike those in the alpha granules, are all small molecules, such as ADP, ATP, Ca^{++}, and serotonin. There are multiple syndromes associated with deficiencies in dense granules, including Chediak-Higashi and Hermansky-Pudlak.

    QCCP2, **Normal platelet function,** p 322

4. C. **GPIIB/IIIA.**

    The GPIb/V/IX complex (CD42) serves as the receptor for platelet adhesion through vWF. GPIIb/IIIa then comes to assist with platelet aggregation through the binding of fibrinogen. Deficiencies in Ib lead to Bernard-Soulier syndrome, while mutation of GPIIb/IIIa accounts for the weakened ("thrombasthenia") platelet binding in Glanzmann.

    QCCP2, **Normal platelet function,** p 322

5. A. **SHEAR FORCE, RISTOCETIN.**

    GPIb along with GPV/IX acts as a receptor for vWF on the exposed basement membrane of the endothelium. Shear forces from the circulation activate the GPIb. Ristocetin is an antibiotic with the side effect of promoting platelet adhesion.

    QCCP2, **Normal platelet function,** p 322

6. B. **FIBRIN.**

    Thrombin released from platelet alpha granules activates fibrinogen by cleaving propeptide to yield fibrin, which, in addition to helping start coagulation, also contributes to platelet aggregation.

    QCCP2, **Normal platelet function,** p 322

7. C. **VII.**

    Factor VIIa functions as a "tenase," activating Factor X, as well as a "ninase," activating Factor IX, leading into the intrinsic pathway.

    QCCP2, **Normal coagulation,** p 322

5: Coagulation and Thrombosis Answers

8.   B.   **ATP.**

The activation of Factor X is central coagulation because active Factor X is responsible for activating thrombin with Factor V as a cofactor. The platelets are involved with coagulation through increased phosphatidyl inositol on their surfaces, thus facilitating factor interaction.

QCCP2, **Normal coagulation,** p 323

9.   A.   INHIBITION OF TISSUE FACTOR-FACTOR VIIa-FACTOR Xa COMPLEX.

TFP1, also know as lipoprotein-associated coagulation inhibitor, anticonvertin, or extrinsic pathway inhibitor, depending who you ask, functions predominantly by inhibiting the critical first step of coagulation, the formation of the tissue factor-Factor VIIa-Factor Xa complex.

QCCP2, **Control of coagulation,** p 324

10.   E.   FACTOR Va.

Antithrombin functions mainly by inactivating thrombin (really!) and Factor Xa, a process that is facilitated by heparin. In addition to Factors II and X, antithrombin also inactivates Factors IX, XII, and XI. Factors V and VIII, on the other hand, are not enzymes, but rather cofactors, inhibited by the action of Protein C and catalyzed by Protein S.

QCCP2, **Control of coagulation,** p 324

11.   A.   **ATP.**

While arachidonate is used less often that the others, ATP is not used. ADP is used as a stimulant of aggregation through its receptor. Ristocetin is an antibiotic that stimulates adhesion.

QCCP2, **Platelet aggregometry,** p 325

12.   B.   PLATELET DEGRANULATION.

Degranulation of platelet dense granules which are full of small molecules, such as ATP, Ca^{++}, and serotonin, leads to further stimulation of platelet aggregation. Initial stimulation (first wave) is due to the direct action of low-dose ADP or low-dose epinephrine.

QCCP2, **Platelet aggregometry,** p 325

13.   D.   **A & B.**

Glanzmann thrombasthenia is characterized by the opposite pattern - response to only ristocetin - and is due to mutation of the GPIIb/IIIa receptor. Bernard-Soulier is due to a defect in GPIa, while von Willebrand disease is due to defects in von Willebrand Factor, which, due to their interactions, can present with overlapping clinical symptoms.

QCCP2, **Platelet function tests,** p 326

14.   B.   GLANZMANN THROMBASTHENIA.

Clot retraction requires functional GPIIb/IIIa receptor in order to begin wound healing after the process of thrombus formation has begun. Since clot retraction requires GPIIB/IIIa, it will be aberrant in individuals with Glanzmann thrombasthenia.

QCCP2, **Abnormal aggregometry,** p 326

5: Coagulation and Thrombosis Answers

15.   C.   MONITORING HEPARIN THERAPY.

The activated clotting time assay is used primarily to monitor heparin in patients on supratherapeutic amounts of heparin where the PTT may exceed the reportable range. Since it is a point-of-care test, it is rapid and most useful in pre-operative or pre-procedure (dialysis) settings.
QCCP2, **Activated clotting time,** p 326

16.   D.   SHORTEN PTT.

Factor VIII, a constituent of the intrinsic pathway, is most sensitively monitored by PTT. The PTT is responsive to changes in factors involved in either the intrinsic or common pathways. For this reason, elevated Factor VIII causes a shortening of the PTT.
QCCP2, **aPTT,** p 327

17.   D.   ANTI-FACTOR VIII ANTIBODIES.

An antibody against Factor VIII presents as a prolongation of aPTT with a relatively normal PT due to Factor VIII being required for the intrinsic pathway but not the extrinsic pathway of coagulation.
QCCP2, **T5.3,** p 328

18.   C.   4:1.

Weak inhibitors can be overwhelmed with too much normal plasma. For that reason, it is recommended that a smaller amount is used. The greater ratio has shown to have a much greater sensitivity for detecting inhibitors while remaining relatively specific.
QCCP2, **aPTT,** p 329

19.   B.   FACTOR V.

Inhibition of coagulation by Protein C involves the cleavage of Factor V at a conserved sequence. The mutation of that site on Factor V (Leiden) results in a protein that is resistant to degradation and cleavage by activated Protein C. Hence, the patient is at risk for thrombosis.
QCCP2, **Activated Protein C resistance screening assay,** p 329

20.   D.   ANTI-CARDIOLIPIN ANTIBODY.

The vast majority of cases of antiphospholipid syndrome are due to anticardiolipin antibody with the remainder of cases due to lupus anticoagulant.
QCCP2, **Anticardiolipin antibody,** p 329

21.   C.   MONITORING LOW MOLECULAR WEIGHT HEPARIN.

Low molecular weight and unfractionated heparin are difficult to monitor. Since they selectively inhibit Factor X, the aPTT is less reliable than it is for monitoring heparin, which also inhibits Factor II. Anti-Xa provides an alternative assay.
QCCP2, **Anti-Xa assay,** p 330

5: Coagulation and Thrombosis Answers

22. C. **60%.**

Anything over 60% is considered normal. Neonates often have lower levels than adults, and as such, normal values can be anything >40%. Antithrombin assays can be either for protein levels or protein activity, with the functional assays being preferred for screening purposes.
QCCP2, **Antithrombin,** p 330

23. B. **FACTOR VIII.**

The specialized Bethesda assay is utilized to determine and quantify the titer of a suspected Factor VIII inhibitor. The assay is based on the premise that, with dilution Factor VIII, deficiency will lead to a progressive prolongation of PTT, while the converse occurs with Factor VIII inhibitors. That is, as the patient serum is diluted, there will be more Factor VIII activity.
QCCP2, **Bethesda assay,** p 330

24. E. **FACTOR XIII.**

The clot stability assay tests whether or not fibrin dimers are cross-linked - the modification that gives the clot its stability. Urea (a denaturant) is added to an *in vitro* formed clot from a patient sample. This assay is very insensitive and is only positive in a patient with virtually no Factor XIII.
QCCP2, **Clot stability test,** p 331

25. A. **PRODUCTS OF PLASMIN-MEDIATED DEGRADATION OF FIBRIN.**

D-dimers are a specific plasmin degradation product. They are only formed when plasmin degrades a formed clot, meaning fibrinogen must have been converted to fibrin. This means the assay is specific for fibrin; fibrinogen is not assayed.
QCCP2, **D-dimer,** p 331

26. C. **FACTOR VII.**

Most commonly, Factor VII deficiency will produce a normal PTT with a prolonged PT. However, the PTT is less sensitive than the PT at detecting deficiencies of common pathway factors, such as Factor I, II, X, and V, and can therefore present in a similar fashion.
QCCP2, **Factor assays,** p 332

27. B. **1 WEEK, 1 MONTH.**

For the most part, assays of Protein C levels can be used as a surrogate for activity. However, there are some patients with dysfunctional Protein C with seemingly normal levels.
QCCP2, **Protein C activity,** p 333

28. E. **THROMBIN.**

The PT is used to assay for defects in the extrinsic pathway of coagulation. Because most of the factors in the extrinsic pathway are vitamin K-dependent, the PT is the preferred assay for monitoring coumadin therapy.
QCCP2, **PT,** p 334

5: Coagulation and Thrombosis Answers

29. A. **THROMBOPLASTIN.**

The sensitivity to inactivation of thromboplastin (tissue factor + phospholipid) by coumadin can vary greatly. As a result, a normalized ratio comparing thromboplastin to a standard was proposed. Because it is the interaction of coumadin with thromboplastin that varies, the INR is useful only in the analysis of coumadin effects, not coagulation in general.
QCCP2, **PT,** p 334

30. C. **HEPARIN.**

Often the thrombin time is used to distinguish a prolonged PTT due to factor deficiencies or inhibitors from one due to heparin in the specimen. Reptilase or heparinase can either be used to further work up a prolonged thrombin time.
QCCP2, **Thrombin time,** p 334

31. B. **WORKUP OF A SUSPECTED VON WILLEBRAND DISEASE, TYPE 2B.**

When a patient's platelets and plasma are mixed in the presence of a low dose of ristocetin, a patient with type 2B vWD will show a characteristic increased aggregation. Similarly, platelet-type vWD will also behave likewise - unlike the other types of vWD. which will show decreased platelet aggregation.
QCCP2, **vWF assays,** p 335

32. B. **MULTIMER ASSAYS.**

von Willebrand disease can be subtyped into several categories - type 1, or mild deficiency; type 3, or severe deficiency; and then type 2, which is due to functional or structural defects in the protein. Type 2 is further subdivided by which type of multimers are missing - 2A has deficiency or high and intermediate multimers; 2B is missing high molecular weight multimers. Types 2M and 2N are due to structural mutations in vWF - type 2M can't bind GPIb but can bind Factor VIII; the opposite is true for type 2N. Type 2N often presents like hemophilia because the interaction between vWF and Factor VIII stabilizes Factor VIII levels.
QCCP2, **vWF assays,** p 335

33. A. **O.**

The choices are organized in order of the relative amount of von Willebrand Factor. There can be an almost 50% difference in the amount of vWF between type O and types B or AB.
QCCP2, **vWF assays,** p 335

34. A. **MUCOSAL BLEEDING.**

Certain characteristics of platelet-type bleeding disorders include mucosal bleeding, petechiae, and a female predominance. Bleeding due to defects in coagulation presents with the other choices in the question
QCCP2, **Causes of excessive bleeding, T5.5 Clinical Manifestations of Bleeding Disorders,** p 336

35. B. **GIANT PLATELETS.**

The platelets seen in the peripheral smear of patients with Bernard-Soulier syndrome are typically larger than normal. There is also usually a thrombocytopenia, but it's a non-specific finding. Otherwise, the clinical presentation of von Willebrand disease (especially platelet-type, and types 2M and 3) and Bernard-Soulier are strikingly similar.
QCCP2, **Platelet disorders,** p 336

5: Coagulation and Thrombosis Answers

36. D. OCULOCUTANEOUS ALBINISM.

Both Hermansky-Pudlak and Chediak-Higashi are due to defects in dense granule storage, where platelets store small molecules in order to initiate the secondary wave of aggregation. Inclusion granules are more common in Chediak-Higashi, while ceroid-like inclusions are more common in Hermansky-Pudlak. Alpha granule defects are not usually seen in either.
QCCP2, **Platelet disorders,** p 336

37. B. A PUERTO RICAN ISLANDER.

Hermansky-Pudlak is most commonly seen in a specific location in Puerto Rico, presumably due to founder effect. A number of genes are involved in Hermansky-Pudlak; the most common in the Puerto Rican population is due to a duplication event in the gene HPS1.
QCCP2, **Platelet disorder,** p 336

38. C. ABSENT RADII.

A similar syndrome of thrombocytopenia with absent radii is most commonly seen in patients without radii and thumbs. Wiskott-Aldrich also presents with platelet-type bleeding, like Hermansky-Pudlak and Chediak-Higashi.
QCCP2, **Platelet disorders,** p 337

39. E. CD62.

In addition to decreased CD62, there is also decreased PF4 expression on the surface of platelets. Grey platelet syndrome, due to defects in alpha granules, are grey-blue staining with Wright-Giemsa.
QCCP2, **Platelet disorders,** p 337

40. A. VON WILLEBRAND DISEASE.

von Willebrand Factor has a role in both coagulation as a carrier protein for Factor VIII, as well as in facilitating platelet adhesion by binding GPIb on platelet surfaces. There are certain subtypes of von Willebrand disease, namely types 2M and 2N, that have defects in either coagulation or clotting.
QCCP2, **Platelet disorders,** p 337

41. A. TYPE 1.

By far, the majority of cases of von Willebrand disease are type 1, which is due to decreased levels of von Willebrand Factor. Type 3 is an absence of von Willebrand Factor, while type 2 (and its subclasses) are due to functional defects in vWF.
QCCP2, **von Willebrand Factor,** p 338

42. D. A & B.

DDAVP stimulates the release of vWF and Factor VIII from Weibel-Palade bodies. Type 2B vWD reacts to DDAVP with enhanced platelet aggregation, leading to potentially dangerous thrombosis, while type 3 doesn't react at all.
QCCP2, **vWD,** p 338

5: Coagulation and Thrombosis Answers

43. B. **AUTOSOMAL DOMINANT.**

    The particular defect associated with type 2N vWD levels leads to defective vWF that can bind GPIb, but not Factor VIII. Because of the stabilizing influence of vWF on Factor VIII in the circulation, a defect in the ability of vWF to bind Factor VIII would present with decreased Factor VIII levels. For this reason, type 2N vWD looks like hemophilia A. However, unlike the X-linked recessive inheritance pattern of hemophilia A, type 2N vWD is autosomal dominant.
    QCCP2, **vWD,** p 339

44. A. **VIRUS INACTIVATION.**

    The ability to remove virus, especially HCV and HIV is of particular importance and provides a considerable benefit for Humate-P (purified Factor VIII and vWF) over other products such as cryoprecipitate and plasma.
    QCCP2, **vWD,** p 340

45. D. **THROMBOXANE A$_2$.**

    Thromboxane stimulates platelets to release dense granules, stimulating the second wave of platelet aggregation. Irreversible inhibition of COX-1 by aspirin leads to decreased thromboxane and, consequently, decreased platelet aggregation.
    QCCP2, **Aspirin and NSAIDs,** p 340

46. C. **INHIBITING ADP-MEDIATED PLATELET AGGREGATION.**

    Ticlopidine and clopidogrel both inhibit ADP-mediated aggregation and present with blunted ADP response with aggregometry studies, but normal results with other agonists. Another class of inhibitors, like abciximab, blocks platelet function through GPIIb/IIIa.
    QCCP2, **Acquired platelet defects,** p 340

47. E. **A, B, C.**

    Patients with uremia tend to present with lab results out of proportion to the clinical presentation. While the *in vitro* aggregation studies can often be abnormal, patients usually don't show evidence of an increased bleeding risk.
    QCCP2, **Acquired platelet defects,** p 341

48. A. **ITP.**

    In adults and children, ITP is the most common cause of thrombocytopenia. Interestingly, neonates can also suffer from ITP but usually because of maternal antibodies capable of crossing the placenta and binding the fetal platelets.
    QCCP2, **Thrombocytopenia,** p 341

49. E. **ITP.**

    Microangiopathic hemolytic anemia can be caused by a number of disorders. HUS, TTP, DIC, and HELLP usually have evidence of intravascular damage to red blood cells (schistocytes) as well as thrombocytopenia. ITP usually presents with isolated thrombocytopenia.
    QCCP2, **Thrombocytopenia,** p 341

5: Coagulation and Thrombosis Answers

50. B. **METHYLPREDNISOLONE AND IVIg.**

     While the definitive therapy for ITP involves splenectomy, it is not the preferred initial therapy, which usually involves methylprednisolone to calm down the immune system with or without IVIg, which functions as a non-specific competitor for platelet binding, effectively decreasing splenic sequestration.
     QCCP2, **ITP,** p 342

51. B. **ANTIBODIES DIRECTED AGAINST PLA-1 ANTIGEN.**

     While the antibody and antigens are the same, the mechanism of antibody formation is different. In neonatal alloimmune thrombocytopenic purpura (NATP), the mother has the unusual platelet phenotype lacking the PLA-1 antigen. As a result of carrying a child whose platelets express PLA-1, the mother makes an antibody in response to fetal platelets. It makes sense that the treatment is washed maternal platelets, since they lack the antigen. In post-transfusion purpura, a PLA-1 (-) recipient makes antibodies to PLA-1 after receiving a transfusion of PLA-1 (+) platelets. Interestingly, not only are the transfused PLA-1 (+) platelets destroyed by the antibody, but so too are the patient's own PLA-1 (-) platelets.
     QCCP2, **NATP, PTP,** p 342

52. D. **HEPARIN-INDUCED THROMBOCYTOPENIA, TYPE II.**

     It is important to distinguish non-immune, early onset type 1 HIT from the more severe delayed onset, immune-mediated type II HIT. While patients who experience type I HIT can receive heparin again at a later time, patients with type II cannot.
     QCCP2, **HIT,** p 342

53. E. **A, B, C.**

     While the assay for anti-PF4 antibody is the most commonly performed confirmatory test, it is less specific than either the gold standard serotonin release assay or the heparin-induced platelet aggregation assay.
     QCCP2, **HIT,** p 343

54. B. **LACTATE DEHYDROGENASE.**

     LDH tends to be very high in TTP. Its levels provide a marker for tracking the course of the disease as well as the response to therapy.
     QCCP2, **TTP,** p 343

55. D. **LIVER FAILURE.**

     The classic pentad of symptoms for TTP can be remembered with the insensitive "FAT RN" mnemonic - Fever, Anemia, Thrombocytopenia, Renal Failure, Neurological symptoms. Clinically, TTP can overlap with HUS except for neurological changes, which are fairly specific for TTP.
     QCCP2, **TTP,** p 343

56. E. **DAILY PLASMA EXCHANGE.**

     Replacement of the patient's plasma which is deficient in ADAMTS-13 with ADAMTS-13-replete plasma has drastically improved the former 90% mortality associated with TTP. Plasma exchange has not been effective in the treatment of HUS, although the clinical pictures often that overlap the etiologies are distinctly different.
     QCCP2, **TTP,** p 343

5: Coagulation and Thrombosis Answers

57. B. **WISKOTT-ALDRICH SYNDROME.**

     Wiskott-Aldrich, along with thrombocytopenia with absent radii, and congenital amegakaryocytic thrombocytopenia all present with thrombocytopenia and small platelets. Sebastian syndrome is a member of a family of diseases of which the May-Hegglin anomaly is the prototype.
     QCCP2, **Inherited thrombocytopenias, T5.8,** p 344

58. A. **<1%.**

     For spontaneous bleeding to occur, there must be a severe deficiency of Factor VIII. Even small amounts of Factor VIII are protective - patients with Factor VIII levels of 5-10% will only present with excessive bleeding following trauma or surgery. The PTT is relatively insensitive in detecting Factor VIII deficiency, demonstrating normal values until there is less than 30% Factor VIII.
     QCCP2, **Hemophilia A,** p 345

59. C. **AN INVERSION MUTATION.**

     While numerous different mutations have been described as causing hemophilia A, almost half of the cases are due to an inversion of intron 22 in the Factor VIII gene.
     QCCP2, **Hemophilia A,** p 345

60. C. **10-25%.**

     While the majority of patients who receive Factor VIII do not make antibodies to Factor VIII, a significant proportion do. This is important because these patients may be refractory to therapy. Spontaneous anti-Factor VIII antibodies have been reported in non-hemophiliacs, usually with a provoking condition, such as malignancy, autoimmune disease, or post-partum status.
     QCCP2, **Hemophilia A,** p 346

61. B. **THERE IS LESS THAN 50% RECOVERY OF FACTOR IX DUE TO DISTRIBUTION INTO INTRA- AND EXTRAVASCULAR SPACE.**

     The half-life of Factors VIII and IX are fairly similar - 12 hrs and 8 hrs, respectively. DDAVP can be used to treat mild hemophilia A and works in a similar fashion as when it is used to treat type 1 vWD - stimulation of endothelial cells to spill the contents of Weibel-Palade bodies. Factor IX is distributed in both the intravascular and extravascular space, which accounts for its less than optimal response to therapy.
     QCCP2, **Hemophilia B,** p 346

62. D. **FACTOR VII.**

     Factor VII deficiency affects both the intrinsic and extrinsic pathways. However, usually only the PT is abnormal.
     QCCP2, **Factor VII deficiency,** p 347

63. D. **FACTOR X.**

     The direct activation of Factor X by dilute Russell viper venom is one assay used to determine whether a prolonged PTT is due to heparin. Factor X activates thrombin so a deficiency of Factor X will present with prolonged PT, PTT, DRVVT, and thrombin time.
     QCCP2, **Factor X deficiency,** p 347

5: Coagulation and Thrombosis Answers

64.   B.   **DELAYED BLEEDING TENDENCY.**

Factor XIII deficiency causes a mild bleeding disorder where patients initially clot but later start to bleed. This makes sense in respect to the role of Factor XIII in the stabilization of the formed clot.
QCCP2, **Factor XIII deficiency,** p 347

65.   B.   **FACTOR V AND FACTOR VIII.**

The combined deficiency of both Factor V and Factor VIII is due to a mutation in an endoplasmic reticulum transport protein, resulting in ineffectual transport of the factors.
QCCP2, **Inherited combined factor deficiency,** p 348

66.   A.   **CIRRHOSIS.**

Similar to alpha-1 antitrypsin deficiency, patients with defects in transportation of fibrinogen often develop cirrhosis.
QCCP2, **Fibrinogen,** p 348

67.   E.   **FACTOR X.**

Amyloid fibrils in the vasculature can selectively adsorb Factor X, leading to an acquired Factor X deficiency. It presents with a prolonged PT and PTT that corrects with mixing studies.
QCCP2, **Acquired factor deficiencies,** p 348

68.   B.   **PROTEIN C.**

Remember that, in addition to a number of pro-coagulation factors, the vitamin K-dependent factors include Protein C and Protein S. The half-life of Factor VII is 2-5 hours, Protein C is approximately twice as long lived with a half-life of 6-8 hours. Protein C deficiency can lead to isolated skin necrosis when the patient is treated with warfarin.
QCCP2, **Acquired factor deficiency,** p 349

69.   A.   **PT.**

The most sensitive tests for DIC include D-dimers and PF1+2.   The PT and PTT are relatively insensitive and often are normal, even in the face of widespread microclot formation.
QCCP2, **DIC,** p 349

70.   D.   **MYOCARDIAL INFARCTION IN A YOUNG PERSON.**

While arterial thromboses can occur in almost any artery, including cerebral, mesenteric, or carotids, the most commonly affected are the coronary arteries, with patients often as young as in their thirties presenting with acute myocardial infarction.
QCCP2, **Thrombophilia,** p 350

71.   D.   **A & B.**

Anti-cardiolipin antibody and the antiphospholipid syndrome as well as the mutation of prothrombin can cause both arterial and venous thrombosis. Deficiency of antithrombin tends to present with isolated venous thrombosis only.
QCCP2, **T5.10, Thrombophilia,** p 350

5: Coagulation and Thrombosis Answers

72.   C.   FACTOR V LEIDEN.

Activated Protein C resistance is almost always due to a mutation in Factor V that prevents Protein C-dependent cleavage and inhibition of Factor V. This is the so-called Factor V Leiden mutation due to a K506Q substitution. The second most common inherited thrombophilia is due to prothrombin G20210A mutation.
QCCP2, **Activated Protein C resistance,** p 350

73.   B.   FACTOR V LEIDEN.

While overall, prothrombin G20210A mutation is seen most commonly in people of European ancestry (~1-2%), it is seen in up to 10% of people with Factor V Leiden.
QCCP2, **Prothrombin variant,** p 351

74.   B.   ANTITHROMBIN DEFICIENCY.

Antithrombin deficiency most often presents this way and can be treated in counterintuitive fashion by administering fresh frozen plasma to the patient with thromboses. Plasma contains antithrombin in addition to all the requisite clotting and patients subsequently respond to heparin. It is also possible to use antithrombin concentrate to treat antithrombin deficiency.
QCCP2, **Antithrombin deficiency,** p 352

75.   D.   A & B.

Factors V and VIII are unique among coagulation factors in that they are specifically inhibited by Protein C and they are not serine proteases, but rather cofactors for activation of other factors.
QCCP2, **Protein C and S deficiency,** p 352

76.   C.   PURPURA FULMINANS.

Purpura fulminans is a very severe intravascular coagulopathy with a significant risk for poor outcomes unless rapidly treated with plasma and heparin.
QCCP2, **Protein C deficiency,** p 352

77.   B.   METHIONINE.

Hyperhomocysteinemia is an increased level of homocysteine (as detected by HPLC on serum samples) in the blood. It is an independent risk factor for atherosclerosis and thrombosis. Mutations in two enzymes have been implicated in causing the disease - cystathionine-beta-synthase and methylenetetrahydrofolate reductase.
QCCP2, **MHTFR gene mutation and hyperhomocysteinemia,** p 353

78.   B.   FACTOR XII.

Hageman Factor (XII) is involved in the initiation of the intrinsic (contact-dependent) pathway of coagulation. Contact with glass can correct the PTT as can a 1:1 mixing study. After a 10-minute incubation however, the PTT can start to become prolonged again.
QCCP2, **Elevated PAI-1 Activity,** p 353

5: Coagulation and Thrombosis Answers

79.   A.   **ARTERIAL THROMBOSIS.**

Arterial thrombosis is usually not seen with lupus anticoagulant, but rather is seen in anti-cardiolipin cases. There are a number of other dissimilarities. Lupus anticoagulant responds to warfarin, and is not associated with livedo reticularis, unlike anti-cardiolipin.
QCCP2, **T5.11 - Anti-cardiolipin antibody v. lupus anticoagulant,** p 354

80.   B.   **PRIMARY PULMONARY HYPERTENSION.**

A substantial proportion of PPH cases (10%) are in patients with coexistent anti-phospholipid antibodies, which may actually directly cause the hypertension and characteristic histological features of the disease.
QCCP2, **Antiphospholipid syndrome,** p 355

81.   A.   **PLATELET MEMBRANE PHOSPHOLIPIDS.**

The platelet neutralization procedure is used as a diagnostic modality for lupus. The phospholipids of the platelets are not inhibited by lupus anticoagulant and, when added to patient serum, will correct a prolonged PTT due to lupus anticoagulant.
QCCP2, **Lupus anticoagulant,** p 355

82.   D.   **STICKY PLATELET SYNDROME.**

Sticky platelet syndrome is a poorly understood autosomal dominant disorder where an individuals present at a young age with vaso-occlusive events such as CVA, MI, and venous thromboses usually precipitated by stress.
QCCP2, **Sticky platelet syndrome,** p 355

83.   E.   **A, B, C.**

Myeloproliferative causes of thrombocytosis, such as chronic myelogenous leukemia and essential thrombocytosis, tend not to perturb C-reactive protein or the erythrocyte sedimentation rate, while iron-deficiency anemia has been shown to cause a reactive secondary thrombocytosis. Additional studies such as the leukocyte alkaline phosphatase (LAP) score and examination of a bone marrow biopsy may help distinguish reactive from neoplastic thrombocytosis.
QCCP2, **Reactive thrombocytosis,** p 356

84.   B.   **INFECTION.**

Thrombocytosis is an acute phase reaction, which in children is most commonly due to infection. Kawasaki disease is an important cause of thrombocytosis in the East, while in the West, malignancy causes a sizable portion of cases of thrombocytosis.
QCCP2, **Reactive thrombocytosis,** p 356

85.   E.   **90%.**

Very high platelet counts are strongly associated with myeloproliferative causes. As the platelet count drops so does the correlation, but not much. At a platelet count of 600,000/dL, there is still a 70% chance that it is due to a myeloproliferative condition.
QCCP2, **Myeloproliferative disorders,** p 356

5: Coagulation and Thrombosis Answers

86.   **B.**   CHOLESTYRAMINE.

The agents that enhance the function of warfarin do so by interfering with the hepatic metabolism, effectively prolonging the half-life of the drug. Drugs like cholestyramine, which binds bile acids, prevent the absorption of warfarin and decrease the drug concentration.

QCCP2, **Coumadin,** p 356

87.   **C.**   HEPARIN.

Warfarin skin necrosis is a noted risk of treating a patient with Protein C deficiency with warfarin. This hypercoagulable state is due to warfarin inhibiting Protein C (a vitamin K-dependent factor) when there are already suboptimal levels of the factor to start with. Heparin prevents this hypercoagulable state by inhibiting Factors V and VIII.

QCCP2, **Coumadin,** p 356

88.   **C.**   1 WEEK.

At least 4 days, if not a week prior to surgery, coumadin should be stopped and heparin started. Heparin has a much shorter half-life and can be stopped the night before the surgery. Emergent reversal of coumadin usually starts with parenteral vitamin K, then plasma as needed. Reversal of heparin can be achieved with protamine.

QCCP2, **Coumadin,** p 357

Chapter 6

Immunology and Autoimmunity

1. All of the following are derived from myeloid stem cells, <u>except</u>:
   A. NK cells
   B. histiocytes
   C. monocytes
   D. eosinophils
   E. dendritic cells

2. What type of immunoglobulin receptor do mast cells express?
   A. Fc alpha
   B. Fc beta
   C. Fc gamma
   D. Fc delta
   E. Fc epsilon

3. Which chromosome bears the genes for the heavy chains?
   A. 2
   B. 22
   C. 14
   D. 16
   E. it depends on which heavy chain you are talking about

4. What is the next step in B cell development for a cell that produces a self-reactive immunoglobulin?
   A. the heavy chain undergoes class-switching
   B. the light chain redoes VDJ recombination
   C. only the variable portion of the light chain is removed
   D. the variable portion undergoes somatic hypermutation to change its specificity
   E. the cell undergoes apoptosis and dies

5. Which of the following stages is the <u>last</u> in B cell development to express CD34 and TdT?
   A. lymphoid stem cell
   B. pro-B-cell
   C. pre-B-cell
   D. B cell
   E. plasma cell

6. Which of the following is required for isotype switching?
   A. antigen stimulation
   B. Th stimulation
   C. migration from bone marrow to spleen
   D. A & B
   E. A, B, C

7. Which of the following antibodies activates complement through the alternative pathway?
    A. IgG
    B. IgA
    C. IgM
    D. IgD
    E. IgE

8. What additional signal is required for T cells to bind to antigen-presenting cells through the T cell receptor?
    A. CD44
    B. CD16
    C. MHC
    D. IgE
    E. complement C3

9. T cell receptor is presented on the T cell surface bound in a noncovalent fashion to this marker:
    A. CD2
    B. CD3
    C. CD5
    D. CD4
    E. CD8

10. Which of the following markers acts as the NK cell receptor for the constant region of the IgG heavy chain?
    A. CD16
    B. CD56
    C. CD57
    D. CD68
    E. CD1a

11. Which of the following antigen-presenting cells express S100 and CD1a?
    A. Langerhans cell
    B. interdigitating reticulum cell of the interfollicular portion of lymph nodes
    C. monocyte-macrophage
    D. A & B
    E. A, B, C

12. What cytokine secreted by T lymphocytes stimulates eosinophilic development?
    A. IL-1
    B. TNF alpha
    C. IFN gamma
    D. IL-5
    E. IL-6

13. Which of the following complement proteins is an opsonin, promoting opsonization through binding cells?
    A. C1a
    B. C3b
    C. C3a
    D. C5a
    E. C9

6: Immunology and Autoimmunity Questions

14. At what point do the classical and alternative pathways of complement activation coalesce?
     A.   the association of C4 with C2
     B.   the conversion of C3 to C3a and C3b
     C.   the association of C4b2b with C3b
     D.   the conversion of C5 to C5a and C5b
     E.   they are completely separate at all times

15. Which of the following byproducts of complement activation function as anaphylatoxins increasing vascular permeability?
     A.   C5a
     B.   C3a
     C.   C2a
     D.   A & B
     E.   A, B, C

16. What chromosome is home to the major histocompatibility complex?
     A.   3
     B.   6
     C.   11
     D.   13
     E.   17

17. What is the chance that two siblings are of identical HLA haplotypes?
     A.   0%
     B.   25%
     C.   50%
     D.   75%
     E.   100%

18. Which of the following infections is suggestive of a terminal complement deficiency?
     A.   mucocutaneous candidiasis
     B.   recurrent encapsulated organism infections
     C.   staphylococcal infections
     D.   recurrent bacterial upper respiratory infections
     E.   persistent *Giardia* infection

19. Which of the following is the preferred methodology for assessing HLA haploptype?
     A.   microlymphocytotoxicity assay
     B.   mixed lymphocyte culture assay
     C.   direct PCR DNA testing
     D.   serology panel antibody detection
     E.   direct antibody screening with control antibodies

20. How many HLA loci are usually matched for transplantation?
     A.   one
     B.   two
     C.   three
     D.   four
     E.   five

6: Immunology and Autoimmunity Questions

21. What does a poor response to *S. pneumoniae* vaccination potentially indicate?
     A.   B cell defect
     B.   T cell defect
     C.   B or T cell defect
     D.   B and T cell defect
     E.   complement deficiency

22. What is the most common specific antibody deficiency?
     A.   IgA
     B.   IgD
     C.   IgE
     D.   IgG
     E.   IgM

23. Which of the following scenarios is the most appropriate use of RAST testing?
     A.   screening for allergens, especially inhaled ones
     B.   identifying a specific allergen, especially an inhaled one
     C.   confirmation of hereditary angioedema
     D.   confirmation of chronic urticaria
     E.   diagnosis of systemic mastocytosis

24. All of the following modalities are examples of tests of T cell function, <u>except</u>:
     A.   delayed-type hypersensitivity skin testing
     B.   enumeration from peripheral blood smear
     C.   flow cytometric CD3+ analysis
     D.   nitroblue tetrazolium assay
     E.   phytohemagglutinin proliferation assay

25. All of the following flow cytometric marker patterns are associated with NK cells, <u>except</u>:
     A.   CD3-
     B.   CD4+
     C.   CD16+
     D.   CD56+
     E.   CD57+

26. What is the expected nitroblue tetrazolium assay reaction in patients with chronic granulomatous disease?
     A.   red color (non-reactive)
     B.   <10% f-
     C.   <10% f+
     D.   >50% purple
     E.   <10% yellow

27. Which complement factor levels are assayed for defects in the alternate pathway of activation?
     A.   C1q
     B.   C3
     C.   C4
     D.   C5
     E.   C9

6: Immunology and Autoimmunity Questions

28. All of the following are associated with B-cell defects, <u>except</u>:
    A. recurrent bacterial sinopulmonary infections
    B. resistant *Giardia* infections
    C. presentation after 6 months of age
    D. recurrent staph and strep infections
    E. opportunistic viral infections

29. What is the most common presentation of Bruton X-linked agammaglobulinemia?
    A. recurrent pneumonia in middle-aged women
    B. persistent sepsis in elderly men
    C. resistant upper respiratory tract infections in adolescents
    D. meningitis in a neonate
    E. chronic diarrhea in a young boy

30. What is the most commonly inherited immunodeficiency?
    A. Bruton X-linked agammaglobulinemia
    B. common variable immunodeficiency
    C. selective IgA deficiency
    D. Job syndrome
    E. severe combined immunodeficiency

31. All of the following are associated with diGeorge syndrome, <u>except</u>:
    A. autosomal recessive inheritance pattern
    B. defective T cell function
    C. hypocalcemia
    D. deletion of chromosome 22q11.2
    E. depletion of lymph node paracortical areas

32. What is the <u>most</u> <u>frequent</u> cause of severe combined immunodeficiency?
    A. autosomal recessive Jak3 deficiency
    B. autosomal recessive defect in adenosine deaminase
    C. autosomal recessive purine nucleosidase phosphorylase deficiency
    D. X-linked recessive defect in IL-2 receptor
    E. autosomal recessive CD3 deficiency

33. The presenting symptoms/signs of Wiskott-Aldrich syndrome include all of the following, <u>except</u>:
    A. microcytic anemia
    B. eczema
    C. small, uniform platelets
    D. thrombocytopenia
    E. immunodeficiency

34. Which of the following disorders is characterized by cerebellar ataxia, telangiectasias, and recurrent infections?
    A. Duncan disease
    B. ataxia telangiectasia
    C. chronic granulomatous disease
    D. Bruton agammaglobulinemia
    E. chronic mucocutaneous candidiasis

6: Immunology and Autoimmunity Questions

35. Duncan disease usually presents as a severe hemophagocytic response to this virus:
    A. HIV
    B. HHV8
    C. HHV6
    D. HTLV-I
    E. EBV

36. Which of the following is a suitable screening test for chronic granulomatous disease?
    A. nitroblue tetrazolium test
    B. NAD-coupled oxidation
    C. catalase-positive bacterial provocative infection
    D. sweat chloride test
    E. Benedict's reagent assay

37. Which of the following treatments can clear the Dohle bodies seen in May-Hegglin anomaly?
    A. DNase
    B. RNase
    C. iron chelation
    D. calcium phosphate precipitation
    E. sodium dithionate treatment

38. Which of the following is/are associated with homozygous Pelger-Huet anomaly?
    A. Dohle bodies
    B. pince-nez cells
    C. Jordan anomaly
    D. Stodtmeister cells
    E. giant platelets

39. What type of disorder usually follows defects in components of the classical pathway of complement activation?
    A. recurrent gram-positive infections
    B. hereditary angioedema
    C. hematolymphoid neoplasms
    D. autoimmune disease
    E. recurrent systemic encapsulated organism infections

40. Which of the following cell types is used most commonly to screen for antinuclear antibody pattern staining?
    A. Vero E6
    B. Hep-2
    C. HeLa
    D. human diploid fibroblasts
    E. primary monkey kidney

41. Which of the following staining patterns is most consistent with CREST syndrome?
    A. speckled with mitoses
    B. nucleolar with mitoses
    C. cytoplasmic
    D. centromeric with mitoses
    E. homogeneous with mitoses

42. What is the use of the microorganism *Crithidia luciliae* in the screening of antibodies?
    A. it is a positive source of many antibodies
    B. it contains giant mitochondria that stain with anti-dsDNA antibodies
    C. it is used to produce recombinant proteins that are used as antigens in many tests
    D. it effectively blocks interfering antibodies
    E. used in the "*Crithidia* interference assay" to selectively identify most autoantibodies

43. What is the effect of age on the detection of anti-nuclear antibody?
    A. decreased false positive rate
    B. increased false positive rate
    C. decreased false negative rate
    D. increased false negative rate
    E. no change in the rate of detection

44. Increases in the titer of which of the following antibodies can be used to predict lupus flares?
    A. anti-histone
    B. anti-Smith
    C. anti-SSA
    D. anti-dsDNA
    E. anti-RNP

45. All of the following conditions are associated with anti-mitochondrial antibodies, except:
    A. primary biliary cirrhosis
    B. syphilis
    C. ulcerative colitis
    D. collagen vascular disease
    E. cardiomyopathy

46. What antigen is c-ANCA responsive to?
    A. proteinase 3
    B. lipoprotein lipase
    C. myeloperoxidase
    D. gluteraldehyde dehydrogenase
    E. pyruvate kinase

47. How is a "lupus erythematosus" cell defined?
    A. a phagocytic cell with an engulfed denatured nucleus
    B. a dessicated cell surrounded by a wreath of T-cells
    C. a binucleate giant cell with a prominent nucleolus
    D. a ghost cell after incubation with patient serum
    E. an opsonized clumped red blood cell in the peripheral smear

48. What feature do all conditions associated with increased angiotensin-converting enzyme have in common?
    A. all form granulomas
    B. all are in the kidney
    C. all present with cholestasis
    D. all affect the seminiferous tubules
    E. all have a characteristic very high white blood cell count

6: Immunology and Autoimmunity Questions

49. All of the following are associated with HLA-DR3, except:
    A. insulin-dependent diabetes mellitus
    B. ankylosing spondylitis
    C. systemic lupus erythematosus
    D. myasthenia gravis
    E. celiac sprue

50. Which of the following drugs is/are associated with drug-induced lupus?
    A. hydralazine
    B. procainamide
    C. isoniazid
    D. A & B
    E. A, B, C

51. What type of hypersensitivity is responsible for a positive reaction to a tuberculin skin test?
    A. Type I
    B. Type II
    C. Type III
    D. Type IV
    E. Type V

52. All of the following are associated with celiac sprue, except:
    A. unexplained short stature and iron-deficiency anemia
    B. HLA-DQ2/8
    C. IgA deficiency
    D. dermatitis herpetiformis
    E. increased intraepithelial neutrophils in the duodenum

53. All of the following are useful in the diagnosis of autoimmune thyroiditis, except:
    A. anti-microsomal antibodies
    B. TSH receptor antibodies
    C. anti-thyroglobulin antibodies
    D. thyroglobulin levels
    E. long-acting thyroid stimulating antibodies

54. What's the most specific serum assay for the diagnosis of lymphoplasmacytic sclerosing pancreatitis?
    A. carbonic anhydrase antibodies
    B. IgG4 levels
    C. anti-smooth muscle antibodies
    D. angiotensin-converting enzyme levels
    E. anti-liver/kidney microsomal antibody

55. All of the following antibodies have been associated with autoimmune hepatitis, except:
    A. ANA
    B. anti-SLA/LP
    C. anti-smooth muscle antibody
    D. c-ANCA
    E. anti-LKM1

6: Immunology and Autoimmunity Questions

56. What is the gold standard of diagnosis for giant cell arteritis?
     A.   confirmation of concurrent polymyalgia rheumatica
     B.   temporal artery biopsy
     C.   increased serum anti-CRP antibody
     D.   aortic biopsy
     E.   increased erythrocyte sedimentation rate

57. Which of the following antibodies is associated with poor prognosis, myositis, high frequency of cardiac manifestations, and HLA-DR5?
     A.   anti-titin
     B.   anti-SRP
     C.   anti-Mi-2
     D.   anti-SS-A
     E.   anti-MuSK

58. Which of the following antibodies is most associated with the majority of types of myasthenia gravis?
     A.   anti-AChR
     B.   anti-MuSk
     C.   anti-titin
     D.   anti-synaptophysin
     E.   anti-cholinesterase

59. Which of the following assays best reflects mast cell degranulation?
     A.   serum total tryptase
     B.   serum mature tryptase
     C.   serum histamine
     D.   urinary histamine
     E.   urinary HIAA

6: Immunology and Autoimmunity Answers

1.   A.   **NK CELLS.**

Lymphocytes, including B, T, and NK cells, are all derived from a common lymphoid stem cell. Cells of the reticuloendothelial system, such as macrophages, histiocytes, and dendritic cells, as well as the granulocytes, monocytes, megakaryocytes, and erythrocytes, are all derived from myeloid precursors.
QCCP2, **Immune system components,** p 364

2.   E.   **FC EPSILON.**

Mast cells are capable of binding IgE through the Fc epsilon receptor.
QCCP2, **B cells,** p 364

3.   C.   **14.**

The genes for mu, gamma, alpha, delta, and epsilon are all on the same chromosome. This is important for the mechanism of class-type switching.
QCCP2, **B cells,** p 364

4.   E.   **THE CELL UNDERGOES APOPTOSIS AND DIES.**

Part of the high level of variety that is generated through the development of B cells is a subset of cells that produce self-reacting immunoglobulins. Alas, a cell that produces a self-reacting immunoglobulin is scheduled to undergo apoptosis and die.
QCCP2, **B cells,** p 364

5.   B.   **PRO B-CELL.**

In the development of a pro-B-cell to a pre-B-cell, the immature markers CD34 and TdT are lost. The equivalent in the T cell is the transition from prothymocyte to mature thymocyte. Note that there is an intermediate stage of T-cell development, the immature thymocyte that still expresses TdT, but not CD34.
QCCP2, **B and T cell maturation sequences, T6.1,** p 364

6.   D.   **A & B.**

Isotype switching, the process whereby the IgM immunoglobulin originally produced is able to become IgG, IgA, or another subclass, requires both the surface IgM to bind to its cognate epitope as well as stimulation by helper T cells. There is no mass migration of isotype-switched B cells from the marrow to the spleen. That's just crazy.
QCCP2, **B cells,** p 365

7.   B.   **IGA.**

There are only three isotypes of immunoglobulin capable of activating complement: IgG, IgA, and IgM. Of these three, only IgA activates complement through the alternative, rather than the classical pathway of complement activation. Of note are that there are subclasses of several immunoglobulins and that IgG3 is unable to activate complement.
QCCP2, **B cells, T6.2,** p 365

6: Immunology and Autoimmunity Answers

8.   C.   **MHC.**

While immunoglobulin both soluble and on the surface of the B cell is able to recognize antigenic isotopes on presenting cells, the T cell receptor requires the antigens to be present complexed to either Class I MHC, which is expressed on almost all nucleated cells in the case of CD8+ T cells, or Class II MHC, which is present on dedicated antigen presenting cells and is recognized by CD4+ T cells.

QCCP2, **T cells,** p 365

9.   B.   **CD3.**

As a member of the signaling complex with the T-cell receptor, CD3 helps transmit the activating signal when the TCR binds a MHC-bound antigen.

QCCP2, **T cells,** p 366

10.   A.   **CD16.**

Antigen-dependent cellular cytotoxicity (ADCC) works through the CD16 binding of IgG constant regions for immunoglobulin-coated opsonized cells. This accounts for one of the primary means that NK cells facilitate the removal of virus-infected and tumor cells.

QCCP2, **NK cells,** p 366

11.   D.   **A & B.**

When CD1a positivity is discussed, often Langerhans cells are considered alone in the differential diagnosis. But it is important to note (especially in the case of some neoplasms) that CD1a is not a specific marker for Langerhans cells. In fact, almost all "professional" antigen-presenting cells including Kuppfer cells in the liver, Hoffbauer cells in the placenta, and the dendritic reticulum cell found in lymph node germinal centers can all be CD1a (+).

QCCP2, **NK cells,** p 366

12.   D.   **IL-5.**

T_H2 cells secrete IL-4 to stimulate the production of IgE and IL-5 to stimulate eosinophils, especially in response to parasite infection.

QCCP2, **Granulocytes,** p 366

13.   B.   **C3b.**

Both C3b and Ig act as opsonins, coating cells and targeting their destruction through several means, including through antigen-dependent cellular cytotoxicity (ADCC) pathway (IgG) or through direct lysis by the membrane attack complex of complement proteins (C3b).

QCCP2, **Complement C3b,** p 366

14.   D.   **THE CONVERSION OF C5 TO C5A AND C5B.**

The alternate and classical pathways of complement activation use different means and factors to achieve the same goal - the creation of a C5 convertase, which is the driving force behind the formation of the C5-C9 membrane attack complex. Some memorable complement factoids: The classical pathway most often is activated by IgG (with the notable exception of IgG4). The alternate pathway is most often directly activated. The alternate pathway relies on low levels of C3 convertase activity to make a C3 convertase of its own, whereas the classical pathway makes a C3 convertase *de novo.*

QCCP2, **Complement,** p 367

6: Immunology and Autoimmunity Answers

15.   D.   **A & B.**

Some of the products of the complement cascade perform functions outside of their role in creating the membrane attack complex. C3b is an opsonin like IgG and both C2a and C5a function as anaphylatoxins.
QCCP2, **Complement,** p 367

16.   B.   **6.**

MHC Classes I, II, and III are all located on the short arm of chromosome 6. Class I encodes receptors found on almost all nucleated cells. Class II encodes receptors found on antigen-presenting cells. Class III encodes a hodge-podge of important and varied proteins, such as 21-hydroxylase, HFE, and TNF-alpha.
QCCP2, **HLA,** p 367

17.   B.   **25%.**

The MHC genes are extremely polymorphic, composed of numerous alleles. It is important to remember that despite the size of the complex, there is very rare crossing over and recombination and therefore the entire region is inherited as a haplotype (barring sporadic mutation). Given that it is simply a matter of independent assortment, with each sibling having a 50% chance of getting one haplotype each from their mother and father, multiply the chances together to get 25%.
QCCP2, **HLA,** p 368

18.   B.   RECURRENT ENCAPSULATED ORGANISM INFECTIONS.

Each of the presented choices is suggestive of a particular deficiency. Mucocutaneous candidiasis suggests defective T cells, Staph infections suggest a possible problem with phagocytes, bacterial URIs and giardiasis - a B cell failure.
QCCP2, **Lab tests of immune function,** p 368

19.   C.   DIRECT PCR DNA TESTING.

Nowadays, many of the laborious assays previously utilized to determine HLA haplotypes, such as the options presented in choices A and B, have been replaced by DNA-based assays, such as PCR. Direct DNA analysis is faster, easier, and more precise, allowing for determination of split antigens and other antigens that were not detected by old techniques.
QCCP2, **Lab tests of immune function, screening tests,** p 368

20.   C.   THREE.

Of course the more the better, but for major antigens a 3 locus (HLA-A, HLA-B, and HLA-DR) match is considered good. In addition *in vitro* crossmatch is still required because DNA testing does not address antibodies or minor HLA antigens, which could appear to match, but still be incompatible.
QCCP2, **Lab tests of immune function, screening tests,** p 369

21.   A.   B CELL DEFECT.

Encapsulated organisms, such as *S. pneumoniae* and *N. meningitidis* with carbohydrate capsule antigens are opsonized and cleared through the spleen. Therefore, poor response to pneumococcal vaccine is a fairly specific assay for B cell defects.
QCCP2, **Testing B cell function,** p 369

6: Immunology and Autoimmunity Answers

22.   A.   IgA.

Overall, IgA deficiency is the most common. IgG deficiency can be hidden if only a selected subtype is affected.
QCCP2, **Testing B cell function,** p 369

23.   B.   IDENTIFYING A SPECIFIC ANTIGEN, ESPECIALLY AN INHALED ONE.

In order to perform RAST testing, patient serum is added to a specific antigen pre-complexed with solid phase to which radiolabeled anti-IgE is added. If patient serum has an antigen-specific IgE, then the result would be positive. Since specific antigens are required, it is a poor screening test. The last three choices offered are all independent of IgE, so RAST testing would not be helpful.
QCCP2, **Testing B cell function,** p 369

24.   D.   NITROBLUE TETRAZOLIUM ASSAY.

The NBT test provides an assessment of oxidative burst, a function of macrophages and neutrophils. The rest of the tests all provide some indication of T cell number or function. Remember that 3/4 of circulating lymphocytes are usually T cells, so that a peripheral smear usually gives a rough indication of T cell number.
QCCP2, **Testing T cell function,** p 370

25.   B.   CD4+.

NK cells in their function as mediating cellular immunity do not express CD4, a marker more associated with helper T cells, which modulate B cell and humoral immunity.
QCCP2, **Testing NK cell function,** p 370

26.   C.   <10% F+.

The NBT test of oxidative burst assays the catalysis from a yellow color to a purple/blue. A positive test is therefore purple, a pattern referred to as f+ (formazan precipitate positive). Normal neutrophils will be nearly all positive. In chronic granulomatous disease, usually there is less than 10% positivity.
QCCP2, **Testing neutrophil function,** p 370

27.   B.   C3.

Low level C3 activation is required in order to kick off the alternate pathway in direct response to lipopolysaccharide. For that reason, it is a sensitive, though non-specific, marker for defects in the alternate pathway. An overall screening assay is CH50, which is a functional assay.
QCCP2, **Testing complement,** p 370

28.   E.   OPPORTUNISTIC VIRAL INFECTION.

For the most part, viral and fungal infections are dealt with by cellular immunity and T cells. B cell deficiencies usually present after a few months due to the protection afforded by maternal IgG. Opportunistic recurrent infections with encapsulated bacterial organisms tend to be a major problem.
QCCP2, **Immunodeficiency, B cell defects,** p 370

6: Immunology and Autoimmunity Answers

29. E. **CHRONIC DIARRHEA IN A YOUNG BOY.**

Most often, GI disease with *Giardia* is the earliest presentation of Bruton agammaglobulinemia. The characteristic histological finding on GI biopsy is the lack of plasma cells in the interstitium of the mucosa.
QCCP2, **Bruton X-linked agammaglobulinemia,** p 371

30. C. **SELECTIVE IgA DEFICIENCY.**

There is a very high prevalence (1/700) of IgA deficiency that usually presents with recurrent respiratory and gastrointestinal infections. Patients with IgA deficiency can develop an anti-IgA antibody, which can cause anaphylactic reactions when exposed to IgA-containing products. An important blood bank pearl for IgA deficiency is that patients should get washed products (to remove the IgA against which they could react) or IgA-deficient products.
QCCP2, **Selective IgA deficiency,** p 371

31. A. **AUTOSOMAL RECESSIVE INHERITANCE PATTERN.**

Velocardiofacial, or diGeorge syndrome, is due to third and fourth pharyngeal pouch fusion and presents with neck, heart, and facial dysfunction/dysmorphia. Because of the neck issues, both the thymus and parathyroids are hypoplastic, leading clinically to T cell defects and hypocalcemia, respectively. The syndrome is due to a sporadic rather than inherited deletion of chromosome 22q11.2.
QCCP2, **T cell defects,** p 371

32. D. **X-LINKED RECESSIVE DEFECT IN IL-2 RECEPTOR.**

All of the choices presented are causes of SCID. However, the defects in the X-linked gene, IL-2 receptor, account for the majority of cases with ADA deficiency a close second. All lead to severe defects in both humoral (B cell) and cellular (T cell) responses.
QCCP2, **SCID,** p 371-372

33. A. **MICROCYTIC ANEMIA.**

The X-linked disorder, Wiskott-Aldrich syndrome (WAS), is characterized by all of the signs and symptoms presented in the question, with the exception of anemia. The WAS gene product, WASP, has been implicated in the disorder. WAS is also one of the causes of platelet dense granule deficiency and bleeding.
QCCP2, **Wiskott-Aldrich syndrome,** p 372

34. B. **ATAXIA TELANGIECTASIA.**

Sometimes the obvious answer is correct! A defect in the DNA mismatch repair gene, ATM leads to a combined T cell and B cell disorder with ataxia and vascular telangiectasias. Since the defect in humoral immunity is primarily IgA, there is usually a history of sinopulmonary infections. There is also a very high (~40%) risk of malignancy, especially hematolymphoid.
QCCP2, **ATM,** p 372

35. E. **EBV.**

There are several less severe prodromal signs associated with Duncan disease, but it is the intense response to EBV that defines the disorder. In addition, there are usually subsequent B cell lymphoid malignancies and hepatic failure.
QCCP2, **Duncan disease,** p 372

36. A. **NITROBLUE TETRAZOLIUM TEST.**

Chronic granulomatous disease is due to defects in oxidative burst microbial killing, secondary to a defect in NADPH oxidase. As a result, catalase positive organisms tend to cause severe granulomatous infections due to the immune system's inability to remove the organisms. Nitroblue tetrazolium is a direct assay of the respiratory burst (see question 26 for more).
QCCP2, **Chronic granulomatous disease,** p 372-373

37. B. **RNASE.**

Dohle bodies are large, pale blue inclusions composed of rough endoplasmic reticulum, and are seen in granulocytes and monocytes of the May-Hegglin anomaly. Treatment of cells with ribonuclease can destroy these bodies. Remember that rough endoplasmic reticulum contains numerous ribosomes, which are mostly composed of ribosomal RNA.
QCCP2, **May-Hegglin anomaly,** p 373

38. D. **STODTMEISTER CELLS.**

Heterozygous Pelger-Huet is associated with the more familiar bilobed, or pince-nez, nuclei found in segmented neutrophils. With a homozygous case of Pelger-Huet, monolobated, or Stodtmeister, cells are often seen.
QCCP2, **Pelger-Huet anomaly,** p 373

39. D. **AUTOIMMUNE DISEASE.**

The vast set of disorders associated with deficiencies of complement proteins reflects the multifaceted role of complement in the body. All of the choices presented (with the exception of hematolymphoid neoplasms) are due to defects in various complement proteins and activation pathways. Recurrent gram positive infections are seen with deficiency of C2 and C3, hereditary angioedema is due to deficiency of C1q esterase inhibitor, autoimmune disease is due to defects in the classical pathway (C1q, C2, and C4) and systemic encapsulated organism infections occur due to deficiencies of membrane attack complex (MAC) components (C5-C9).
QCCP2, **Complement deficiency,** p 373

40. B. **HEP-2.**

Diluted patient serum is added to Hep-2 cells in culture followed by detection with fluorescently-labeled anti-human globulin and a nuclear (DNA) counterstain. From this assay, the classic staining patterns are interpreted.
QCCP2, **Screening for anti-nuclear antigen with Hep-2,** p 374

41. D. **CENTROMERIC WITH MITOSES.**

There's no way around it. The staining patterns are classic, so they have to be memorized. At least c̲entromeric and C̲REST begin with the same letter. Table 6.3 provides the most common antibody/clinical presentations, including the antinuclear antibodies. It would be worthwhile to spend some time incorporating the chart into your mind!
QCCP2, **Screening for ANA with Hep-2,** p 374

42. B. **IT CONTAINS GIANT MITOCHONDRIA THAT STAIN WITH ANTI-DSDNA ANTIBODIES.**

Either the *Crithidia* test or an ELISA test can be used to screen for anti-dsDNA antibodies. Given the novelty of the *Crithidia* test, it tends to be asked about more often than the ELISA.
QCCP2, **Anti-dsDNA,** p 374

6: Immunology and Autoimmunity Answers

43. B. **INCREASED FALSE POSITIVE RATE.**

With age, there is decreased test specificity manifested as an increased false positive rate. In addition, the prevalence of autoimmune disease increases with age, which means that, for the positive predictive value of the test to increase with prevalence, the number of true positives must increase <u>more</u> than false positives, relatively....quite confusing. Bottom line - both true and false positive rates of the ANA assay increase with age, true positive a little more than false positive.
QCCP2, **ANA,** p 376

44. D. **ANTI-DSDNA.**

All of the choices are associated with lupus: histone, dsDNA, and RNP mostly with drug-induced lupus, anti-Smith with systemic lupus, and SSA both with lupus and Sjogren syndrome. Anti-RNP is also associated with mixed connective tissue disease. Of all of the antibodies, anti-dsDNA is the most sensitive to changes in lupus status, while anti-Smith is the most specific for SLE.
QCCP2, **ANA,** p 376

45. C. **ULCERATIVE COLITIS.**

There are many antigens in mitochondria against which antibodies can be raised. Different anti-mitochondrial membrane antibodies are associated with different diseases - M2 with primary biliary cirrhosis, M1 with syphilis, M5 with collagen vascular disease, M7 with cardiomyopathy. Ulcerative colitis is often seen with primary sclerosing cholangitis (more often PSC is seen with ulcerative colitis than the converse) and is associated with p-ANCA.
QCCP2, **Antibodies to cytoplasmic constituents,** p 377

46. A. **PROTEINASE 3.**

So called because of its cytoplasmic staining pattern, c-ANCA is directed against the cytoplasmic protein, c-ANCA. It is most specific for Wegener granulomatosis. p-ANCA, or perinuclear ANCA, is directed against the predominant perinuclear myeloperoxidase antigen, and is less specific than c-ANCA.
QCCP2, **ANCA,** p 377

47. A. **A PHAGOCYTIC CELL WITH AN ENGULFED DENATURED NUCLEUS.**

The LE cell assay has a high sensitivity for lupus, nearly 70%. The assay is performed by agitating tissue or body fluids in a tube and then looking for the characteristic LE cell - a phagocytic cell with an engulfed denatured nucleus.
QCCP2, **Other markers of autoimmune disease,** p 377

48. A. **ALL FORM GRANULOMAS.**

While all granulomatous diseases are not associated with increased ACE, most disorders associated with increased ACE are granulomatous in nature - sarcoidosis, leprosy, primary biliary cirrhosis, and Gaucher disease. In the case of sarcoidosis, ACE levels are useful in diagnosing a flareup of disease.
QCCP2, **ACE,** p 377-378

6: Immunology and Autoimmunity Answers

49. B.   **ANKYLOSING SPONDYLITIS.**

HLA haplotypes are more strongly associated with disease than would be expected by chance. HLA-DR3 is associated with all of the choices except ankylosing spondylitis, which is associated with HLA-B27. Several other HLA haplotypes, especially HLA-DR ones are associated with a number of other autoimmune disorders.
QCCP2, **Autoimmune disease pathophysiology,** p 378

50. E.   **A, B, C.**

All are associated with drug-induced lupus, which in turn is highly associated with anti-dsDNA and anti-histone antibodies.
QCCP2, **Autoimmune disease pathophysiology,** p 378

51. D.   **TYPE IV.**

First of all, there is no Type V. The hypersensitivity reactions can be remembered with the mnemonic "ACID." Type I is Antigen-Antibody-mediated and immediate, like in anaphylaxis. Type II is Cell-mediated when antibody binds antigen to activate cellular toxicity, like in myasthenia gravis. Type III is Immune complex-mediated when antibody-antigen-complement complexes are deposited, like in SLE. Finally, Type IV is Delayed, where antibodies bind antigen and active cellular immunity, like in a positive skin tuberculin test.
QCCP2, **Autoimmune disease pathophysiology,** p 379

52. E.   **INCREASED INTRAEPITHELIAL NEUTROPHILS IN THE DUODENUM.**

Often, the earliest histological manifestation of sprue will be increased intraepithelial lymphocytes. This change often precedes the characteristic villous blunting and crypt elongation. There are many other conditions and findings associated with sprue, including diabetes mellitus, dermatitis herpetiformis, cystic fibrosis, enteropathy-associated T cell lymphoma, arthritis, and malnutrition.
QCCP2, **Celiac sprue,** p 381

53. D.   **THYROGLOBULIN LEVELS.**

For the most part, the diagnosis of autoimmune thyroiditis depends on demonstration of some anti-thyroid antibodies, whether it's Hashimoto, which is associated with anti-thyroglobulin and anti-microsomal antibodies, or Graves, which is associated with LATS or TSH receptor antibodies.
QCCP2, **Anti-thyroid autoantibodies,** p 381

54. B.   **IgG4 LEVELS.**

The majority of cases of LPSP present with an increased serum IgG4 fraction, which is often identified by increased IgG4-expressing plasma cells within the lesion. Anti-carbonic anhydrase, though less sensitive, is also associated with LPSP.
QCCP2, **Autoimmune pancreatitis,** p 381-382

55. D.   **c-ANCA.**

Anti-smooth muscle antibody is the most commonly associated antibody with autoimmune hepatitis, but it is important to note that there are several other antibodies also commonly associated with autoimmune hepatitis. In fact, there may be several subgroups of the disease with different antibodies associated with each.
QCCP2, **Autoimmune hepatitis,** p 382

6: Immunology and Autoimmunity Answers

56.   B.   TEMPORAL ARTERY BIOPSY.

Giant cell arteritis was previously called temporal arteritis, but due to its more widespread presentation, it was renamed. However, the temporal artery is still the most commonly affected with headache, and visual changes are the most common presentation. There are often increased ESR and CRP levels, but the temporal artery biopsy is the gold standard. An aortic biopsy? Are you kidding?
QCCP2, **Giant cell arteritis**, p 382

57.   B.   ANTI-SRP.

The myositis diseases are an assortment of anti-muscle autoimmune disorders with various antibodies and presentations. In addition to being *de novo* autoimmune disorders, they are also frequently seen as paraneoplastic conditions or associated with other autoimmune disorders. The anti-SRP antibody has the worst prognosis and is most commonly associated with polymyositis.
QCCP2, **Inflammatory myopathies**, p 383

58.   A.   ANTI-AChR.

MG presents with the characteristic progressive muscle weakness/fatigue that is relieved by cholinesterase inhibitors (the basis of the Tensilon test). There are several subtypes of MG, including those cases associated with thymoma, each associated with different antibodies. The anti-AChR antibodies tend to be found in almost all types of MG with the exception of the so-called seronegative cases, which are more commonly associated with anti-MuSK antibodies.
QCCP2, **Myasthenia gravis**, p 383

59.   B.   SERUM MATURE TRYPTASE.

Both tryptase and histamine are released into the serum in cases of anaphylaxis. Histamine is less specific than tryptase and can be also seen in scombrodic fish poisoning. Both total and mature tryptase are produced by mast cells with total representing the overall amount of mast cells and mature more a reflection of mast cell degranulation.
QCCP2, **Laboratory diagnosis of anaphylaxis**, p 383

Chapter 7

Molecular Methods

1. What type of specimens can be utilized for classical cytogenetic karyotyping?
   A. fresh, viable tissue
   B. formalin-fixed unembedded tissue
   C. formalin-fixed paraffin-embedded tissue
   D. A & B
   E. A, B, C

2. Which characteristic of chromosomes is responsible for obtaining staining contrast in banded karyotyping?
   A. GC-rich areas
   B. AT-rich areas
   C. euchromatin
   D. heterochromatin
   E. A & B

3. Which of the following specimens can be utilized for molecular cytogenetic testing, such as fluorescent in situ hybridization?
   A. fresh, viable tissue
   B. frozen tissue
   C. formalin-fixed paraffin-embedded tissue
   D. all of the above
   E. none of the above, FISH requires specially-prepared tissue

4. Which of the following is NOT one of the most common types of probes used in molecular cytogenetics?
   A. allele-specific probes
   B. telomeric probes
   C. centromeric probes
   D. painting probes
   E. all are commonly used

5. Which is more sensitive, PCR or FISH?
   A. PCR
   B. FISH
   C. it depends on the assay
   D. they are equally sensitive

6. Which type of FISH translocation probe starts with a single color signal that becomes two signals with a positive test result?
   A. fusion probe
   B. chromosome enumeration probe
   C. break-apart probes
   D. allele-nonspecific probe
   E. none of the above

7: Molecular Methods Questions

7.   Which of the following is NOT a common source of artifact in FISH assays?
   A.   FISH "bait" - homologous sequence binding probes
   B.   truncation artifact - underrepresentation of chromosomal material
   C.   aneuploidy and polyploidy
   D.   autofluorescence leading to increased background signal
   E.   all of the above are common sources of artifact

8.   In addition to the following reagents - template DNA, primers, magnesium or another divalent cation, pH buffer, and heat-stable DNA polymerase - what other component must be added to a PCR reaction for amplification to occur?
   A.   denaturing agent
   B.   blocking agent
   C.   reverse transcriptase
   D.   dNTPs (nucleotide triphosphates)
   E.   restriction endonuclease

9.   What is the major disadvantage of nested PCR?
   A.   lack of suitable primers
   B.   requirement for large amounts of nucleotide precursors
   C.   use of denaturing agents
   D.   high rate of contamination
   E.   extremely slow (days to weeks) turnaround

10.   Which two processes are coupled in real-time PCR (choose two)?
   A.   PCR product subcloning
   B.   protein expression/translation
   C.   product detection
   D.   target amplification
   E.   reverse transcription

11.   To what does "multiplex" PCR refer?
   A.   a staggered array process
   B.   transcription-coupled PCR
   C.   multistep amplification using secondary primers internal to a primary set of primers
   D.   isothermal amplification of DNA
   E.   use of two or more primer sets to simultaneously amplify multiple products in a single reaction tube

12.   Which of the following detection systems is NOT an example of a target amplification technique?
   A.   branched DNA
   B.   strand displacement
   C.   multiplex PCR
   D.   nested PCR
   E.   reverse transcription (RT)-PCR

13.   Which of the following is NOT one of the advantages of PCR over Southern blot analysis?
   A.   rapid turnaround
   B.   ability to analyze small amounts of DNA
   C.   ability to simultaneously analyze multiple DNA sequences in a single assay
   D.   ability to analyze products in a single tube assay
   E.   all of the above are advantages of PCR over Southern blot

7: Molecular Methods Questions

14. Mutations of portions of chromosomes 1p and 19q are important in the diagnosis and prognosis of oligodendroglioma. The mutations are examples of which of the following phenomena?
    A. microsatellite instability
    B. loss of heterozygosity
    C. DNA methylation
    D. histone acetylation
    E. single nucleotide polymorphism

15. Which of the following nucleotides is most often methylated in silenced DNA?
    A. adenine
    B. cytosine
    C. guanine
    D. thymidine
    E. uracil

16. What criterion is used to enumerate and order chromosomes?
    A. length
    B. GC content
    C. centromere location
    D. extent of histone acetylation
    E. hetero-/euchromatin ratio

17. What is the reference point for numbering chromosome bands?
    A. telomere
    B. depends on the chromosome
    C. differs for the p arm and the q arm
    D. centromere
    E. none of the above

18. Which of the following directly results in excess complements of the 23 chromosomes such that the total number of chromosomes is divisible by 23 (eg, 69)?
    A. aneuploidy
    B. monosomy
    C. trisomy
    D. polyploidy
    E. none of the above

19. What is the best definition of an isochromosome?
    A. a chromosome with only short or long arm genetic material on either side of the centromere
    B. a chromosome that results from two breaks occurring on a single arm, leading to the loss of genetic material
    C. a chromosome that results from two breaks occurring on a single arm with inversion of genetic material
    D. an abnormal chromosome formed from portions of two or more chromosomes
    E. a chromosome that results from a break in two chromosomes where material is traded between the chromosomes involved

20. Which of the following is the best description of a Mendelian disorder?
    A. a disorder inherited solely from the maternal lineage
    B. a disorder due to a series of inherited mutations in multiple genes
    C. a disorder without a clear genetic causal relationship
    D. a disorder that results from alterations in a single gene
    E. a disorder that results from sporadic mutation

7: Molecular Methods Questions

21.   In which type(s) of inheritance patterns can phenotypically normal individuals pass on the disorder to their offspring?
    A.   autosomal dominant
    B.   autosomal recessive
    C.   X-linked recessive
    D.   A & B
    E.   B & C

22.   In order to calculate allele frequencies for a particular gene with two major alleles, which of the following is NOT needed?
    A.   homozygote frequency of the first allele
    B.   heterozygote frequency of both alleles
    C.   homozygote frequency of the second allele
    D.   all are needed
    E.   only the frequency for one of the alleles is needed; it doesn't matter which

23.   What's the best definition of a missense mutation?
    A.   a mutation that alters the codon so that a different amino acid is encoded
    B.   a mutation that alters the codon without changing the encoded amino acid
    C.   a mutation that changes a codon into a translation stop codon
    D.   a mutation that affects the mRNA splice site
    E.   a mutation where the base is inserted and, in doing so, alters the reading frame

24.   Which is the preferred target for evaluating a clonal B-cell process?
    A.   Ig kappa
    B.   Ig lambda
    C.   Ig heavy chain
    D.   T-cell receptor beta chain
    E.   T-cell receptor gamma chain

25.   Approximately what percentage of clonal processes detected by Southern blot analysis are detected by PCR?
    A.   >100% (ie, PCR detects more clonal processes than Southern blot)
    B.   100%
    C.   85%
    D.   50%
    E.   10%

26.   What is the preferred technology for the detection of minimal residual disease?
    A.   PCR
    B.   FISH
    C.   Southern blot analysis
    D.   ELISA
    E.   immunohistochemistry

27.   Which of the following presentations is suspicious for a hereditary cancer or tumor syndrome?
    A.   the presence of a particular tumor type
    B.   an unusually young age at presentation
    C.   a characteristic histological appearance of a tumor
    D.   all of the above
    E.   none of the above

7: Molecular Methods Questions

28. What is the underlying mechanism that causes hereditary nonpolyposis colorectal carcinoma (HNPCC)?
    A. autosomal dominant mutations in tumor suppressor genes
    B. autosomal recessive mutations in tumor suppressor genes
    C. germline mutations that result in defective mismatch repair
    D. sporadic mutations proto-oncogenes
    E. autosomal dominant mutations in proto-oncogenes

29. What's the most common gene that is hypermethylated in sporadic colorectal and gastric carcinomas that display microsatellite instability?
    A. MLH1
    B. MSH2
    C. MSH6
    D. PMS2
    E. MSH3

30. Which of the following techniques is used to diagnose syndromic HNPCC (hereditary non-polyposis colorectal cancer)?
    A. amplification of specific mononucleotide and dinucleotide repeats from tumor and non-tumor tissue from an affected individual
    B. immunohistochemical staining of neoplastic and non-neoplastic tissue from an affected individual
    C. Southern blot analysis of microsatellites in tumor and non-tumor tissue
    D. A & B
    E. A, B, C

31. Where are MSI (microsatellite instability)-H (high) tumors usually located in the colon?
    A. ascending colon
    B. transverse colon
    C. descending colon
    D. sigmoid colon
    E. rectum

32. What is the gold standard for the diagnosis of HNPCC (hereditary non-polyposis colorectal cancer)?
    A. fulfillment of Amsterdam Criteria
    B. fulfillment of Amsterdam II Criteria
    C. fulfillment of Bethesda Criteria
    D. microsatellite instability (MSI) testing and immunohistochemistry
    E. DNA-based testing for germline mutations

33. Which of the following genes or gene products is mutated in familial adenosis polyposis (FAP)?
    A. retinoblastoma gene (Rb)
    B. p53
    C. assorted DNA mismatch repair genes
    D. APC
    E. SMAD4

7: Molecular Methods Questions

34. Which of the following tumors has a high association with von Hippel-Lindau syndrome, as well as a strong association with chromosome 3p deletions in sporadic cases?
    A. pheochromocytoma
    B. hemangioblastoma
    C. papillary neoplasm of endolymphatic sac origin
    D. clear cell renal cell carcinoma
    E. cystadenomas of ovary or epididymis.

35. Which of the following gene products and their chromosomal location are associated with tuberous sclerosis?
    A. Ret, 10q
    B. hamartin, 9q34
    C. tuberin, 16q13.3
    D. A & B
    E. B & C

36. Which of the following mutations of BRCA genes is not one of the predominant mutations in the Ashkenazi Jewish population?
    A. a deletion for the codon for phenylalanine 508 in BRCA1
    B. a two base-pair deletion (185delAG) of BRCA1
    C. a 5382insC mutation in BRCA1
    D. a 6174delT mutation of BRCA2
    E. all of the above are found in BRCA-associated breast cancer

37. Which of the following lesions is NOT commonly associated with MEN 1 (multiple endocrine neoplasia 1)?
    A. paragangliomas
    B. pituitary adenoma
    C. parathyroid adenoma
    D. pancreatic islet cell tumor
    E. all of the above are associated with MEN1

38. What is the gene, locus, and protein product that is mutated in multiple endocrine neoplasia, type 1 (MEN 1)?
    A. MEN1, 11q13, Ret
    B. MEN1, 11q13, menin
    C. MEN1, 10q, Ret
    D. MEN1, 10q, MTC
    E. MEN1, 9p21, p16

39. Which tumor is most strongly associated with MEN2A and MEN2B?
    A. medullary thyroid cancer
    B. medullary breast cancer
    C. mucosal neuroma
    D. parathyroid adenoma
    E. ganglioneuroma

40. Although MEN2A, MEN2B, Hirschprung disease, and familiar medullary thyroid carcinoma (FMTC) are all associated with mutations of the *RET* gene, why are the manifestations of each of them different?
    A. each is also associated with an additional gene mutation
    B. the age of onset determines the course of the disease
    C. gender determines which disease affects the individual
    D. they are each associated with mutations in different parts of the gene
    E. the process is stochastic and has not been sufficiently elucidated

7: Molecular Methods Questions

41.   Which of the following best describes Carney Complex?
      A.   gastric gastrointestinal stromal tumor (GIST), pulmonary chondroma, extra-adrenal paraganglioma
      B.   hamartomatous intestinal polyps, mucocutaneous lesions, Lhermitte-Duclos
      C.   cutaneous lentigos, atrial myxomas, endocrine tumors, blue nevi
      D.   mucocutaneous pigmentation, hamartomatous gastrointestinal polyps, sex cord tumors
      E.   fibrofolliculomas, pneumothorax, renal tumors

42.   Which of the following syndromes is NOT associated with mutations in the *PTEN* gene?
      A.   Cowden syndrome
      B.   Peutz-Jeghers syndrome
      C.   Bannayan-Riley-Ruvalcaba syndrome
      D.   Proteus syndrome
      E.   all of the above are associated with *PTEN* mutations

43.   Which of the following genes is/are associated with juvenile polyposis?
      A.   *BMPR1A* (10q22.3)
      B.   *SMAD4* (18q11.1)
      C.   *PTEN* (10q23)
      D.   all of the above
      E.   none of the above

44.   What is the most common site for gastrointestinal hamartomatous polyps in patients with Peutz-Jeghers syndrome?
      A.   stomach
      B.   duodenum
      C.   jejunum
      D.   ileum
      E.   colon

45.   Which of the following is NOT one of the cardinal features of Birt-Hogg-Dube syndrome?
      A.   pseudohermaphroditism
      B.   fibrofolliculomas
      C.   pneumothorax
      D.   renal tumors
      E.   all of the above are features of BHD syndrome

46.   What percentage of cases of neurofibromatosis, type 1 (NF1) are due to new sporadic mutations?
      A.   90%
      B.   50%
      C.   10%
      D.   1%
      E.   0%

47.   What changes in neurofibromas have been associated with pregnancy in affected female patients?
      A.   increased number and size
      B.   decreased number and size
      C.   increased malignant transformation rate
      D.   decreased malignant transformation rate
      E.   decreased penetrance in offspring

7: Molecular Methods Questions

48. Which of the following molecular tests detects the highest percentage of neurofibromatosis, type 1 (NF1) cases?
    A. *in vitro* protein assay
    B. cytogenetic testing
    C. FISH analysis
    D. protein truncation testing
    E. direct sequencing analysis

49. What is the most consistent lesion seen with neurofibromatosis, type 2 (NF2)?
    A. cafe au lait spots
    B. meningioma
    C. bilateral vestibular nerve schwannomas
    D. ependymoma
    E. peripheral schwannomas

50. Match the gene with the locus.
    A. NF1
    B. NF2
    C. VHL
    D. TSC1
    E. TSC2

    1. 3p25-26
    2. 22q11.2
    3. 17q
    4. 16p13.3
    5. 9q34

51. What is the most common genetic anomaly associated with conventional clear cell renal cell carcinoma?
    A. loss of the Y chromosome
    B. Xp11.2 translocations
    C. t(6;11)(p11.2;q12)
    D. t(X;17)
    E. del(3p)

52. Which of the following is a feature commonly associated with Her2-overexpression breast tumors?
    A. good outcome, independent of other markers
    B. low nuclear grade
    C. good response to adriamycin-based adjuvant chemotherapy
    D. good response to tamoxifen, independent of ER/PR status
    E. poor response to anti-Her2 antibody

53. What is the mechanism underlying increased expression of Her-2 in affected breast tumors?
    A. increased gene expression due to upregulation of transcription
    B. increased gene expression due to gene amplification
    C. decreased protein degradation
    D. increased protein stability at membrane
    E. increased gene expression due to translational upregulation

7: Molecular Methods Questions

54. Which of the following chromosome pairs are most commonly (and specifically) LOST in oligodendrogliomas and assist in differentiating them from other similar-appearing tumors, such as dysembryoblastic neurectodermal tumor (DNET), protoplasmic astrocytoma, and central neurocytoma?
    A. 1p, 9p
    B. 1p, 19q
    C. 9p, 10q
    D. X, 19p
    E. 1q, 19p

55. Which of the following is associated with a good prognosis in oligodendrogliomas?
    A. loss of heterozygosity 10q
    B. del (16p)
    C. EGFR amplification
    D. loss of 9p21
    E. loss of 1p and 19q

56. What's the most common type of mutation associated with retinoblastoma?
    A. frame shift mutations of the retinoblastoma gene
    B. point mutations of the retinoblastoma gene
    C. deletion mutations of the retinoblastoma gene
    D. trinucleotide repeat expansion in the retinoblastoma gene
    E. insertion mutation in the retinoblastoma gene

57. All of the following tumors are associated with germline mutations of the *RB1* gene, except:
    A. pineal gland tumors
    B. peripheral neurectodermal tumor
    C. retinoblastoma
    D. meningioma
    E. osteosarcoma

58. What is the gene product and its function that is mutated in neurofibromatosis, type 2 (NF2)?
    A. merlin, cell-cell contact and cell contact inhibition
    B. merlin, receptor tyrosine kinase
    C. neurofibromin, transcription factor
    D. neurofibromin, tumor suppressor
    E. none of the above are accurate

59. All of the following are high-grade (WHO II/III) types of meningioma, except:
    A. meningothelial
    B. papillary
    C. rhabdoid
    D. chordoid
    E. anaplastic

60. All of the following translocations are associated with Ewing sarcoma/peripheral neurectodermal tumor (PNET), except:
    A. t(11;22)
    B. t(21;22)
    C. t(7;22)
    D. t(17;22)
    E. t(12;22)

7: Molecular Methods Questions

61. What is the nature of the *MYCN* alteration most commonly seen in neuroblastoma?
    A. deletion
    B. translocation
    C. amplification
    D. point mutation
    E. a complex combination of mutations

62. Which gene(s) is/are involved with WAGR (Wilms' tumor, aniridia, genitourinary anomalies, retardation) syndrome?
    A. *WT1*
    B. *PAX6*
    C. *WT2*
    D. A & B
    E. A, B, C

63. Which two tumors are seen at a higher frequency in patients affected by Beckwith-Wiedemann syndrome (pick 2)?
    A. Wilms' tumor
    B. meningioma
    C. extraskeletal osteosarcoma
    D. hepatoblastoma
    E. synovial sarcoma

64. What subtype of rhabdomyosarcoma is associated with the translocation t(2;13)?
    A. embryonal
    B. sarcoma botyroides
    C. alveolar
    D. spindle cell
    E. pleomorphic

65. Synovial sarcoma is associated with the translocation t(X;18) resulting in a *SYT-SSX* fusion. Which of the following statements is correct?
    A. *SYT-SSX2* is associated more with biphasic synovial sarcoma
    B. *SYT-SSX1* is associated more with monophasic synovial sarcoma
    C. *SYT-SSX2* is associated more with monophasic synovial sarcoma
    D. *SYT-SSX1* is associated more with biphasic synovial sarcoma
    E. none of the above are true

66. Which of the following disorders is due to a single conserved point mutation?
    A. alpha-thalassemia
    B. beta-thalassemia
    C. sickle cell anemia
    D. A & B
    E. A, B, C

67. Which of the following tests can be performed with amniocentesis but not with chorionic villus sampling (CVS)?
    A. chromosomal status
    B. AFP (alpha-fetoprotein) levels
    C. enzyme levels
    D. mutation status
    E. all of the above tests can be performed on samples from amniocentesis and CVS.

7: Molecular Methods Questions

68. All of the following specimens have been used for fetal *in utero* diagnosis, except:
    A. umbilical cord blood
    B. fetal cystic hygroma fluid
    C. fetal vesicular urine
    D. fetal skin
    E. all of the above have been used for fetal diagnosis

69. What is the most common indication for prenatal cytogenetic studies?
    A. advanced maternal age
    B. family history of genetic disease
    C. non-reassuring ultrasound findings
    D. positive triple test results
    E. none of the above

70. Aneuploidies of all of the following chromosomes are among the common causes of spontaneous abortion, except:
    A. 21
    B. 1
    C. 13
    D. 18
    E. X

71. All of the following are associated with Alzheimer disease, except:
    A. mutations in lipoprotein L gene
    B. mutations in *PSEN1, APP,* & *PSEN2* genes
    C. Down syndrome
    D. mutations in ApoE4 gene
    E. all of the above are associated with Alzheimer disease

72. Which class of mutation is associated with Huntington disease?
    A. frame shift
    B. deletion
    C. trinucleotide repeat expansion
    D. point mutation
    E. there is a heterogeneous collection of mutations associated with Huntington disease

73. Mutations of which gene are associated with cerebral autosomal dominant arteriopathy with subcortical infarctions and leukoencephalopathy (CADASIL)?
    A. *NOTCH3*
    B. patched
    C. Ret
    D. *CAD1*
    E. all of the above are associated with CADASIL

74. Which of the following set of symptoms best describes McLeod syndrome?
    A. giant platelets, Dohle bodies
    B. peripheral RBC acanthocytosis, decreased expression of Kell antigen, basal ganglia dysfunction
    C. motor and sensory neuropathy due to demyelination
    D. resting tremor, bradykinesia, and rigidity
    E. eczema and immune dysfunction

7: Molecular Methods Questions

75. Of the subtypes of Charcot-Marie-Tooth disease, which is more readily characterized with genetic means?
    A. *CMT1*
    B. *CMT2*
    C. *CMT5/6*
    D. autosomal recessive CMT
    E. Hallervorden-Spatz syndrome

76. Familial amyloidosis, senile cardiac amyloidosis, and cerebral amyloid angiopathy - similar, overlapping diseases - share in common mutations of which of the following proteins?
    A. albumin
    B. CFTR
    C. kappa light chain
    D. transthyretin
    E. presenilin

77. Which of the following diseases is due to mutation of the *DMD* gene located on chromosome Xp21.2?
    A. Becker muscular dystrophy
    B. Duchenne muscular dystrophy
    C. familial dysautonomic dystrophy
    D. A & B
    E. A, B, C

78. Which of the following modalities is used in the molecular diagnosis of DMD-related disease?
    A. multiplex PCR
    B. quantitative PCR
    C. direct sequence analysis
    D. Southern blot
    E. all of the above

79. What critical process is required for the visualization of the granular basophilic rimmed vacuoles of inclusion body myositis?
    A. rapid formalin fixation of tissue
    B. acid pretreatment prior to formalin fixation of tissue
    C. freezing of tissue
    D. protease digestion
    E. nothing special - the vacuoles show up with standard formalin fixation/processing

80. Genetically speaking, which of the following conditions has the most in common with myotonic muscular dystrophy (Steinert disease)?
    A. inclusion body myositis
    B. Duchenne muscular dystrophy
    C. Nemaline body myopathy
    D. familial dysautonomia
    E. Huntington disease

81. Which protein is defective in malignant hyperthermia?
    A. *RYR1* calcium channel
    B. pyruvate kinase
    C. ornithine decarboxylase
    D. cytochrome p450 2CA
    E. methylmalonyl CoA mutase

7: Molecular Methods Questions

82. Which of the following symptoms are associated with Brugada syndrome?
    A. EKG abnormalities
    B. cardiac rhythm disturbances
    C. sudden unexpected nocturnal death syndrome
    D. sudden infant death syndrome
    E. all of the above

83. What is the single best sign that distinguishes the Jervell and Lange-Neilsen syndrome from Romano-Ward syndrome?
    A. long QT
    B. fasciculations
    C. short QT
    D. sensorineural hearing loss
    E. torsades de pointe

84. What is the hallmark hepatic histologic feature of medium-chain-acyl-coenzyme A dehydrogenase (MCAD) deficiencies?
    A. cirrhosis
    B. interface hepatitis
    C. macrovesicular steatosis
    D. Mallory bodies
    E. microvesicular steatosis

85. What the most clinically effective means of testing for medium-chain-acyl-coenzyme A dehydrogenase (MCAD) deficiencies?
    A. histology of liver biopsy
    B. tandem mass spectrophotometric acylcarnitines in blood
    C. FISH analysis of *ACADM* gene
    D. direct sequencing of the *ACADM* gene
    E. clinical symptoms and family history

86. What is the approximate gene frequency of cystic fibrosis in the Caucasian population?
    A. 1/5
    B. 1/20
    C. 1/100
    D. 1/2000
    E. 1/17000

87. Cystic fibrosis can present with all the following symptoms, except:
    A. recurrent pneumonia
    B. meconium ileus
    C. male infertility
    D. chronic, recurrent pancreatitis
    E. all of the above are symptoms associated with cystic fibrosis

88. What is the most common disease-associated *CFTR* mutation?
    A. C282Y
    B. deltaF508
    C. H63D
    D. W1282X
    E. G542X

7: Molecular Methods Questions

89. What is the preferred newborn screening test for cystic fibrosis?
    A.   molecular test for homozygosity of CFTR mutations
    B.   abnormal pilocarpine iontophoresis sweat chloride test
    C.   elevated immunoreactive trypsinogen
    D.   abnormal transepithelial nasal potential difference measurements
    E.   clinical symptomatic criteria

90. Which ethnic group has the lowest prevalence of hereditary hemochromatosis?
    A.   Northern European Caucasians
    B.   American Caucasians
    C.   American Hispanics
    D.   African-Americans
    E.   Asian-Americans

91. What genetic alteration(s) is/are responsible for the vast majority of HFE-associated hemochromatosis?
    A.   C282Y
    B.   H63D
    C.   S65C
    D.   A & B
    E.   A, B, C

92. Mutations in which of the following genes is responsible for Wilson disease?
    A.   ceruloplasmin
    B.   *HFE*
    C.   *ATP7B*
    D.   major cuprotransferrin
    E.   a regulated chloride channel

93. All of the following are common presenting symptoms of Wilson disease, except:
    A.   diabetes
    B.   liver disease
    C.   neuropsychiatric disease
    D.   hemolysis
    E.   decreased serum ceruloplasmin

94. Which of the following genotypes of the *SERPIN1A* gene is most commonly associated with alpha-1-antitrypsin deficiency?
    A.   PiMM
    B.   PiMZ
    C.   PiZZ
    D.   PiMS
    E.   PiSZ

95. Which two organ systems are most commonly affected by alpha-1-antitrypsin (pick 2)?
    A.   neural
    B.   renal
    C.   pulmonary
    D.   hepatic
    E.   musculoskeletal

7: Molecular Methods Questions

96. What is the typical serum protein electrophoresis (SPEP) pattern appearance of patients with alpha-1-antitrypsin disease?
    A. decreased alpha 1 region
    B. decreased alpha 2 region
    C. beta-gamma bridging
    D. decreased gamma region
    E. sharp peak in the gamma region

97. Which of the following presentations is most compatible with Alagille syndrome?
    A. normal number of bile ducts at birth
    B. noninflammatory paucity of interlobular bile ducts
    C. triangular facies
    D. A & B
    E. A, B, C

98. Mutations of which gene are most commonly associated with Alagille syndrome?
    A. *ALA1*
    B. *JAG1*
    C. *NOTCH1*
    D. *NOTCH2*
    E. *NOTCH3*

99. Which type of Hirschprung disease is more common in males than in females?
    A. short segment aganglionosis
    B. long segment aganglionosis
    C. total colonic aganglionosis
    D. all of the above are more common in males than females
    E. all types of Hirschprung disease are more common in females than males

100. Which of the following syndromes is <u>NOT</u> associated with Hirschprung disease?
    A. trisomy 21
    B. MEN2A
    C. NF1
    D. Smith-Lemli-Opitz syndrome
    E. all of the above are associated with Hirschprung disease

101. Which enzyme is most commonly deficient in congenital adrenal hyperplasia?
    A. 11-hydroxylase
    B. 17-hydroxylase
    C. 21-hydroxylase
    D. 20,22-hydroxylase
    E. 3-hydroxysteroid-dehydrogenase

102. What is the gene and chromosomal location associated with androgen-insensitivity syndrome?
    A. estrogen receptor, X chromosome
    B. estrogen receptor, Y chromosome
    C. androgen receptor, X chromosome
    D. androgen receptor, Y chromosome
    E. none of the above

7: Molecular Methods Questions

103. Alport syndrome and thin basement membrane disease are inherited nephritic syndromes due to deficiencies in which of the following:
    A. nephrin
    B. collagen, type II
    C. collagen, type IV
    D neurofilaments
    E. tubulin

104. Which of the following genes is mutated in autosomal recessive polycystic kidney disease?
    A. *NPHP1*
    B. *PKD1*
    C. *PKD2*
    D. *PKHD1*
    E. *PKHD2*

105. Which of the following genes is associated with cystic renal dysplasia?
    A. *MCDK1*
    B. *NPHP1*
    C. *NPHP2*
    D. *PKD1*
    E. none of the above

106. What is the primary difference phenotypically between juvenile and adult-onset nephronophthisis?
    A. extrarenal anomalies
    B. the presence of cartilage
    C. the size of the cysts
    D. sensorineural hearing loss
    E. tuberous sclerosis

107. What is the <u>most common</u> presentation of autosomal dominant polycystic kidney disease?
    A. renal stones
    B. hypertension
    C. liver cysts
    D. intracranial Berry aneurysms
    E. mitral valve prolapse

108. Autosomal dominant polycystic kidney disease (ADPKD) is associated with a contiguous gene syndrome which presents with features overlapping those of multiple syndromes due to deletions in two or more closely adjacent genes. Match the two genes that are often comutated.
    A. *PKD1/TSC1*
    B. *PKD2/TSC2*
    C. *PKD1/VHL*
    D. *PKD2/VHL*
    E. *PKD1/TSC2*

109. Fabry disease, Lesch-Nyhan, and Hunter disease are all metabolic diseases inherited in this fashion:
    A. autosomal recessive
    B. autosomal dominant
    C. X-linked recessive
    D. X-linked dominant
    E. maternal (mitochondrial)

7: Molecular Methods Questions

110. Which two metabolic diseases are screened for in EVERY state (pick 2)?
    A. Hunter disease
    B. phenylketonuria
    C. Tay-Sachs
    D. galactosemia
    E. congenital hypothyroidism

111. What are the two most critical times for the regulation of phenylalanine intake in order to minimize morbidity (pick 2)?
    A. infancy
    B. early childhood
    C. early adulthood
    D. pregnancy
    E. menopause/later adulthood

112. Which one of the following infections are children with galactosemia at the highest risk of contracting?
    A. cryptococcal meningitis
    B. *E. coli* sepsis
    C. *Burkholderia* pneumonia
    D. subacute bacterial endocarditis
    E. *Actinomyces* cervicitis

113. What is the enzyme deficient in Tay-Sachs disease?
    A. galactose-1-phosphate uridyl transferase
    B. tay-saccharidase I
    C. glycosphingolipid
    D. hexosaminidase A
    E. glucocerebrosidase

114. All of the following syndromes are associated with accumulations of very long chain fatty acids (VLFCA), except:
    A. Gaucher disease
    B. classic Zellweger syndrome
    C. neonatal adrenoleukodystrophy
    D. infantile Refsum disease
    E. all of the above are VLCFA diseases

115. What is the enzyme deficient in Gaucher disease?
    A. galactose-1-phosphate uridyl transferase
    B. gacheridase
    C. glycosphingolipid
    D. hexosaminidase A
    E. glucocerebrosidase

116. Which of the following features do organic acidemias and urea cycle disorders have in common?
    A. autosomal recessive inheritance
    B. hyperammonemia
    C. typically normal appearance at birth
    D. A & B
    E. A, B, C

117. Which of the following is NOT a sphingolipidosis?
    A. Gaucher disease
    B. Hurler disease
    C. Niemann-Pick disease
    D. Fabry disease
    E. Tay-Sachs disease

118. In which of the following disorders does the affected individual exhibit self-mutilating behavior, such as finger/lip-biting and head banging?
    A. Krabbe disease
    B. Fabry disease
    C. Lesch-Nyhan disease
    D. Hunter disease
    E. cystinosis

119. Deficiency of which of the following enzymes is associated with angiokeratomas and blindness?
    A. hypoxanthine guanine phosphoribosyl transferase (HGPRT)
    B. galactocerebrosidase
    C. phenylalanine hydroxylase
    D. alpha-galactosidase
    E. galactose-1-phosphate uridyl transferase

120. Which of the following metabolic disorders presents with characteristic hexagonal and birefringent crystals deposited in the cornea, bone marrow, and kidney?
    A. cystinuria
    B. alkaptonuria
    C. maple syrup urine disease
    D. Krabbe disease
    E. none of the above

121. Which of the following is the most common chromosome abnormality in LIVE births?
    A. monosomy X
    B. triploidy
    C. trisomy 16
    D. trisomy 21
    E. trisomy 18

122. Which population demographic accounts for the majority of parentage of Down syndrome offspring?
    A. fathers >25 years old
    B. fathers >35 years old
    C. mothers <35 years old
    D. mothers >35 years old
    E. there is no age preference

123. What is the most common outcome of monosomy X?
    A. spontaneous abortion
    B. Turner syndrome
    C. Edward syndrome
    D. Down syndrome
    E. Patau syndrome

7: Molecular Methods Questions

124. Which of the following most closely phenotypically resembles Turner syndrome?
    A.   Patau syndrome
    B.   Edward syndrome
    C.   Down syndrome
    D.   Noonan syndrome
    E.   Klinefelter syndrome

125. What are the two causes of Prader-Willi syndrome (pick 2)?
    A.   microdeletion in paternal 15q11.2
    B.   microdeletion in maternal 15q11.2
    C.   uniparental (maternal) disomy
    D.   uniparental (paternal) disomy
    E.   methylation of maternal 15q11.2

126. All of the following are examples of trinucleotide repeat expansions, except:
    A.   Huntington disease
    B.   Bloom syndrome
    C.   Fragile X syndrome
    D.   Friedreich ataxia
    E.   all of the above are examples of trinucleotide repeat expansions

127. All of the following disorders demonstrate increased sensitivity to ionizing radiation, except:
    A.   Friedreich ataxia
    B.   xeroderma pigmentosa
    C.   ataxia telangiectasia
    D.   Bloom syndrome
    E.   all of the above demonstrate increased sensitivity to ionizing radiation

128. Which of the following syndromes is most consistent with aplastic anemia and absent radii?
    A.   xeroderma pigmentosa
    B.   Fanconi anemia
    C.   Nijmegen breakage syndrome
    D.   Bloom syndrome
    E.   ataxia telangiectasia

129. True or false: Mitochondrial disease is due exclusively to mutations in mitochondrial DNA.

130. Which of the following accounts for the clinical variability of mitochondrial disease?
    A.   homoplasmy
    B.   heteroplasmy
    C.   nuclear genes, exclusively
    D.   mitochondrial membrane thickness
    E.   gender

131. All of the following are examples of mitochondrial disease, except:
    A.   Kearns-Sayre syndrome
    B.   mitochondrial encephalopathy with lactic acidosis and stroke-like episodes (MELAS)
    C.   myoclonic epilepsy with ragged red fibers (MERRF)
    D.   Leber hereditary optic neuropathy
    E.   Nijmegen breakage syndrome

7: Molecular Methods Answers

1.   A.   **FRESH, VIABLE TISSUE.**

One of the critical limitations of cytogenetic karyotyping is the absolute requirement for viable tissue. This is necessary (and makes sense) because actively-dividing cells are arrested in metaphase of the cell cycle (the point of maximal condensation of chromosomes) to obtain chromosomes for analysis.
QCCP2, **Cytogenetics,** p 388

2.   E.   **A & B.**

Rather than the protein and epigenetic modifications of DNA that lead to the formation of heterochromatin and euchromatin, it is the intrinsic deoxyribose base sequences that are responsible for the highly reproducible banding contrast patterns.
QCCP2, **Cytogenetics,** p 388

3.   D.   **ALL OF THE ABOVE.**

Unlike classical cytogenetics, molecular cytogenetic techniques do not routinely require the use of viable cells. In addition, cells in any phase, not just metaphase, can be studied by molecular cytogenetics.
QCCP2, **Cytogenetics,** p 388

4.   B.   **TELOMERIC PROBES.**

Allele-specific probes are used to target particular DNA sequences of interest. Centromeric probes and painting probes are used to enumerate and identify whole chromosomes.
QCCP2, **Cytogenetics,** p 388

5.   C.   **IT DEPENDS ON THE ASSAY.**

If the appropriate primers are available, PCR is more sensitive. FISH, however, can be more sensitive than PCR in detecting polymorphous mutations or mutations spanning a larger distance where specific PCR primers may not be available.
QCCP2, **Cytogenetics,** p 388

6.   C.   **BREAK-APART PROBES.**

This is a fairly straightforward question that helps to elucidate the difference between the two more commonly used types of FISH probes for translocation analysis. One can think of these probes as being directed toward each of the two broad "phases" of translocation. First, the gene of interest "breaks away" from its native locus. Break-apart probes span two sides of a break point in a locus. Before the initial break, there is a single signal. After the initial break, the signal splits into two signals. Fusion probes monitor the second step of translocation - the formation of a novel fusion gene. For a fusion probe, two signals come together to form a new single signal.
QCCP2, **Cytogenetics,** p 388

7.   A.   **FISH "BAIT" - HOMOLOGOUS SEQUENCES BINDING PROBES.**

The non-specific binding of the probe to homologous sequences is less of a problem in FISH than many other nucleic acid-based assays, due to the extreme specificity of the large probes. The other three choices are the most common sources of artifact in FISH analysis.
QCCP2, **Cytogenetics,** p 389

7: Molecular Methods Answers

8.   D.   dNTPs (NUCLEOTIDE TRIPHOSPHATES).

While some PCR reactions can utilize a denaturing agent in modest amounts to increase stringency, it is not an absolute requirement like the presence of dNTPS is.
QCCP2, **Polymerase chain reaction (PCR),** p 389

9.   D.   HIGH RATE OF CONTAMINATION.

If the sequence to be amplified is known, then finding suitable primers is usually not a problem. Reactions are run typically with excess dNTPs, so that is usually not a problem, either. Nested PCR involves a two-step process of subjecting a first amplicon to a second round of amplification. Therefore, non-specific amplification is further amplified and contaminating sequence, even in very small amounts, runs a greater risk of being amplified.
QCCP2, **Polymerase chain reaction,** p 389

10.   C.   PRODUCT DETECTION.

   D.   TARGET AMPLIFICATION.

The power of real-time PCR is the simultaneous amplification and detection of PCR products. The limitation is that, to run a real-time PCR reaction, there is a requirement for a special thermal cycler with optics capable of monitoring the small amounts of fluorescence produced.
QCCP2, **Polymerase chain reaction,** p 389

11.   E.   USE OF TWO OR MORE PRIMER SETS TO SIMULTANEOUSLY AMPLIFY MULTIPLE PRODUCTS IN A SINGLE REACTION TUBE.

Multiplex PCR uses more than one set of primers in order to amplify multiple amplicons in parallel (at the same time). This is useful, for example, in microbiology for the detection of multiple agents in a single patient specimen.
QCCP2, **Polymerase chain reaction,** p 389

12.   A.   BRANCHED DNA.

Along with hybrid capture, branched DNA is a technique that aims to amplify the signal in the detection of a particular sequence rather than amplify the amount of target sequence. A sequence-specific probe with multiple signals binds to a target of interest.
QCCP2, **Polymerase chain reaction,** p 390

13.   E.   ALL ARE ADVANTAGES OF PCR OVER SOUTHERN BLOT.

For the most part, the Southern blot is bested by PCR. Southern blot is still utilized in some labs and provides useful information, predominantly in the analysis of immunoglobulin gene and T-cell receptor clonal rearrangements. However, many labs use PCR now for gene rearrangement assays - unsurprisingly, given all the advantages of PCR. Southern blot, however, is still the gold standard due to a limitation of PCR - the sequence to be amplified must be defined and appropriate primers designed. (See question 25 for more.)
QCCP2, **PCR and Southern blot analysis,** p 390

14.   B.   **LOSS OF HETEROZYGOSITY.**

Another example is retinoblastoma where the affected individual inherits a heterozygous state of the retinoblastoma gene - one defective copy and one normal one. When the normal copy is lost - the "second hit" - the heterozygous state is lost, too. Single nucleotide polymorphism may be considered under certain circumstances to be a specific example of loss of heterozygosity.
QCCP2, **Loss of heterozygosity,** p 390

15.   B.   **CYTOSINE.**

If you can remember that CpG islands (cytosine phosphate guanine) are a major site for methylation and silencing, you're halfway there. In my mind, silencing and methylation are consistent with each other, which helps me to remember that "Cy"tosine and "Si"lencing start with the same sound.
QCCP2, **DNA Methylation,** p 390

16.   A.   **LENGTH.**

Autosomes are numbered based on the length of the metaphase chromosomes, with chromosome 1 as the longest, through chromosome 22, followed by the sex chromosomes, according to convention.
QCCP2, **Cytogenetic nomeclature,** p 391

17.   D.   **CENTROMERE.**

Bands (and sub-bands) are numbered from the centromere outward to the ends for both the short (petite, or p) arm and the long q arm.
QCCP2, **Cytogenetic nomenclature,** p 391

18.   D.   **POLYPLOIDY.**

The three other terms refer to losses or gains of chromosomes leading to a chromosome number that is an uneven multiple of 23. Monosomy and trisomy are specific examples of aneuploidy.
QCCP2, **Cytogenetic nomenclature,** p 391

19.   A.   **A CHROMOSOME WITH ONLY SHORT OR LONG ARM GENETIC MATERIAL ON EITHER SIDE OF THE CENTROMERE.**

An example of an isochromosome is the i(12p) associated with the majority of germ cell tumors where only the short arm of chromosome 12 is represented. Choice B refers to a deletion, C is an inversion, D is a derivative, and E is a translocation.
QCCP2, **Cytogenetic nomenclature,** pp 391-392

20.   D.   **A DISORDER THAT RESULTS FROM ALTERATIONS IN A SINGLE GENE.**

Many of the genetic diseases and their inheritance patterns are considered Mendelian disorders. That is, they are the result of a single gene mutation transmitted in a single reproducible pattern.
QCCP2, **Mendelian disorders,** p 392

7: Molecular Methods Answers

21. E. **B & C.**

The point of this question is to help define the term "carrier." It's a bit tricky with traits passed in an x-linked recessive manner, as only phenotypically normal females can pass on the disorder, and then usually only to male offspring. An affected male and a carrier female can have an affected female child. However, since many of the x-linked recessive conditions adversely affect fertility, this is very unlikely (though of course not impossible) to happen.
QCCP2, **Mendelian disorders,** p 392

22. E. IT'S ONLY THE FREQUENCY FOR ONE OF THE ALLELES IS NEEDED; IT DOESN'T MATTER WHICH.

It's a misleading question! I admit this isn't the best question I have written, especially for a subject as confusing as Hardy-Weinberg equilibrium. You really only need the frequency for one allele. We can calculate the frequency of alleles from observed phenotypes with the Hardy-Weinberg equation. The frequency of homozygotes for one allele is represented by p^2. Heterozygotes are 2pq, and homozygotes for the other allele are represented by q^2. The sum of all gene frequencies at the locus is equal to 1. For each allele $(p + q)^2 = 1$ or $p^2 + 2pq + q^2 = 1$. Because we can calculate the allele frequencies from the binomial expansion of the Hardy-Weinberg, we only need the frequency of one allele. $p = 1 - q$.
QCCP2, **Mendelian disorders,** pp 392-393

23. A. A MUTATION THAT ALTERS THE CODON SO THAT A DIFFERENT AMINO ACID IS ENCODED.

Choice B is the definition of a silent mutation, C is a nonsense mutation, D is a splice site mutation, and E is a frameshift mutation.
QCCP2, **Mutations,** p 393

24. C. IG HEAVY CHAIN.

For T-cell processes, both the T-cell receptor beta and gamma genes can be examined. Usually, beta is examined with Southern blot analysis, while gamma is examined with PCR.
QCCP2, **Demonstration of lymphoid clonality,** p 393

25. B. **85%.**

PCR requires knowledge of specific primer sites, some of which may not amplify. By this comparison, PCR is <u>less</u> sensitive than Southern blot analysis. If there are appropriate primers available and a sequence can be amplified, PCR can detect clonal rearrangements with less starting material. In this case, PCR is <u>more</u> sensitive than Southern blot analysis.
QCCP2, **Demonstration of lymphoid clonality,** p 393

26. A. **PCR.**

If defined probes are available, PCR is theoretically the most sensitive detection for minimal residual disease. One important caveat is that the molecular abnormality must be characterized pre-treatment by PCR or else the target for the detection for minimal residual disease would be unknown. FISH and Southern blot can be used, but are most useful in the initial characterization and detection of the molecular anomalies associated with the disease.
QCCP2, **Demonstration of gene rearrangements,** p 394

27.   D.   **ALL OF THE ABOVE.**

All are suspicious for hereditary tumor syndromes.
QCCP2, **Hereditary Cancer and Tumor Syndromes,** p 394

28.   C.   **GERMLINE MUTATIONS THAT RESULT IN DEFECTIVE MISMATCH REPAIR.**

Microsatellite instability is the result of defective mismatch repair. Lynch syndrome is the manifestation of defective mismatch repair.
QCCP2, **Hereditary nonpolyposis colon cancer (HNPCC, Lynch syndrome),** p 394

29.   A.   **MLH1.**

The majority of germline MSI-associated tumors are associated with mutations in MLH1 or MSH2. Sporadic MSI-associated tumors are most commonly associated with hypermethylation of MLH1.
QCCP2, **Hereditary nonpolyposis colon cancer (HNPCC, Lynch syndrome),** p 394

30.   D.   **A & B.**

The National Cancer Institute recommends a series of five microsatellite markers to screen for microsatellite instability in hereditary non-polyposis colon cancer. Two are mononucleotide repeats (BAT25 and BAT26) and three are dinucleotide repeats (D25123, D55346, D175250). Screening should be done in tandem on lesional and non-lesional tissue from the patient. If there are differences between the tumor and non-tumor of two or more of the markers, the tumor is classified as MSI-high, 1 marker is classified as MSI-low, and no changes is classified as MSS (microsatellite stable). Immunohistochemical analysis of MLH proteins can also be used, but does not directly demonstrate microsatellite instability, nor does it offer a hierarchical graded classification scheme.
QCCP2, **Hereditary nonpolyposis colon cancer (HNPCC, Lynch syndrome),** p 394

31.   A.   **ASCENDING COLON.**

There is a statistically significant high number of MSI-high tumors found in the right (ascending) colon. The tumors also tend to be poorly-differentiated, mucinous, and have a prominent lymphoid component.
QCCP2, **Hereditary nonpolyposis colon cancer (HNPCC, Lynch syndrome),** p 395

32.   E.   **DNA-BASED TESTING FOR GERMLINE MUTATIONS.**

The criteria were developed to guide screening test administration. Of each set of criteria, the Bethesda criteria are the most recent and the most liberal. MSI testing and IHC are used for screening. Definitive diagnosis is made with DNA-based testing.
QCCP2, **Hereditary nonpolyposis colon cancer (HNPCC, Lynch syndrome),** p 395

33.   D.   **APC.**

Located on the long arm of chromosome 5, APC mutations are inherited in an autosomal dominant fashion.
QCCP2, **Familial adenomatous polyposis (FAP),** p 395

34.   D.   **CLEAR CELL RENAL CELL CARCINOMA.**

All of the above tumors are associated with von Hippel-Lindau syndrome, which is due to deletion of the VHL gene on chromosome 3p25-26. However, the clear cell renal cell carcinoma is also commonly seen outside of von Hippel-Lindau in sporadic cases where it is associated with deletion of 3p.
QCCP2, **von Hippel-Lindau disease,** p 395

35.   E.   **B & C.**

TSC1 on chromosome 9q34 and TSC2 on 16q13.3 encode hamartin and tuberin, respectively.
QCCP2, **Tuberous sclerosis,** p 396

36.   A.   **A DELETION IN THE CODON FOR PHENYLALANINE 508 IN BRCA1.**

This is really hard - you can't memorize everything! The mutations listed in B, C, and D account for 90% of the cases of BRCA-associated breast cancer in the Ashkenazi Jewish population, despite the characterization of over 2000 different disease-associated mutations in BRCA1 and BRCA2. Choice A is misleading. It juxtaposes the most common mutation of CFTR(deletion of the phenylalanine 508 codon) to the BRCA1 gene.
QCCP2, **BRCA1 and BRCA2,** p 396

37.   A.   **PARAGANGLIOMAS.**

The three "P's" of MEN1 - pituitary adenoma, parathyroid adenoma, pancreatic islet cell tumor - do not include paragangliomas, which are much more commonly associated with MEN2.
QCCP2, **Multiple endocrine neoplasia Type 1 (MEN1),** p 396

38.   B.   **MEN1, 11Q13, MENIN.**

This is simply rote memorization. The MEN1 gene encodes the tumor supressor menin. 90% of families with MEN1 have germline mutations of the MEN1 gene. In single MEN1-associated tumors, germline mutations are rare.
QCCP2, **Multiple endocrine neoplasia Type 1 (MEN1),** p 396

39.   A.   **MEDULLARY THYROID CANCER.**

The listed syndromes, as well as familial medullary thyroid carcinoma (FMTC), are all associated with mutations in the ret gene. Ret encodes a receptor tyrosine kinase. Of the tumors listed, medullary thyroid carcinoma is most strongly associated with MEN2. In MEN2B, there is also a strong association with mucosal neuromas and ganglioneuromas.
QCCP2, **Multiple endocrine neoplasia Type 2 (MEN2, Sipple syndrome),** p 396

40.   D.   **THEY ARE EACH ASSOCIATED WITH MUTATIONS IN DIFFERENT PARTS OF THE GENE.**

Over 95% of individuals affected by MEN2, as well as a large percentage of those affected by Hirschprung disease and FMTC, have mutations in the gene encoding ret. The appearance of the distinct syndromes is dependent on whether or not there are germline mutations and on the location of the specific mutations.
QCCP2, **Multiple endocrine neoplasia Type 2 (MEN2, Sipple syndrome),** p 396

41.　C.　**CUTANEOUS LENTIGOS, ATRIAL MYXOMAS, ENDOCRINE TUMORS, BLUE NEVI.**

Carney complex is also known by the acronymic LAMB or NAME syndrome. LAMB stands for lentigines, atrial myxomas, mucocutaneous myxomas, and blue nevi, while NAME stands for nevi, atrial myxomas, myxoid neurofibromas, and ephelides. Choice A describes the Carney triad, B is Cowden syndrome, D is Peutz-Jeghers, and E is Birt-Hogg-Dube.

QCCP2, **Carney complex,** p 397

42.　B.　**PEUTZ-JEGHERS SYNDROME.**

Along with all the manifestations of Cowden syndrome (hamartomatous polyps, lipomas, fibromas, facial trichilemmomas, palmoplantar pits, and Lhermitte-Duclos), there is an increased risk of certain malignancies, especially of the breast, follicular thyroid, colon, and endometrium.

QCCP2, **Cowden syndrome and other PTEN-related disorders,** p 397

43.　D.　**ALL OF THE ABOVE.**

Several genes have been associated with cases of juvenile polyposis, including *BMPR1A, SMAD4,* and *PTEN.* Nearly 1/2 of all cases of juvenile polyposis are not associated with mutations of any of these genes.

QCCP2, **Juvenile polyposis,** p 397

44.　C.　**JEJUNUM.**

While the polyps occur also in both the stomach and the colon, the most common site is the jejunum. PJS manifests at an early age with mucocutaneous pigmentation, followed by sex cord-stromal tumor annular tubules and adenoma malignum in women, and calcifying Sertoli cell tumors of the testis in men. The majority of cases are associated with mutations in the gene *STK11* (also known as *LKB1*) on chromosome 19q.

QCCP2, **Peutz-Jeghers syndrome (PJS),** p 398

45.　A.　**PSEUDOHERMAPHRODITISM.**

Birt-Hogg-Dube is not associated with pseudohermaphroditism and renal tumors, but Denys-Drash syndrome is.

QCCP2, **The Birt-Hogg-Dube syndrome,** p 398

46.　B.　**50%.**

Approximately 1/2 of NF1 cases are due to new mutations.

QCCP2, **Neurofibromatosis Type 1 (von Recklinghausen disease, NF1),** p 398

47.　A.　**INCREASED NUMBER AND SIZE.**

A rapid increase in the number and size of neurofibromas has been demonstrated in a small subset of patients with NF1.

QCCP2, **Neurofibromatosis Type 1 (von Recklinghausen disease, NF1),** p 398

48.　E.　**DIRECT SEQUENCING ANALYSIS.**

Selections B through E are listed in order of increasing sensitivity, with direct sequence analysis detecting almost 90% of the mutations.

QCCP2, **Neurofibromatosis Type 1 (von Recklinghausen disease, NF1),** p 398

7: Molecular Methods Answers

49. C. **BILATERAL VESTIBULAR NERVE SCHWANNOMAS.**

By age 30, nearly all NF2 patients have developed bilateral vestibular nerve schwannomas. Café au lait spots are more commonly associated with NF1. The three other tumors mentioned are all seen at a higher rate in NF2 than in the general population, but not nearly as high as the vestibular nerve schwannoma.

QCCP2, **Neurofibromatosis Type 2 (bilateral acoustic neuromas, NF2),** p 398

50. A-3, B-2, C-1, D-5, E-4.

QCCP2, **Tuberous Sclerosis, von Hippel-Lindau, NF1, NF2,** p 396-398

51. E. **DEL(3P).**

Deletion of portions of the short arm of chromosome 3 is among the most common mutations in conventional renal cell carcinoma, though it is rarely the sole mutation. It is important to note that some of these mutations are in the region associated with von Hippel-Lindau (3p25-26) and that conventional clear cell renal cell carcinoma is associated with von Hippel-Lindau syndrome. Loss of the Y chromosome is commonly seen in papillary renal cell carcinoma, while Xp11.2 translocations, such as t(X;17) ASPL-TFE3, are associated with a subset of renal cell carcinoma that tends to affect younger patients. t(6;11) affects a gene similar to the TFE3 gene and the tumors behave in a similar fashion to the TFE3 translocation-associated tumors.

QCCP2, **Renal cell carcinoma,** p 399

52. C. **GOOD RESPONSE TO ADRIAMYCIN-BASED CHEMOTHERAPY.**

All of the other responses are the opposite of the way that HER2+ breast cancer behaves.

QCCP2, **Breast carcinoma,** p 399

53. B. **INCREASED GENE EXPRESSION DUE TO GENE AMPLIFICATION.**

Additional copies of the gene are made in HER2+ tumors. This is the basis of the HER2 FISH analysis, where the ratio of HER2 signals is expressed as a ratio to the chromosome 17 enumeration probe.

QCCP2, **Breast carcinoma,** p 399

54. B. **1P, 19Q.**

I don't care how you do it, but burn those two loci into your brain (so to speak). The combined loss of 1p and 19q is 60-80% sensitive for oligodendroglioma and much more specific, making the combination an excellent marker to distinguish an oligodendroglioma from any other similar tumor.

QCCP2, **Gliomas,** p 400

55. E. **LOSS OF 1P AND 19Q.**

Again, there it is. While this combination is associated with a relatively good prognosis, all the other choices presented are associated with worse prognoses.

QCCP2, **Gliomas,** p 400

56. B. **POINT MUTATIONS OF RETINOBLASTOMA GENE.**

The majority (~70%) of the disease-associated mutations in the Rb gene are due to point mutations.

QCCP2, **Retinoblastoma,** p 400

7: Molecular Methods Answers

57.   D.   **MENINGIOMA.**

Unlike NF2, there is no significant association between meningiomas and Rb.
QCCP2, **Meningioma**, p 400

58.   A.   **MERLIN, CELL-CELL CONTACT AND CELL CONTACT INHIBITION.**

Merlin is encoded by the NF2 gene located on chromosome 22q12.2 and functions as a mediator of cell contact. CD44 is the ligand that binds to merlin and may modulate cell growth.
QCCP2, **Meningioma**, p 400

59.   A.   **MENINGOTHELIAL.**

Clear cell and chordoid subtypes, as well as atypical meningiomas are considered WHO Grade II tumors. Atypical meningioma is defined as any WHO Grade I subtype meningioma with atypical features, such as greater than 4 mitotic figures per 10 HPF, brain invasion, or 3 or more of the following: increased cellularity, small cells with increased nuclear:cytoplasmic ratio, prominent nucleoli, sheet-like growth, and spontaneous or geographic necrosis. Anaplastic features, such as frank malignancy resembling sarcoma, melanoma, or carcinoma, or greater than 20 mitotic figures per 10 HPF, are consistent with a WHO Grade III tumor. In addition the rhabdoid and papillary subtypes of meningioma are considered WHO Grade III.
QCCP2, **Meningioma**, p 401

60.   E.   **T(12;22).**

The translocation most commonly associated with Ewing sarcoma is t(11;22)(q24;a12). This translocation in Ewing sarcoma leads to the formation of an EWS-FLI1 fusion protein. This should not be confused with the predominant translocation in desmoplastic small round cell tumor, t(11;22) (p13;q12), which leads to an EWS-WT1 fusion protein. t(21;22) results in a EWS-ERG fusion protein, while t(12;22) is not associated with Ewing sarcoma, but rather, the EWS-ATF1 fusion protein that results is associated with clear cell sarcoma (malignant melanoma of soft parts).
QCCP2, **Ewing/PNET**, p 401

61.   C.   **AMPLIFICATION.**

Double minutes and homogeneously-stained regions are examples of amplification that can be seen in some cases of neuroblastoma. In general, the amplification results in greater than 10-fold more protein.
QCCP2, **Neuroblastoma**, p 401

62.   D.   **A & B.**

A large germline deletion in chromosome 11p13, spanning the coding region for PAX6 - the loss of which can lead to aniridia and WT1, which causes the Wilms' tumor feature -is responsible for WAGR syndrome. Similar mutations of WT1 can also lead to Denys-Drash syndrome, which is characterized by Wilms tumor, nephropathy, and either true or pseudo hermaphroditism.
QCCP2, **Wilms tumor**, p 402

7: Molecular Methods Answers

63.   A.   **Wilms tumor.**

       D.   **hepatoblastoma.**

       Beckwith-Weidemann syndrome is associated with a protean array of features as well as a complex set of defects leading to aberrant transcription of genes at 11p15.5. Among the features of BWS is an increased risk of Wilms tumor and hepatoblastoma.
       QCCP2, **Wilms tumor,** p 402

64.   C.   **alveolar.**

       The translocation t(2;13)(q35;q14) leads to a fusion protein of PAX3 and FKHR (forkhead). A smaller percentage of cases harbor the t(1;13) PAX7-FKHR translocation. Both translocations juxtapose the DNA-binding domain of PAX with the transcriptional activation domain of FKHR.
       QCCP2, **Rhabdomyosarcoma,** p 402

65.   C.   **SYT-SSX2 is associated with monophasic synovial sarcoma.**

       Several reports have shown that SYT-SSX2 fusions are more commonly seen in monophasic synovial sarcomas and SYT-SSX1 fusions are more commonly seen in biphasic synovial sarcomas.
       QCCP2, **Synovial sarcoma,** p 402

66.   C.   **sickle cell anemia.**

       Alpha-thalassemia is most commonly attributed to deletion mutations of the alpha-globin gene, while beta-thalassemia is usually due to point mutations in the beta-globin gene. Beta-thalassemia, however, unlike sickle cell anemia, is caused by one of a number of different mutations (over 200 published). Sickle cell anemia for the most part is due to a single reproducible point mutation in the beta-globin gene.
       QCCP2, **Diagnosis of Mendelian disorders,** p 402

67.   B.   **AFP (alpha-fetoprotein) levels.**

       AFP levels in pregnancy can be measured in maternal serum (MSAFP) as part of the so-called triple or quadruple tests. AFP can also be measured in amniotic fluid. In order to sample amniotic fluid, the chorioamniotic membranes must be violated, something which chorionic villi sampling does not do. A high level of amniotic AFP is associated with an open neural tube or abdominal wall defect. Below-normal levels of AFP have been demonstrated in patients with trisomy 18 (Edwards syndrome) and trisomy 21 (Down syndrome).
       QCCP2, **Prenatal diagnosis, samples,** p 404

68.   E.   **all of the above have been used for fetal diagnosis.**

       All of the specimens mentioned have been used for prenatal diagnosis. Each has its own inherent limitations. Collecting umbilical cord blood has a relatively high risk of fetal loss and maternal blood contamination. Cystic hygromal fluid can only be used in fetuses with a cystic hygroma. Fetal vesical urine collection increases the risk of oligohydramnios. Fetal skin biopsies are best suited for the diagnosis of a primary skin disease, but can also be used to diagnose systemic disease.
       QCCP2, **Prenatal diagnosis, samples,** p 404

7: Molecular Methods Answers

69. A. **ADVANCED MATERNAL AGE.**

The overall incidence of genetic disease sharply increases after age 35. Beyond age 35 is considered advanced maternal age. The risk of Down syndrome in a 35 year old mother is ~1:270. Invasive screening beyond the standard triple or quadruple maternal serum test is offered for any mother over 35 years or with any predisposition that increases the risks to those of a mother 35 years or older.

QCCP2, **Prenatal diagnosis, indications**, p 404

70. B. **1.**

In addition to being the most common causes of spontaneous abortions, aneuploidies of all of the remaining chromosomes are associated with live birth syndromes - trisomy 21 with Down syndrome, trisomy 13 with Patau syndrome, trisomy 18 with Edwards syndrome, and monosomy X with Turner syndrome. Perhaps due to the size of the chromosome and the number of genes encoded on the large chromosomes, there are almost never live births with aneuploidies of the first dozen chromosomes.

QCCP2, **Prenatal diagnosis, indications**, p 405

71. B. **MUTATIONS IN LIPOPROTEIN L GENE.**

There is no known association between LPL and Alzheimer disease. Mutations in genes encoding pre-senilin proteins (*PSEN1, PSEN2*) and the gene encoding amyloid beta A4 protein (APP) have been associated with cases of early onset familial Alzheimer disease. Patients with Down syndrome account for approximately 1% of cases of Alzheimer disease, while alleles of ApoE4 are usually associated with usual late-onset Alzheimer disease.

QCCP2, **Neurologic and muscular diseases**, p 405

72. C. **TRINUCLEOTIDE REPEAT EXPANSION.**

Huntington disease is a classic example of a mutation due to expansion of a trinucleotide repeat, CAG in this case. Other examples of diseases caused by trinucleotide repeats include Fragile X syndrome and some types of myotonic dystrophy. The gene associated with Huntington disease is located near the telomere of the short arm of chromosome 4. Normal (unaffected non-carrier) individuals usually have more than 26 CAG repeats, carriers have between 26 and 36, while those with more 36 than repeats typically manifest symptoms. Huntington disease exhibits the phenomenon of anticipation, where subsequent generations develop a greater number of repeats and with that the earlier onset of disease.

QCCP2, **Huntington disease**, p 406

73. A. *NOTCH3.*

There is a very strong association between mutations of *NOTCH3* on chromosome 19p and the dementing disease, CADASIL. The findings of multiple lacunar infarctions at the gray-white border as well as eosinophilic granular deposits in the blood vessels of the white matter and basal ganglia.

QCCP2, **CADASIL**, p 406

74. B. **PERIPHERAL RBC ACANTHOCYTOSIS, DECREASED KELL ANTIGEN, BASAL GANGLIA DYSFUNCTION.**

McLeod syndrome is an X-linked recessive condition primarily affecting young males where the Kx antigen is not expressed on the red blood cells. This leads to the so-called McLeod RBC phenotype, where there is decreased Kell antigen expression. In addition, individuals with McLeod syndrome can have skeletal or cardiac myopathy. Choice A describes May-Hegglin, C describes Charcot-Marie-Tooth syndrome, D is Parkinson disease, and E is Wiskott-Aldrich.

QCCP2, **McLeod syndrome**, p 406

7: Molecular Methods Answers

75.   A.   **CMT1.**

There are only two types of Charcot-Marie-Tooth; selections C and D don't exist. Hallervorden-Spatz is a separate entity, also known as pantothenate kinase-associated neurodegeneration unrelated to CMT.
QCCP2, **Charcot-Marie-Tooth disease**, p 406

76.   D.   **TRANSTHYRETIN.**

TTR gene encodes transthyretin and is found on the long arm of chromosome 18. There are several defined patient mutations which account for the majority of cases. Interestingly, there are several geographic regions which exhibit a very high incidence, particularly northern Portugal, where the frequency of familial amyloidosis is 1:500.
QCCP2, **Familial amyloidosis**, p 407

77.   D.   **A & B.**

Both Becker and Duchenne muscular dystrophy are due to mutations in the *DMD* gene, which encodes the protein dystrophin. Becker tends to present later (early 20s) with less severe weakness than Duchenne, which presents in early childhood with the characteristic symmetric proximal limb weakness.
QCCP2, **Dystrophin muscular dystrophies**, p 407

78.   E.   **ALL OF THE ABOVE.**

The majority (~65%) of dystrophinopathies can be diagnosed with multiplex PCR and a small (5%) can be diagnosed with Southern blot or quantitative PCR. Most of the remaining cases (30-35%) can be diagnosed by direct sequencing.
QCCP2, **Dystrophin muscular dystrophies**, p 408

79.   C.   **FREEZING OF TISSUE.**

The skeletal muscle cells of inclusion body myositis demonstrate the basophilic granular rimmed vacuoles on FROZEN tissue. If the tissue is fixed in formalin or gluteraldehyde, the rimmed vacuoles are not apparent.
QCCP2, **Inclusion body myositis**, p 408

80.   E.   **HUNTINGTON DISEASE.**

Steinert disease, like Huntington disease, is a trinucleotide repeat disease. As such, the expansion of repeats, CTG in the case of Steinert disease, is associated with symptomatology. As it is a trinucleotide repeat disease, there is also anticipation. (see question 72.)
QCCP2, **Myotonic muscular dystrophy**, p 408

81.   A.   *RYR1* **CALCIUM CHANNEL.**

Don't let all the giant biochemical compounds scare you! Malignant hyperthermia and all its attendant signs and symptoms are due to lactic acidosis from increased anaerobic metabolism secondary to inappropriate release of calcium for the sarcoplasmic reticulum. The cause? A defective calcium channel.
QCCP2, **Malignant hypothermia**, p 409

7: Molecular Methods Answers

82. E.   **ALL OF THE ABOVE.**

Brugada syndrome has manifold features. Some of the cases have been associated with a mutation in the gene, *SCN5A*, which encodes the alpha subunit of a sodium channel. It is most common in S.E. Asia.
QCCP2, **Brugada syndrome,** p 409

83. D.   **SENSORINEURAL HEARING LOSS.**

Both are types of long QT syndrome. While Romano-Wood is autosomal dominant, Jervell and Lange-Nielsen are autosomal recessive and in addition to prolonged QT demonstrate sensorineural hearing loss.
QCCP2, **Long QT syndromes,** p 410

84. E.   **MICROVESICULAR STEATOSIS.**

Medium-chain-acyl-coenzyme A dehydrogenase (MCAD) is one member of a family of disorders of fatty acid oxidation along with respiratory chain disorders and carnitine transport disorders. They may account for a number of cases of pediatric microvesicular steatosis that were previously diagnosed as Reye syndrome.
QCCP2, **Medium-chain acyl-coenzyme A dehydrogenase (MCAD) deficiency,** p 410

85. B.   **TANDEM MASS SPECTROPHOTOMETRIC ACYLCARNITINES IN BLOOD.**

Since children who have early detection and appropriate frequent feeding (to avoid the hypoglycemia) have an excellent prognosis, the optimal testing clinically is neonatal screening. The detection of acylcarnitines is the screening test of choice.
QCCP2, **Medium-chain acyl-coenzyme A dehydrogenase (MCAD) deficiency,** p 410

86. B.   **1/20.**

Cystic fibrosis is the most common autosomal recessive disease affecting Caucasians. The incidence of disease in that population is 1:2000 live births, compared to the 10-fold lower incidence in the African-American population. Based on the autosomal recessive nature of the disease, the high incidence of disease and carrier frequency explains the gene frequency of 1/20.
QCCP2, **Cystic fibrosis,** p 411

87. E.   **ALL OF THE ABOVE ARE SYMPTOMS ASSOCIATED WITH CYSTIC FIBROSIS.**

Cystic fibrosis has a wide and varied array of symptoms due to the multisystem nature of the disease. Interestingly, some males present with isolated azoospermia due to the congenital bilateral absence of the vasa deferentia.
QCCP2, **Cystic fibrosis,** p 411

88. B.   **DELTAF508.**

By far the most common mutation of the CFTR that is associated with disease is the delta F508. The mutation is an inframe trinucleotide deletion that results in the loss of phenylalanine at codon 508. The second most common mutation is the G542X. In the Ashkenazi Jewish population, the W1282X is the most common. However, overall these cases represent only a small percentage of the total cases.
QCCP2, **Cystic fibrosis,** p 411

7: Molecular Methods Answers

89. C. **ELEVATED IMMUNOREACTIVE TRYPSINOGEN.**

The preferred newborn screening exam is the presence of elevated immunoreactive trypsinogen in blood spots. A positive test is confirmed by one of the other testing modalities mentioned (A, B, D). Waiting for symptoms to appear is a terrible way to screen for disease.
QCCP2, **Cystic fibrosis,** p 411

90. E. **ASIAN-AMERICANS.**

The choices are written in order of frequency, with Northern Europeans having the highest (1:200-1:300 in the U.S.) and the lowest frequency in the Asian-American population, where the frequency is <1/1000000.
QCCP2, **Cystic fibrosis,** p 412

91. D. **A & B.**

While the point mutation C282Y accounts for the majority of cases due to a single mutation, those with the single mutation and compound heterozygotes of C282Y and H63D account for by far most of the cases.
QCCP2, **Hereditary hemochromatosis,** p 412

92. C. *ATP7B.*

While the typical screening test for Wilson disease is a decreased serum ceruloplasmin, the actual gene mutated is the copper transporter, ATP7B.
QCCP2, **Wilson disease (hepatolenticular degeneration),** p 413

93. A. **DIABETES.**

Diabetes is not commonly associated with Wilson disease as it is with hemochromatosis. Liver disease can manifest as hepatitis and progress to fibrosis/cirrhosis. The Kayser-Fleischer iris pigmentation rings often accompany neuropsychiatric symptoms. In addition, there is often a nonimmune hemolytic anemia.
QCCP2, **Wilson disease,** p 413

94. C. **PIZZ.**

There are nearly one hundred alleles of the Pi gene. Of them, homozygosity for the Z allele is most commonly associated with clinical alpha-1-antitrypsin deficiency. The only other allele associated with disease is the S allele, especially when seen as a SZ heterozygote.
QCCP2, **Alpha-1-antitrypsin (AAT) deficiency,** p 414

95. C. **PULMONARY.**

D. **HEPATIC.**

Pan-acinar emphysema with a predilection for the lung bases is the most common pulmonary presentation. In the liver, there is typically neonatal hepatitis that can develop into cirrhosis and hepatocellular carcinoma.
QCCP2, **Alpha-1-antitrypsin (AAT) deficiency,** p 414

96.　A.　DECREASED ALPHA 1 REGION.

Honestly. The name of the disease practically gives it away - alpha-1-antitrypsin deficiency. Choice B could refer to a number of things, such as decreased haptoglobin (intravascular hemolysis) or decreased ceruloplasmin (Wilson disease). C describes a common finding in chronic inflammation. D describes agammaglobulinemia and E describes a potential monoclonal gammopathy.

QCCP2, **Alpha-1-antitrypsin (AAT) deficiency,** p 414

97.　E.　**A, B, C.**

Patients with Alagille syndrome usually have a triangular-shaped face, butterfly or non-fused vertebrae, cardiac defects, and the characteristic disappearing bile ducts where there is a normal number at birth which progressively diminishes, resulting in an increased portal tracts to bile duct ratio.

QCCP2, **Alagille syndrome,** p 414

98.　B.　*JAG1.*

Almost all cases of Alagille syndrome are associated with mutations of *JAG1*. *NOTCH2* mutations account for a small proportion of cases (*JAG1* encodes the NOTCH ligand). *NOTCH1* mutations are found in some cases of T-cell acute lymphocytic leukemia, while mutations of *NOTCH3* are associated with CADASIL (cerebral autosomal dominant arteriopathy with subcortical infarctions and leukoencephalopathy).

QCCP2, **Alagille syndrome,** p 415

99.　A.　SHORT SEGMENT AGANGLIOSIS.

Long segment and total colonic agangliosis have an equal frequency in males and females. Short segment, however, is four times more commonly seen in males than in females.

QCCP2, **Hirschprung disease,** p 415

100.　E.　ALL OF THE ABOVE ARE ASSOCIATED WITH HIRSCHPRUNG DISEASE.

Hirschprung disease is associated with a number of genes and syndromes, including Waardenburg syndrome, Haddad syndrome, and Riley-Day syndrome, in addition to the syndromes mentioned as choices in the question.

QCCP2, **Hirschprung disease,** p 415

101.　C.　21-HYDROXYLASE.

While deficiencies of all the enzymes mentioned are associated with congenital adrenal hyperplasia, the most common by far (~90% of cases) is 21-hydroxylase deficiency. As a result of the enzyme deficiency, a precursor, 17-hydroxyprogesterone (17-OHP), accumulates. Measurement of 17-OHP in dried blood spots is the preferred screening tool.

QCCP2, **Congenital adrenal hyperplasia,** p 415

102.　C.　ANDROGEN RECEPTOR, X CHROMOSOME.

The presentation of a genotypic male with external female genitalia suggests androgen insensitivity, an X-linked recessive condition (makes sense, doesn't it?). There are a variety of androgen insensitivity phenotypes, ranging from complete insensitivity with external female genitalia and a 46,XY karyotype to infertility in an adult male. The defect is due to the inability of the androgen receptor to respond to testosterone.

QCCP2, **Androgen insensitivity syndrome (testicular feminization),** p 416

7: Molecular Methods Answers

103. C. **COLLAGEN, TYPE IV.**

Alport syndrome most commonly is inherited as an X-linked recessive disease and, as such, primarily affects males with sensorineural hearing loss, glomerulonephritis, and ocular lesions. Three genes have been identified as being involved with this family of diseases. One, *COL4A5*, encodes the alpha 5 chain of type IV collagen and is the cause of Alport syndrome.

QCCP2, **Inherited nephritic syndromes (collagen IV-related nephropathies),** p 416

104. D. *PKHD1.*

Mutations in the *NPHP1* gene are associated with juvenile-onset nephronophthsis. *PKD1* and *PKD2* mutations are seen in autosomal dominant polycystic kidney disease. *PKHD1*, or polycystic kidney and hepatic disease gene 1, is located on chromosome 6p12 and encodes a protein of uncertain function, polycystin.

QCCP2, **Inherited polycystic kidney diseases,** p 416

105. E. **NONE OF THE ABOVE.**

Actually, cystic renal dysplasia is non-Mendelian and sporadic. It may be reactive in response to ureteral obstruction - similar to the reactive condition, nephrogenic adenoma.

QCCP2, **Cystic renal dysplasia,** p 417

106. A. **EXTRARENAL ANOMALIES.**

Juvenile-onset nephronophthsis is an autosomal recessive mutation in *NPHP1* and is associated with cortical cysts with occasional extrarenal manifestations, such as hepatic fibrosis and retinal degeneration. The adult forms are associated with mutations in different genes, *NPHP1* and *NPHP2*. While the renal symptoms of adult-onset nephronophthsis are the same as the juvenile form, there is generally an absence of extrarenal disease.

QCCP2, **Nephronophthsis,** p 417

107. B. **HYPERTENSION.**

While all of the choices are associated with ADPKD, hypertension is seen in almost all cases and is often the presenting symptom. Of the remaining choices, liver cysts are seen in almost 3/4 of cases. Renal stones, Berry aneurysms, and mitral valve prolapse are seen in 20-25% of patients.

QCCP2, **Autosomal dominant polycystic kidney disease (ADPKD),** p 417

108. E. *PKD1/TSC2.*

PKD1 and *TSC2* are located immediately adjacent to each other on chromosome 16p13. The majority of cases of autosomal dominant polycystic kidney disease are associated with mutations of *PKD1* (85%). Of these, a small percentage has symptoms that overlap with tuberous sclerosis. The majority of cases of tuberous sclerosis are due to mutations of *TSC2* (80-90%).

QCCP2, **Autosomal dominant polycystic kidney disease (ADPKD),** p 417

109. C. **X-LINKED RECESSIVE.**

While the vast majority of metabolic diseases are inherited in an autosomal recessive fashion, there are at least three notable exceptions - Fabry, Hunter, and Lesch-Nyhan diseases.

QCCP2, **Metabolic diseases,** p 417

110. B. **PHENYLKETONURIA.**

   E. **CONGENITAL HYPOTHYROIDISM.**

   Galactosemia and sickle cell disease are the second most widely screened diseases. Many, many other diseases are screened, but these vary from state to state.
   QCCP2, **Metabolic diseases,** p 417

111. B. **EARLY CHILDHOOD.**

   D. **PREGNANCY.**

   The morbidities associated with elevated phenylalanine include mental retardation and seizures. Removing phenylalanine from the diet of very young affected children can ameliorate many of the sequelae. After early childhood, tight phenylalanine control is not as critical. There is one notable exception - the offspring of affected pregnant women with poor control can be subject to a number of problems, even if the child is not phenylalanine hydroxylase deficient.
   QCCP2, **Phenylketonuria (PKU),** p 418

112. B. *E. COLI* **SEPSIS.**

   Especially in the neonatal period, children with galactosemia are at a higher than normal risk for *E. coli* sepsis. Some of the other infections mentioned in the question are associated with other predisposing conditions - cryptococcal meningitis is a common opportunistic infection in patients with AIDS, *Burkholderia* pneumonia is most commonly seen in patients with cystic fibrosis, subacute bacterial endocarditis is seen in patients with damaged heart valves or patients with high levels of bacteremia, and finally, *Actinomyces* cervicitis is most commonly associated with IUD use.
   QCCP2, **Galactosemia,** p 418

113. D. **HEXOSAMINIDASE A.**

   Choice A is the enzyme deficient in galactosemia (GALacTosemia), while E is deficient in Gaucher disease. In patients affected by Tay-Sachs, glycosphingolipids accumulate in the lysosomes. Choice B, Tay-saccharidase I is something I made up because I like the sound of it. One way to remember that hexosaminidase is deficient in Tay-Sachs is to pronounce the disease, "Tay-Sex" (sex = hex).
   QCCP2, **Tay-Sachs disease (GM2 gangliosidosis),** p 418

114. A. **GAUCHER DISEASE.**

   Classic Zellweger with the dysmorphic features and multiple biochemical anomalies presents earlier than neonatal adrenoleukodystrophy or Refsum disease and is more severe. The characteristic facial features of Zellweger (flattened facies with large fontanelle and broad nasal bridge) are also not present with the other very long chain fatty acid syndromes. A helpful memory aid for Zellweger syndrome is to think of Renee Zellweger, the actress, as a peroxide blonde - Zellweger is due to a peroxisomal defect. Alternatively, imagine her hanging on a very long chain with a football referee (Refsum and Zellweger are diseases due to accumulation of very long chain fatty acids).
   QCCP2, **Zellweger syndrome, Gaucher disease,** p 418

115. E. **GLUCOCEREBROSIDASE.**

The gene encoding the enzyme, glucocerebrosidase *GBA* is located on chromosome 1q. Both Gaucher and glucocerebrosidase have a G and U at the beginning of the word.
QCCP2, **Gaucher disease,** p 418-419

116. E. **A, B, C.**

There are number of diseases lumped under the rubric "organic acidemias," such as maple syrup urine disease and the urea cycle disorders. They are all autosomal recessive disorders that share hyperammonemia in common. As ammonia accumulates, symptoms such as vomiting, lethargy, and neurological deterioration appear.
QCCP2, **Organic acidemias and urea cycle disorders,** p 419

117. B. **HURLER DISEASE.**

Hurler and Hunter disease are mucopolysaccharidoses, characterized by the accumulation of mucopolysaccharides, such as dermatan, heparan, keratan, or chondroitin sulfate. The accumulations can occur in a number of places, especially the spleen, liver, heart, and brain. This sphingolipidoses have accumulations of glycolipids, such as sphingomyelin, gangliosides, or glucocerebrosides.
QCCP2, **Inherited Metabolic Disorders,** p 420, **T7.10**

118. C. **LESCH-NYHAN DISEASE.**

A fairly memorable presentation, Lesch-Nyhan is due to hyperuricemia as a result of a defect in the X-linked gene, hypoxanthine guanine phosphoribosyl transferase (HGPRT). HGPRT is a critical enzyme in the purine salvage biosynthetic pathway. A deficiency of HGPRT leads to overproduction of urate.
QCCP2, **Lesch-Nyhan syndrome,** p 421

119. D. **ALPHA-GALACTOSIDASE.**

Fabry disease is an X-linked recessive condition caused by a mutation in the gene encoding alpha-galactosidase. The manifestations of the disease include distal extremity pain, angiokeratomas, hypohydrosis, corneal opacities, renal failure, cardiovascular or cerebrovascular disease, all due to accumulation of globotriaosylceramide.
QCCP2, **Fabry disease,** p 421

120. A. **CYSTINURIA.**

The characteristic crystals of cystinuria are not only evident in the urine but can also be often visualized by slit lamp illumination of the cornea. The *CTNS* gene on chromosome 17p13 is mutated in cystinuria.
QCCP2, **Cystinosis,** p 421

121. D. **TRISOMY 21.**

Monosomy X (45, X or Turner syndrome), triploidy, and trisomy 16 are more commonly associated with spontaneous abortions (especially trisomy 16, which is the most common mutation seen in spontaneous abortions). Trisomy 18 causes Edwards syndrome and is associated with live births, but is nowhere nearly as common as trisomy 21.
QCCP2, **Structural and numerical chromosomal disorders,** p 421

122. B. **MOTHERS <35 YEARS OLD.**

A little tricky, I admit. While the risk of Down syndrome increases with maternal age from 1/725 for a 32 year-old mother to 1/365 for a 35 year-old mother, a greater number of children are born to women less than 35 years old. As a matter of fact, more than 80% of cases of Down syndrome are in babies born to women less than 35 years old. Paternal age as a risk factor for Down syndrome is controversial, with some large studies showing no correlation while a few small studies have shown a significant effect.

QCCP2, **Down syndrome,** p 421

123. A. **SPONTANEOUS ABORTION.**

45, X is one of the most common abnormalities in spontaneous abortions, with 99% of 45, X conceptuses spontaneously aborting. Those that do live are affected by Turner syndrome and usually live to adulthood.

QCCP2, **Turner syndrome,** p 421

124. D. **NOONAN SYNDROME.**

Superficially, both Noonan and Turner syndromes appear similar - wide-spaced nipples, webbed neck, and short stature. Noonan syndrome is autosomal dominant and linked to mutations in the genes *PTPN11* on chromosome 12q and *KRAS* on 12p.

QCCP2, **Noonan syndrome,** p 422

125. A. **MICRODELETION IN PATERNAL 15Q11.2.**

C. **UNIPARENTAL (MATERNAL) DISOMY.**

Prader-Willi and Angelman syndrome are genotypically, though not phenotypically, related entities caused by microdeletions or inactivations in the same region of chromosome 15q11.2. The difference is that Prader-Willi is due to a loss of paternal activity and Angelman is due to a loss of maternal activity ("Daddy's little angel"). Therefore, loss of parental DNA leads to Prader-Willi.

QCCP2, **Angelman syndrome and Prader-Willi syndrome,** p 422

126. B. **BLOOM SYNDROME.**

Huntington disease is a CAG repeat disorder, Fragile X is a CGG repeat disorder, Friedreich ataxia is a GAA repeat disorder. For each of these disorders, the expansion leads to chromosome instability *in vitro*. The *in vivo* effect of expansion may be due to increased silencing of the involved gene secondary to increased methylation. Of the three disorders, only Friedreich ataxia does not exhibit anticipation!

QCCP2, **Friedreich ataxia,** p 423

127. A. **FRIEDREICH ATAXIA.**

Both xeroderma pigmentosa and Bloom syndrome patients are at risk for cutaneous neoplasms in sun-exposed skin, while patients with ataxia telangiectasia are subject to ionizing radiation and develop hematolymphoid malignancies.

QCCP2, **Friedreich ataxia, xeroderma pigmentosa, Bloom syndrome, ataxia telangiectasia,** p 424

7: Molecular Methods Answers

128. **B. FANCONI ANEMIA.**

   Among the distinctive features of Fanconi anemia, aplastic anemia and forearm malformations, there is also short stature, café au lait spots, an increased risk of malignancy, ocular and renal anomalies, and sensorineural hearing loss. Multiple genes are involved and the cytogenetic assay shows increased chromosome breakage.
   QCCP2, **Fanconi anemia,** p 424-425

129. **FALSE.**

   While mitochondrial disease is due to mutations in mitochondrial proteins, not all mitochondrial proteins are encoded by mitochondrial genes. There are a significant number of mitochondrial proteins that are encoded by nuclear genes.
   QCCP2, **Mitochondrial disease,** p 425

130. **B. HETEROPLASMY.**

   A cell will typically contain a single clonal population of mitochondria, a state known as homoplasmy. Cells affected by mitochondrial disease may contain more than one clone, a condition called heteroplasmy. Variations in the population of normal mitochondria and abnormal mitochondria may account for the differences.
   QCCP2, **Mitochondrial disease,** p 425

131. **E. NIJMEGEN BREAKAGE SYNDROME.**

   Mitochondrial disease tends to manifest at an early age, childhood to early adulthood with the mutations in nuclear genes presenting earliest, mitochondrial genes later. There is usually neuromuscular involvement. The typical muscle biopsy feature is the "ragged red fiber" seen on Gomori trichrome staining.
   QCCP2, **Nijmegen breakage syndrome, Mitochondrial disease,** p 425

Chapter 8

Laboratory Statistics and Quality Control

1. In a normal Gaussian distribution, what percentage of the population falls between -2 and +2 standard deviations?
   A. 68%
   B. 90%
   C. 95.5%
   D. 99.7%
   E. 99.9%

2. Which term describes the most frequently occurring variable in a range of values?
   A. mean
   B. standard deviation
   C. median
   D. mode
   E. accuracy

3. Which of the following equations best describes the coefficient of variation?
   A. $\sum x_i/n$
   B. $\sum (x_i\text{-mean})^2/(n\text{-}1)$
   C. true positives/(true positives - false negatives)
   D. standard deviation/mean $\times$ 100
   E. true positives/(true positives + false positives)

4. Which of the following are affected by pre-test probability? (you can choose more than one)
   A. sensitivity
   B. specificity
   C. positive predictive value
   D. negative predictive value
   E. relative risk

5. Which equation best describes sensitivity?
   A. true positives divided by the sum of true positives plus false negatives
   B. true negatives divided by the sum of true negatives plus false positives
   C. true positives divided by the sum of true positives plus false positives
   D. true negatives divided by the sum of true negatives plus false negatives
   E. none of the above

6. What is the purpose of a receiver operating characteristic (ROC) curve?
   A. to graphically determine the positive predictive value of a given test
   B. to calculate the standard deviation of a set of values
   C. to determine the prevalence of a particular condition
   D. to measure the ability of a test to perform reliably
   E. to determine the performance characteristics of a test at different cut-off values

7. What is the most standardized definition of the reference interval for a test?
   A. +/- 1 SD of the mean
   B. +/- 2 SD of the mean
   C. +/- 3 SD of the mean
   D. sensitivity divided by specificity
   E. a value calculated from the ROC curve

8. All of the following are categories of CLIA-regulated lab tests, <u>except</u>:
   A. waived tests
   B. provider-performed microscopy
   C. low complexity testing
   D. moderate complexity testing
   E. high complexity testing

9. What is the purpose of a Levey-Jennings curve?
   A. to calculate the mean of a new control sample
   B. to calculate the standard deviation of a new control sample
   C. to determine "in control" and "out of control" runs
   D. all of the above
   E. none of the above

10. All of the following are shorthand for Westgard rules, <u>except</u>:
    A. 1:3s rule
    B. 2:2s rule
    C. R:4s rule
    D. 4:1s rule
    E. 10:10s rule

11. Which of the Westgard rules are most sensitive to random error (pick two)?
    A. 1:3s rule
    B. 2:2s rule
    C. R:4s rule
    D. 4:1s rule
    E. 10:10s rule

12. Who is the final approving agency for proficiency testing as mandated by CLIA '88?
    A. College of American Pathologists
    B. Food and Drug Administration
    C. American Society for Clinical Pathology
    D. Department of Health and Human Services
    E. American Association of Blood Banks

13. All the following are considered in calculating the standard deviation index that the College of American Pathologists uses for grading proficiency testing, <u>except</u>:
    A. lab test result
    B. lab reference intervals
    C. mean for peer group
    D. standard deviation for peer group
    E. all of the above are used to calculate the standard deviation index

8: Laboratory Statistics and Quality Control Questions

14. Different kinds of bias are revealed with a correlation study. Which kind of bias is a cause of systemic variability?
    A. constant (offset) bias
    B. analytical bias
    C. proportional bias
    D. all of the above
    E. none of the above

15. All of the following are examples of tests where the analytical sensitivity of the test is extremely important, <u>except</u>:
    A. troponin
    B. D-dimer
    C. microalbumin
    D. human chorionic gonadotropin
    E. all of the above are tests where analytical sensitivity is very important

16. Which of the following scenarios poses the greatest risk of non-linearity?
    A. samples with low analyte concentration
    B. samples with high analyte concentration
    C. mixed samples of several weak analytes
    D. contaminated samples
    E. none of the above

17. Which of the following techniques is useful in avoiding heterophile antibody interference in an assay?
    A. serial sample dilution
    B. removal of immunoglobulins from a sample with polyethylene glycol
    C. assay antibody modification
    D. the use of specialized buffers
    E. all of the above

18. All of the following often increase with changes in posture from supine to sitting, <u>except</u>:
    A. electrolytes
    B. proteins
    C. substances largely bound to proteins
    D. formed elements, such as red blood cells
    E. none of the above change in concentration with changes in posture

19. Which tube top color and additive are usually used for coagulation testing?
    A. red, none
    B. green, heparin
    C. blue, citrate
    D. black, buffered sodium citrate
    E. lavender, EDTA

20. Which phase(s) of testing account for the great majority of laboratory errors?
    A. preanalytic
    B. analytic
    C. postanalytic
    D. A & B
    E. A & C

8: Laboratory Statistics and Quality Control Questions

21. Which of the following is typically NOT used in the calculation of the corrected (platelet) count increment?
     A. pre-transfusion platelet count
     B. post-transfusion platelet count
     C. patient gender
     D. body surface area
     E. number of units of platelets given

22. What is the osmolal gap in a patient with a measured osmolarity of 311 mOsm/L, a sodium of 140, glucose of 180, and a blood urea nitrogen of 2.8?
     A. 10
     B. 20
     C. 100
     D. 200
     E. 0

23. Which of the following is the correct Friedewald equation?
     A. percent fetal cells × maternal blood volume = volume of fetal blood cells in maternal circulation
     B. CCI = ([post-pre] × BSA)/# of units
     C. pH = pKa + log ([base]/[acid])
     D. CV = SD/mean × 100
     E. LDL = total cholesterol - HDL - TG/5

8: Laboratory Statistics and Quality Control Answers

1. C. **95.5%.**

    For an ideal Gaussian distribution, the population is evenly distributed in a bell curve centered on the mean or mathematical average. That is, one half of the values are above the center and one half below, with the greatest frequency occurring at the mean. The standard deviation is the average distance of any value from the mean. In a Gaussian distribution, 68% of values lie between -1 and +1 standard deviation of the mean, 95.5% of values between -2 and +2 standard deviations, and 99.7% between -3 and +3 standard deviations.
    QCCP2, **Gaussian distribution**, p 438

2. D. **MODE.**

    Mean, median, and mode are three statistical terms that often pepper the conversation in a discussion of the distribution of values in a Gaussian population. Mean is the arithmetic average of all the values - simply add up all the values and divide by the number of values. Median is the middle value among all values. The mode is the most commonly occurring value. In a standard Gaussian distribution, the mean, median, and mode are all equal. In cases of skew, the mean, median, and mode may be different.
    QCCP2, **Mean and standard deviation, Median, Mode**, p 438

3. D. **STANDARD DEVIATION/MEAN $\times$ 100.**

    When discussing test results, the concepts of accuracy and precision are frequently encountered and are often confused. Accuracy refers to how close a particular value is to a gold standard reference value. Precision, however, is a description of how reproducible a particular result is. Precision can be mathematically expressed with the coefficient of variation, which compares the deviation from the mean to the mean value, expressed as a percentage. $CV = SD/mean \times 100$.
    QCCP2, **Precision**, p 438

4. C. **POSITIVE PREDICTIVE VALUE, D. NEGATIVE PREDICTIVE VALUE, E. RELATIVE RISK.**

    Pretest probability is a function of the prevalence of a condition. When prevalence is high, the positive predictive value of a test is also usually high, while the negative predictive value is low. When the prevalence of a disease is low, the opposite occurs - low PPV, high NPV. The relative risk is also affected by prevalence in a similar fashion.
    QCCP2, **PPV, Relative risk**, p 439

5. A. **TRUE POSITIVES DIVIDED BY THE SUM OF TRUE POSITIVES PLUS FALSE NEGATIVES.**

    It's easy to get overwhelmed with terms when sensitivity and specificity are brought up. In essence, the sensitivity of a test is the ability of a test to rule out (you can use the mnemonic, SnOUT) a disease. That is, a sensitive test is one that must be able to detect those that have the disease, so it makes sense that sensitivity is defined as the number of people who test positive divided by the number of people who actually have the disease (true positives + false negatives). As a result, a sensitive test is an excellent screening tool. On the other hand, a specific test is one that can "rule in" a disease (SpIN). Specificity is defined as the number of people who test negative for a disease divided by the number of people WITHOUT the disease (true negatives + false positives). For this reason, a specific test is best used as a post-screening test to differentiate false positives from true negatives.
    QCCP2, **Clinical sensitivity, Specificity**, p 439

8: Laboratory Statistics and Quality Control Answers

6.   E.   **TO DETERMINE THE PERFORMANCE CHARACTERISTICS OF A TEST AT DIFFERENT CUT-OFF VALUES.**

If you would have used the classic test-taking skill of choosing the longest answer, you would have nailed this one. If you didn't, maybe the explanation will help. Plotting sensitivity on the Y axis and 1-specificity on the X axis for a set of values, then connecting the values will generate a ROC curve. The purpose of the curve is to determine the specificity or sensitivity of a test at any given value. As sensitivity increases, specificity decreases (or 1-specificity increases), leading to a curve. The area under the curve is a function of the accuracy of the test. *QCCP2*, **Receiver operating characteristic (ROC) curves**, p 439

7.   B.   **+/- 2 SD FROM THE MEAN.**

The central 95% of results (+/- 2 SD) obtained from healthy persons is most commonly used as the reference interval. This means that 5% of healthy individuals will have values that fall out of the reference interval. In addition, a particular reference interval many not apply to another population. *QCCP2*, **Reference intervals**, p 440

8.   C.   **LOW COMPLEXITY TESTING.**

Tests are listed in order of increasing CLIA regulation. Waived tests have the least regulation - follow manufacturer's instructions and good laboratory practices. Similarly, provider-performed microscopy, such as ferning tests must also follow the same guidelines. The vast majority of standard laboratory tests fall under the moderate complexity category. In addition to following the rules for waived tests, labs providing moderate complexity testing must have a standard operating procedure in addition to performing and documenting calibration, controls, and quality control. High complexity testing must adhere to the same rules as moderate complexity testing but must also document the validation of the assay, since most high complexity testing is created in house. *QCCP2*, **Quality control**, p 440-441

9.   D.   **ALL OF THE ABOVE.**

Test runs are made with a new control sample to create a Levey-Jennings plot and determine the mean and standard deviation. From then on, the control is run on a regular basis and the results are plotted on the Levey-Jennings plot created previously. The results of the plot are interpreted according to the Westgard rules to determine if a test is "in control" or "out of control". *QCCP2*, **Quality control**, p 441

10.   E.   **10:10s RULE.**

The missing rule is the 10:mean rule. Each rule is a shorthand means of representation. The "s" in each stands for standard deviation, while the number preceding it stands for the number of values. For example, the 1:3s rule states, "Is one value + or - 3 SD from the mean?", the 2:2s rule: "Are 2 consecutive values + or - 2 SD on the same side of the mean?" R:4s means, "Are any 2 values >4 SD from each other?" and 4:1s: "Are any 4 values >1 SD on the same side of the mean?". Finally, the 10:mean rule asks, "Are any 10 values on the same side of the mean?" Any run that violates one of the Westgard rules is labeled as "out of control." The results from this run should not be reported and the assay re-run. *QCCP2*, **Control specimens, The Westgard rules**, p 441

8: Laboratory Statistics and Quality Control Answers

11.   A.   **1:3s RULE, C. R:4s RULE.**

The rules that address widening result distribution are more sensitive to random error. Drifting or shifting values imply a more systematic error and can be detected with the other 3 Westgard rules, 2:2s, 4:1s, and 10:mean. *QCCP2,* **The Westgard rules,** p 441

12.   D.   **DEPARTMENT OF HEALTH AND HUMAN SERVICES.**

The HHS has the authority to recognize agencies as suitable providers of proficiency testing, while most of the other choices presented in the question represent some of those agencies authorized to provide such testing. *QCCP2,* **Proficiency testing,** p 441

13.   B.   **LAB REFERENCE INTERVALS.**

Each participant in CAP's proficiency testing program is given a standard deviation index calculated by subtracting the lab result from the peer group. In general, the lab must be within 2 standard deviations to be graded as acceptable. Greater than 3 standard deviations is considered unacceptable, while between 2 and 3 is regarded as "needing improvement." *QCCP2,* **Proficiency testing,** p 443

14.   D.   **ALL OF THE ABOVE.**

Constant bias and proportional bias are types of analytical bias. A constant bias is when the value of a new test is off from the standard assay by a predictable constant amount. Proportional bias is when the difference between the two tests is non-linear. The analytical bias can also be mixed. If variability is random, then it cannot be predicted accurately. *QCCP2,* **Analytical correlation,** p 443

15.   E.   **ALL OF THE ABOVE ARE TESTS WHERE ANALYTICAL SENSITIVITY IS VERY IMPORTANT.**

The analytical sensitivity of a test refers to the lowest analyte concentration detectable by the test. All of the tests mentioned share a common characteristic - very low levels of the analyte may be clinically important. For this reason, it is very important to have a high analytical sensitivity for each of these tests. *QCCP2,* **Analytic sensitivity,** p 443

16.   B.   **SAMPLES WITH HIGH ANALYTE CONCENTRATION.**

Typically assays are at the greatest risk of becoming non-linear at high analyte concentrations. In enzymatic assays, when the enzyme is fully saturated by substrate, the rate of the reaction varies only with the concentration of the enzyme (remember that from Chapter 1?). Low analyte samples are at risk of pushing the analytic sensitivity of an assay. Mixed and contaminated samples may pose other risks, such as interference. *QCCP2,* **Linearity,** p 443

17.   E.   **ALL OF THE ABOVE.**

Heterophile antibodies are interfering antibodies present in the sample that bind to the animal antibodies in the assay. Serial dilution will reveal the non-linear changes in the assay due to heterophile antibodies vs. the expected linear changes in a true sample. All of the other techniques have been used to run assays once the presence of heterophile antibodies is recognized. *QCCP2,* **Interference,** p 444

8: Laboratory Statistics and Quality Control Answers

18.   A.   ELECTROLYTES.

Small molecules follow water when hydrostatic pressure increases and drives water into the interstitial space. Large molecules, such as proteins, and cells cannot. Therefore, the concentration of the larger molecules and cells increases when water leaves.
QCCP2, **Interference,** p 444

19.   C.   BLUE, CITRATE.

Each additive has its own special use. Obviously, a tube with no additive cannot be used for coagulation studies as it will likely clot prior to the assay being run on it. Heparin is also a poor choice due to its potential effect on the assay. Samples collected in buffered sodium citrate are used for a fairly specific purpose - determining the erythrocyte sedimentation rate. EDTA inhibits enzymatic assays, so samples containing it are used for non-enzymatic assays, such as obtaining cell counts. It is difficult to remember the tube top colors, the specific additives, and the uses of each. To remember the colors and what additives are used, I put the tube top colors in the same order as the colors of the rainbow - red, yellow, green, blue, purple (more about black and gray later). Once the colors are arranged "rainbowically," I use the mnemonic "NO CHoiCE," which stands for (respectively) none, citrate with dextrose, heparin, citrate, and EDTA. So red tube tops have no additive and therefore the sample will clot. You know that won't be a useful sample for plasma chemistry, but will be useful for serum chemistry. Red tube tops are also used in the blood bank for antibody workups, and for "serology" (remember serum is what's left behind when blood clots.). Yellow tube tops have citrate with dextrose. Remember from your blood banking, if you add adenine to citrate and dextrose, you have one of the most common blood preservation additives. It stands to reason that samples collected in yellow tube tops are used in the blood bank for cell-centered assays and are used for HLA testing. Samples in green tube tops have heparin added; therefore, the blood doesn't clot and the plasma can be assayed. For this reason, they are typically used for plasma chemistry applications. Citrate is an anticoagulant that does not interfere with enzymatic clotting assays and that is why samples in blue tube tops are used. Finally, purple tube tops have EDTA. EDTA will inhibit enzymes, preventing clotting and proteolysis. Therefore the sample is only used for non-enzymatic assays where an unclotted sample is necessary, such as obtaining cell counts. Black tube tops contain buffered sodium citrate and, as mentioned previously, are used specifically for determination of erythrocyte sedimentation rates. Gray tube tops contain sodium fluoride, an enzyme inhibitor, and are used primarily in the measurement of glucose. One can relate that if you don't brush the glucose off your teeth (using a toothpaste with fluoride), your teeth will turn gray. Perhaps, too, that may help you to remember the use and additive of gray tube tops.
QCCP2, **T8.1 Blood Collection Tubes,** p 445

20.   E.   A & C.

Perhaps not a fair question, but something we in pathology should always remember. The majority of errors in testing occur outside the lab. We typically are very good at controlling the analytical phase of the test with controls, quality assurance, proficiency testing, etc. However, we are not as good at controlling errors before the sample arrives at the lab (labeling errors, ordering errors, collection errors, etc) and after the test is performed (delayed or inaccurate reporting, inappropriate response to results, etc).
QCCP2, **Errors in laboratory medicine,** p 445

8: Laboratory Statistics and Quality Control Answers

21.   C.   **PATIENT GENDER.**

The corrected count increment (CCI) measures the response of a patient's platelet count to a platelet transfusion. It is useful in determining whether a patient has platelet refractoriness or not. The CCI is the change in platelet count (post-pre) multiplied by the patient's body surface area (sort of a substitute for the volume of distribution), all divided by the actual number of platelets given. Ideally, if platelet refractoriness is suspected, the platelet count should be measured within an hour of transfusion and again after 12-24 hours. (More in the hematology and blood bank chapters.)
QCCP2, **Corrected (platelet) count increment,** p 446

22.   B.   **20.**

The osmolal gap is the difference between the measured osmolarity and the calculated expected osmolarity based on the concentration of the three major cellular osmolytes - sodium, glucose, and blood urea nitrogen. In the calculation, each osmolyte is normalized for its respective contribution to osmolarity (more in Chapter 1). In this case, the calculated osmolarity would be $(140 \times 2) + (180/18) + (2.8/2.8) = 280 + 10 + 1 = 291$. Subtracting that from the measured osmolarity of 311 gives 20.
QCCP2, **Osmolal gap,** p 446

23.   E.   **LDL = TOTAL CHOLESTEROL - HDL - TG/5.**

The Friedewald equation can be used to calculate the LDL from measured values of total cholesterol, HDL, and triglyceride.
QCCP2, **Friedewald equation,** p 446